líma 1980

# Spinal Injury

# SPINAL INJURY

*David Yashon,* M.D., F.A.C.S., F.R.C.S. (C)

*Professor of Neurosurgery*
*The Ohio State University*
*University Hospitals*
*Columbus, Ohio*

APPLETON-CENTURY-CROFTS/NEW YORK

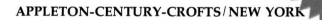

78 79 80 81 82 / 10 9 8 7 6 5 4 3 2 1

Prentice-Hall International, Inc., London
Prentice-Hall of Australia, Pty. Ltd., Sydney
Prentice-Hall of India Private Limited, New Delhi
Prentice-Hall of Japan, Inc., Tokyo
Prentice-Hall of Southeast Asia (Pte.) Ltd., Singapore
Whitehall Books Ltd., Wellington, New Zealand

**Library of Congress Cataloging in Publication Data**

Yashon, David, 1935–
    Spinal injury.

    Bibliography:  p.
    Includes index.
    1.  Spinal cord—Wounds and injuries.  2.  Spine—
Wounds and injuries.  I.  Title.  [DNLM: 1.  Spinal
injuries.  2.  Spinal cord injuries.  WE725 Y29s]
RD594.3.Y37      617'.1      78-7367
ISBN 0-8385-8635-X

Text design: Naomi Feiner
Cover design: Rodelinde Albrecht

PRINTED IN THE UNITED STATES OF AMERICA

*The frog instantly dies
when the spinal cord is pierced;
and previous to this it lived without head,
without heart or any bowels or intestines or skin;
and here therefore it would seem lies the foundation
of movement and life.*

Leonardo da Vinci
(1452–1519)

# Contents

# Preface

This volume is designed to serve as an encyclopedia of all aspects of spinal cord and vertebral injury. Paralysis from spinal cord damage is the costliest infirmity afflicting man and is certainly one of the most devastating in that the victim possesses all his faculties yet cannot exercise motor function nor perceive sensory stimuli. Because of improved care, patients are surviving longer and therefore are encountering more of the problems of chronicity.

The table of contents illustrates the intended breadth of the volume. A brief review of the history and what is known of the epidemiology, as well as the anatomy and the relevant physiology of spinal injury, is presented. Management of the emergency is discussed in detail, along with its rationale. Traction procedures, surgical procedures, and anesthetic technics are described to extend the volume's usefulness into the practical aspects of treatment. Various etiologic factors and radiographic measures to demonstrate the extent of injury are considered, as well as the pathology and the pathogenesis of such injuries thought important at present. It is hoped that in the future pathogenesis will be better understood and many present-day controversies will be resolved. Controversial issues have been presented in this volume as fairly as possible, allowing the reader to make his own judgments.

Special areas such as missile and stab injuries, root injuries, birth injuries, and injuries in children are discussed. Pharmacologic treatment, mostly experimental at this time, is presented with the expectation that in future editions considerable modification will be made in these areas. The injuries most commonly associated with acute spinal injury are discussed, since it is desirable to be familiar with all aspects of the problem. Finally, subacute and chronic complications are presented in several chapters in the hope of giving the reader a precise knowledge of what is known and what to expect in this regard.

Because physical and social rehabilitation are of utmost importance, they are discussed fully. The establishment of centers for total care of the spinally injured is an important new area to be explored in the United States, and an up-to-date appraisal has been made. Some fundamentals concerning biomechanics and regeneration in the experimental animal (and man) are provided so that the reader may have an understanding of the current state of the art. Finally, a brief discussion of medicolegal aspects is provided, along with recommendations. All in all, this volume is intended to provide comprehensive information in many areas in the broad medical fields relating to spinal cord and vertebral injury. Controversies and differences of opinion regarding spinal injury are presented throughout.

In reviewing textbooks and the literature on spinal injury, it became apparent that there was no single volume that presented a multifaceted approach to the problem. This is not to say that there are not many excellent textbooks dealing with aspects of spinal injury, but that no one of these could be counted on to give a complete discussion of the entire spectrum of the disease. For example, in certain volumes there was a nearly complete disregard for surgical procedures commonly employed in treatment; in others, the social and rehabilitative aspects were neglected; and in still others, complications were not included. Many textbooks can be considered only primers lacking a comprehensive bibliography. In preparing this volume, a complete literature search was carried out, utilizing computers and the *Index Medicus*. Additional older material, now considered classic, is included when applicable. Each chapter has a broad bibliography, sometimes numbering over 100 references. The inclusion of such an extensive bibliography is intentional, so that if further details are required, the reference work itself can be examined. For the serious student of spinal injury, this will be a necessity in almost every area, since it is not possible to cover in detail all the important research and clinical reports published in the last several decades. That is not to say that every published research or clinical paper of significance has been included. Unfortunately, not all of these could be included, since there are many thousands of related published papers. What was attempted was an overview of papers in the field. Exclusion of some excellent papers is regrettable, but limitations of space have made it unavoidable.

Illustrations are in many cases original drawings provided by the Department of Medical Illustration of the Ohio State University. In other instances, previously published drawings have been included with the gracious permission of the authors and publishers. It is hoped that the choice of illustrations will be meaningful to the reader in his understanding of the processes involved in spinal injury. Over the past 18 years the author has participated actively in the care of many patients having acute, subacute, and chronic spinal injuries, and most x-ray reproductions are from these cases in the author's files. They have been chosen to illustrate the problems and findings in patients with spinal injury. It is hoped that the reader, after study of the x-rays, can more easily detect the variants and avoid the pitfalls associated with the x-ray diagnosis of spinal injury.

This volume has been designed not only for physicians and medical students, but also for associated professionals who care in some way for patients with a spinal injury. In every area of specialization it is important to know something of the other areas, since a comprehensive overview is important for each individual treating a spinally injured patient. This includes physicians such as orthopaedists and neurosurgeons, emergency room physicians, physiatrists, urologists, anesthesiologists, and neurologists, as well as generalists and physicians in almost every other medical specialty. The spinally injured patient is an excellent laboratory of physiologic, anatomic, and neurologic diagnosis for the medical student. In addition, nursing personnel, physical therapists, occupational therapists, social workers, and other specialists should find areas of interest. The book is meant to be a comprehensive encyclopedic work for individuals caring for spinally injured patients in the hope that care can be improved. It is sincerely hoped that this mission will be accomplished.

DY

# Acknowledgments

There is no way an author can compile a volume of this sort without considerable assistance which requires acknowledgment. The editorial abilities of Mrs. Helene Ayers and the secretarial assistance of Mrs. Cynthia Griest have been invaluable. Miss Sara McKinley, Mrs. Karen Martin, Mrs. Pam Engler, and Mrs. Anita Black were all of great assistance in typing the various chapters. Bibliographic help was provided by Mr. Henry Penner and Mr. Ronald Yates, both of whom were extremely thorough. Dr. John A. Jane reviewed the manuscript and suggested many beneficial changes in format. Several physicians acquainted with areas in question reviewed the chapters and made useful suggestions. These are Dr. Nicholas Checkles (Physical and Social Rehabilitation), Dr. Henry Wise (Urology), and Dr. Thomas Beach (Anesthesiology). Mr. Robert McGrath of Appleton-Century-Crofts has been very easy to work with and most cooperative in this venture. Lastly, such an undertaking requires an enormous amount of time and indulgence for which I am thankful to my family, consisting of my wife Myrna; children Jaclyn, Lisa, and Steven; and parents Samuel and Dorothy. They provided considerable encouragement when the going became rough and at those times that I felt the project could not be accomplished. Their understanding and encouragement has been wonderful.

# Spinal Injury

# 1

## History

The history of neurosurgery is as long as the history of medicine. The operation of trephining the skull is undoubtedly the oldest known surgical procedure, and trephined skulls from the neolithic period of the Stone Age have been found in nearly all parts of the world. From the prehistoric and Egyptian eras to the advent of neurosurgery as a specialty with the work of Sir Victor Horsley and Harvey Cushing in the late nineteenth century, physicians have sought to treat spinal injury.

In this volume we make no attempt to do more than touch upon historical facts that have been set forth and documented by others. The interested reader is advised to consult the *Historical Sketch of Neurosurgery* by Dr. Gilbert Horrax and *A History of Neurological Surgery* edited by Dr. A. Earl Walker,[8] as well as the other references at the end of this chapter.[1,2,4-7]

### EGYPTIAN AND MESOPOTAMIAN PERIOD
#### (4000–500 B.C.)

The earliest known document concerning surgical procedures is the Edwin Smith papyrus. It was translated in 1930, with careful detailed commentaries on each case by the famous Egyptologist, Professor J. H. Breasted, who believed that although the papyrus itself was written about 1700 B.C., it was a copy of an original manuscript written between 3000 and 2500 B.C. The ancient Egyptian surgeons classified injuries into three categories:

1. An ailment which I will treat (favorable cases)
2. An ailment with which I will contend (cases that might be cured)
3. An ailment not to be treated (hopeless cases)

1

Spinal injuries were listed in the hopeless category. The Edwin Smith papyrus lists six cases of injury to the spine including sprain in a spinal vertebra, dislocated vertebrae, and crushed vertebrae. It was recognized that vertebral injuries with cord damage caused paralysis of the arms and legs, bowel and bladder incontinence, and loss of erection.

The Egyptian surgeon treated patients with signs of spinal cord injury by application of meat and honey to the neck and maintenance of the seated position. The Breasted translation of Case 32 from the Smith papyrus states, "Thou should bind it with meat the first day, thou shall loose his bandages and apply grease to his head as far as his neck, and thou shall bind it with ymrw (sic). Thou shouldst treat it afterwards with honey every day and his relief of sitting until he recovers."

## THE GREEK OR HIPPOCRATIC AND GALENIC PERIOD
### (500 B.C.–500 A.D.)

Hippocrates (460–377 B.C.) discussed the nature of dislocation of vertebrae and its relation to paralysis of the limbs, but it is not clear that the role of the spinal cord was appreciated. Celsius (30 B.C.) noted that death followed quickly when the spinal injury involved the cervical area. Aretaeus (150 B.C.) made the observation that in injuries involving the spinal cord, the resulting paralysis originated in some cases at the site of injury. Galen (130–201 A.D.) proved experimentally that interruption of the spinal cord caused paralysis and loss of sensation below the level of injury.

Paraplegia, questionably of traumatic origin, was reported in the Talmud. An account in the Talmud reported by Leibowitz describes signs and symptoms of paraplegia as well as a differential diagnosis and verification of the diagnosis by postmortem examination. The case properly belongs in the veterinary medicine literature because it deals with sheep. The reason for the discussion in the Talmud is that the case necessitated a ritual decision, since consumption of meat of certain animals suffering from certain diseases, such as bony lesions, is not permitted according to the Hebraic ritual code. In addition to the case of the sheep, mention is also made of an animal sustaining similar injuries to the spine in a fall from a roof.

Hippocrates had observed the results of traumatic spinal cord injury, but did not believe that anything could be done to correct spinal deformity in a living person. Oribasius (325–403 A.D.) illustrated a stretching-type traction frame for treating fractured spinal columns. In spite of the observations of these and other writers, progress was very slow toward an accurate and detailed knowledge of spinal cord function and treatment of injury.

## MEDIEVAL PERIOD (ca. 500–1500 A.D.)

Paul of Aegia (625–690 A.D.) was one of the outstanding medieval figures whose writings on spinal injuries are translated thus: "but if any of the processes of the vertebrae of the spine, as it is called, be broken off, it will readily be felt upon examination with the finger, the broken piece yielding and returning again to its position, and therefore we must make an incision of the skin externally and extract it and having united the wounds with sutures, pursue the treatment for recent wounds." Lanfranc (1296) said that the prognosis of dislocation of the spine was hopeless, but was the first to report peripheral nerve suture. Guy de Chauliac (1300–1368) dismissed the matter by saying that one should not labor to cure paralysis from spinal injury. de Chauliac has been called the father of modern surgery and his great book on surgery was completed in 1363.

## RENAISSANCE (ca. 1500–1700 A.D.)

Ambrose Paré advocated the cure of spinal dislocations by traction. He recognized the seriousness of operating on spinal injuries and said, "you may make an incision so as to take forth the splinters of the broken vertebrae which driven in pressed the spinal marrow and the nerves thereof." The diagnosis was made by palpation and evidence of crepitation.

Petrus L'Argelata (1531) described reduction of a cervical fracture dislocation by pressure applied to the point of angulation. Fabricus Hildanus (1646) described treatment of fracture-dislocations of the cervical spine by grasping soft tissues of the neck with forceps and applying pressure. If this procedure of apparent reduction was unsuccessful, the surgeon was advised to explore the spinous processes and vertebral arch and extricate fragments of bone.

## THE PRE-LISTERIAN PERIOD (ca. 1700–1846 A.D.)

In 1745, James advocated operative intervention for fracture of the spine. Heister, in 1768, advocated surgical removal of fragments in cases of fractured spine. Geraud described attempts to remove a musket ball from the body of the third lumbar vertebra in a patient who had paraplegia and bladder paralysis. He finally removed the missile on the fifth attempt, and the wound drained. The patient did recover some strength in his legs. Markham[8] described several other surgical procedures during this period including an operation by Louis during the war of 1762 in which a metallic fragment was removed from the lumbar spine and the patient made a complete functional recovery. Chopart and Desault, writing in 1796, advocated removal of depressed fragments of bone in spinal injury and also suggested trephining the laminae. Cline, in 1814, resected fractured spines and laminae for a thoracic fracture-dislocation associated with signs of a complete transverse lesion of the spinal cord. He operated within 24 hours of the injury but was unable to reduce the dislocation and the patient died soon thereafter. In 1827, Tyrrell reported several cases of spinal dislocation with cord compression treated with operation, but all patients died. Rogers, in 1835, also reported discouraging results. In 1828, Alban Smith of Kentucky operated on a man who had fallen from a horse and suffered immediate paralysis of the legs. Smith removed the spinous processes and depressed laminae, inspected the dura, and closed the incision. The patient survived and improved somewhat.

## DISCOVERY OF ANESTHESIA AND ANTISEPSIS (1846–1890)

The use of ether in 1846 and chloroform in 1848 as anesthetic agents initiated a new epoch in surgery. Lister introduced antisepsis in 1867. Spinal tumors were removed by Macewen on May 9, 1883, and by Horsley on June 9, 1887. During the middle and latter part of the nineteenth century, debate concerning suture of the severed spinal cord in cases of trauma was heated. The practice did not survive, although in 1905, Fowler and Harte performed this operation and claimed good results. It was apparent, however, that the improvement was return of spinal reflexes. Chipault, in 1895, suggested that nerve roots might be anastomosed for renervation of structures below the level of the spinal lesion. In 1912, Frazier anastomosed the roots of the cauda equina and noted some improvement in the patient.

## NEUROSURGERY AS A SPECIALTY (1890–THE PRESENT)

Cushing, in 1905, described indications and contraindications for operation in spinal injuries which, with slight modification, are largely those still considered at this time.[3] Corning introduced lumbar puncture in 1885, and it was popularized by Quincke in 1891. The Queckenstadt test was described in 1916, and a cisternal puncture in 1919 by Wegefarth et al. Lipiodol was used as an intraspinal contrast medium by Sicard and Forestier in 1921, and myelography with air by Dandy in 1922.

In this period many surgeons were concerned that laminectomy would weaken the postoperative stability of the spine. For that reason, osteoplastic laminectomy was performed and was the most popular operation for about 30 years. According to that technique, the laminae, posterior portion of the pedicles, and spinous processes, as well as a considerable amount of muscle, was lifted off in toto, exposing the dura-invested spinal cord. Various rongeurs and drills were utilized for modification of these methods. For details of the various surgical procedures, consult the chapter by Markham.[8]

In the nineteenth century, after reducing a fracture-dislocation of the spine by mechanical means, Wilkins used silver wire to make a figure-of-eight ligature about the pedicles for fixation. Chipault used a similar method in 1895. Fixation by plaster of paris cast was carried out in 1852 by Mathijsen, and Burrell also suggested and utilized a plaster cast. The modern era to be described in later chapters was thus ushered in.

## REFERENCES

1.   Bedbrook GM: Injuries of the thoracolumbar spine with neurological symptoms. In Vinken PJ, Bruyn GW (eds): Handbook of Clinical Neurology. New York, American Elsevier, 1976

2. Bennett G: Historical chapter. In Howorth MB, Petrie JG (eds): Injuries of the Spine. Baltimore, Williams & Wilkins, 1964

3. Cushing H: The special field of neurological surgery. Bull J Hopkins Hosp 16:168, 1905

4. Horrax G: Neurosurgery–An Historical Sketch. Springfield Ill, Charles C Thomas, 1952

5. Horworth MB: Petrie JG: Injuries of the Spine. Baltimore, Williams & Wilkins, 1964

6. Leibowitz JO: Traumatic (?) paraplegia as reported in the Talmud. Med Hist 4: 350–351, 1960

7. Loeser JD: History of skeletal traction in the treatment of cervical spine injuries. J Neurosurg 33:54–59, 1970

8. Markham JW: Surgery of the spinal cord and vertebral column. In Walker AE (ed): A History of Neurological Surgery. Baltimore, Williams & Wilkins, 1951, pp 364–394

# 2

## Epidemiology

Accidents are the fourth leading cause of death in the United States after heart disease, cancer, and stroke, accounting for about 50 deaths per 100,000 population each year. Of these, some 3 percent are caused directly by spinal cord injury due to trauma, and an additional 2 percent from spinal cord injury as a part of multiple systemic trauma. The death rate in males is three times that in females, and motor vehicle accidents and falls are responsible for 2/5 and 1/5 respectively of accidental deaths. Prevalence of complete or partial paralysis caused by accidents is nearly 80 per 100,000 population. The prevalence of either complete paraplegia or quadriplegia due to accidents is about 20 per 100,000 population.[3] An estimate of the prevalence of traumatic spinal cord injury including not completely paralyzed patients approximates 60 per 100,000 population. All figures are valid for any given time per 100,000 population.[3]

In industrialized countries, the incidence of traumatic spinal cord injury is approximately 3 per 100,000 population. Men are affected five times more often than women. Half the injuries are due to motor vehicle accidents, and one-fourth are due to falls. One in 10 is a consequence of sports or recreational injuries, with diving accidents by far the commonest. The automobile accident carries a higher risk factor for death than a diving accident, but both are responsible for a large number of spinal cord injuries each year. The most prevalent ages for traumatic spinal cord damage are 15 through 34 years, but such injury can occur in any age group. Elderly persons are more prone to spinal injury from a fall, since there is a higher incidence of cervical spondylosis in that group. In California, incidence of spinal injury in blacks was twice that in whites.[2]

According to Kurtzke,[3] early survivors of spinal cord injury showed neurologic improvement in one-fifth of cases during acute and short-term hospitalization; late survivors in one-third of cases after intensive rehabilitation in a spinal cord injury center. Patients with incomplete paralysis were more likely to improve, while only one in six paraplegics with complete sensory loss showed any neurologic recovery after rehabilitation.

Kurtzke[3] reports survival after spinal cord injury from life-expectancy tables analyzed in two series and calculated in a third. About four in five spinal cord injury patients now live 10 years after injury, compared with a normal expectancy of 97 percent survival for 10 years. He calculated median survival from a British series as almost 18 years, contrasted with a normal life-expectancy of about 40 years. Survival rates were much worse for complete lesions: 50 percent in the fourteenth year after injury for complete quadriplegics, and in the seventeenth year for complete paraplegics. For incomplete quadriplegics, the estimated 50 percent survival rate was calculated to occur in the nineteenth year; for incomplete paraplegics in the twentieth year; and for cauda equina injuries in the twenty-eighth year after trauma. Survival was also a function of age, but the observed/expected survival rates declined with age for the cord-injured patients much less than did the survival rates themselves. He found that four of five survivors of any spinal injury in England were employed, as was true of Norway; but only half of neurologically complete quadriplegics had some gainful occupation.

If prevalence of traumatic spinal cord injury is as high as 50 per 100,000 population, based on an annual incidence rate of 3 per 100,000 population, and survival figures are as described, it can be estimated that in the United States there are now 100,000 patients with traumatic spinal cord injury alive, of whom approximately 40,000 have complete paralysis. Of the latter, 35,000 have paralysis of the lower extremities and 5000 of all four limbs.

An interesting relationship is seen between incidence and socioeconomic status as measured by the educational level of the head of the family.[3] Generally speaking, there is a steady decrease in rates of spinal cord injury in each age group with increasing educational levels. Rates of spinal cord injury for residents of nonmetropolitan areas exceed those of metropolitan areas 7.6 to 6.5, and rates in the southern United States are notably higher than in the other three regions.

Death rates for spinal cord injury patients were examined.[3] In Scotland in 1971, there were 62 deaths due to fracture of the spine in 50 men and 12 women. Scotland's population is 5.29 million, so the mortality rate was 1.2 per 100,000 persons. The death rate in England was lower by approximately one-third, at 0.4 per 100,000. In the study by Kraus et al.[2] of 18 northern California counties, the death rates were 2.6 per 100,000 (3.6 male to 1.6 female) for the years 1970 and 1971. These were patients having multiple trauma. If only those patients are considered in whom spinal cord injury was the underlying and most contributory cause of death, the death rate was 1.4 per 100,000, which is close to that of Scotland.

Many spinal cord injuries are associated with ingestion of alcohol and/or drugs. The National Spinal Cord Injury Registry established by Ducker and Perot[1] reports that 40 percent of spinal injuries are due to vehicular accidents, 20 percent due to falls, and 40 percent due to gunshot wounds, sporting accidents, industrial accidents, and agricultural accidents in that order. During peacetime, the prevalence of sporting accidents and gunshot wounds is reversed. Approximately 85 percent of injured patients are male, with the peak age range from 15 to 28 years. The most frequent time of occurrence is between 12 midnight and 5:00 AM, with a lower peak near midafternoon. Seasonally, there is a rise in incidence in summer from diving accidents and another rise in winter due to skiing and snowmobiling.

Ducker and Perot[1] found the most frequent level of injury to be the mid-to-low cervical lesion (C5–6), with the next being the thoracolumbar junction (T12–L1). These are also the areas of the greatest mobility of the spinal column. According to the National Spinal Cord Registry, 43 percent of patients had complete neurologic deficit below the level of injury, 18 percent had partial deficits, 3 percent had a Brown-Sequard-type syndrome, 3 percent had a central cervical cord syndrome, 12 percent had nerve root injury only, and 23 percent had vertebral fractures, of which two-thirds were compression fractures and one-sixth laminar fractures. Fracture-dislocations were also seen in two-thirds of patients; 7 percent had significant preinjury degenerative changes in the vertebral column, usually older persons with spondylosis.

Associated injuries included fractures of the limbs and jaw in 26 percent, lacerations and somatic contusions in 28 percent; a large number had ruptured abdominal viscera, abrasions, and burns. Associated severe injury to an extremity was noted in 21 percent of patients, and 14 percent had an associated head injury. The most frequent injuries were to the face, thoracic cavity, ribs, and shoulders; 60 percent of patients had abnormal bladder function. It was estimated that there are approximately 200,000 patients with spinal cord injury presently living in the United States, and 10,000 to 12,000 new injuries occur each year.[1] The cost of supporting such a patient injured in the prime of life may exceed one million dollars during his lifetime.

It is very difficult to arrive at accurate figures for incidence and prevalence of spinal cord injury patients. Kraus et al.[2] did an admirable job in their study of 18 California counties. Still, one need only review the paper to appreciate the difficulty presented to them and the inaccuracies that may exist in any analysis of such injuries in the United States. They estimated that 4200 of these patients will die before they reach a hospital and an additional 1150 will die during hospitalization. Kraus et al.[2] found that the risk of spinal cord injury was highest for divorced or separated persons or those who have never been married.

Riggins and Kraus[4] assessed risks of neurologic damage with fractures of vertebrae. They found that the incidence of spinal cord injury with spine fractures and dislocations is about 14 percent of the patients studied in northern California. No overt radiographic evidence of vertebral injury was noted in 17 percent of traumatic spinal cord injuries: the vertebral bodies and elements were normal by x-ray. Patients with fracture-dislocations with at least a slight degree of malalignment of the vertebral bodies had a 61 percent incidence of neurologic deficit. Therefore, 39 percent did not have neurologic deficit, even with fracture-dislocation. Injuries to the cervical spine resulted in an incidence of neurologic deficit of 39 percent, which was higher than that in thoracic and lumbar injuries.

## REFERENCES

1. Ducker T, Perot P: National spinal cord injury registry. U.S. Department of Defense, Charleston, South Carolina, 1974–1975
2. Kraus JF, Franti CE, Riggins RS, Richards D, Borhani NO: Incidence of traumatic spinal cord lesions. J Chron Dis 28:471–492, 1975
3. Kurtzke JF: Epidemiology of spinal cord injury. Exper Neurol 48:163–236, 1975
4. Riggins RS, Kraus JF: The risk of neurologic damage with fractures of the vertebrae. J Trauma 17:126–133, 1977

# 3

# Anatomy and Physiology

This chapter includes sections on anatomy relating to the neurologic examination, embryology,[2,3] the vertebral column,[9] including the nucleus pulposus and ligaments,[6] and the spinal cord and nerve roots and its blood supply.[1,4,5,7] Neurophysiology is emphasized only as it relates to spinal injury.

## ANATOMY RELATING TO THE NEUROLOGIC EXAMINATION

A knowledge of the dermatomes of man (Fig. 1) is essential for the sensory examination of the injured patient to determine the segmental level of injury.[20] Tables 1 and 2 present the myotomal (segmental) or root level associated with muscle function. Examination of muscle strength aids in determination of the level of injury as well as estimation of future functional ability.[20]

The following data are useful in determining the level of cord damage. Significant disruption of cord segments C3–C5 invariably destroys the phrenic innervation, causing diaphragmatic paralysis and respiratory difficulty. Injury to the cervical or upper thoracic cord also affects respiration by abolishing intercostal muscular function. The C5 and C6 nerve roots supply the muscles concerned with abduction (deltoid, supraspinatus), external rotation (infraspinatus, teres minor), flexion of the elbow (biceps, brachialis), and supination of the forearm (biceps, brachioradialis). The C6–C7 roots serve the muscles that extend the elbow and wrist (triceps, wrist extensors) and pronate the forearm. Flexion of the wrist is a function of C7 and C8; C8 and T1 supply the small muscles of the hand (Table 1).[18]

In general, a lesion between T10 and T12 will abolish the lower abdominal reflexes; in such a case Beevor's sign will be demonstrable because of con-

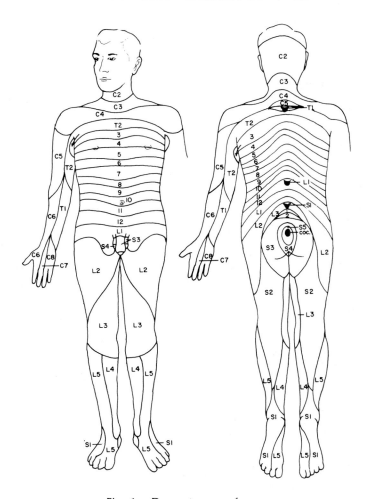

*Fig. 1.* Dermatomes of man.

traction of the upper abdominal muscles and paralysis of the lower ones. A lesion of L1 is revealed by absence of the cremasteric reflex. Hip flexion is mediated by L1–L3 roots (Table 2), extension by L5–S2, while abduction is controlled by the L4–S1 motor segments. Extension of the knee (quadriceps) is mediated by L2–L4 roots; the patellar reflex is absent in lesions involving these segments or roots. The flexors of the knee are controlled by L4–S2. Adduction of the hip is mediated by L2–L4. Dorsiflexion and eversion of the foot and extension of the toes are dependent on L5–S1. Inversion of the foot is a function of L4–L5. Plantar flexion of the ankle, flexion of the toes, as well as contraction of the small muscles of the foot, are mediated by S1 and S2. The perianal muscles are innervated by S3–S5. A lesion of S1 or S2 will depress or abolish the ipsilateral Achilles reflex. Lesions of the conus medullaris and cauda equina cause a flaccid paralysis. Since the cauda equina hangs loosely

## TABLE 1.
## SEGMENTAL INNERVATION OF MUSCLES (C1–T1)

| MUSCLES | C1 | C2 | C3 | C4 | C5 | C6 | C7 | C8 | T1 |
|---|---|---|---|---|---|---|---|---|---|
| STERNOMASTOID | • | • | • | • | | | | | |
| TRAPEZIUS | | • | • | • | | | | | |
| LEVATOR SCAPULAE | | | • | • | • | | | | |
| DIAPHRAGM | | | • | • | | | | | |
| TERES MINOR | | | | • | • | | | | |
| SUPRASPINATUS | | | | • | • | | | | |
| RHOMBOIDS | | | | • | • | | | | |
| INFRASPINATUS | | | | • | • | • | | | |
| DELTOID | | | | | • | • | | | |
| TERES MAJOR | | | | | • | • | | | |
| BICEPS | | | | | • | • | | | |
| BRACHIALIS | | | | | • | • | | | |
| SERRATUS ANTERIOR | | | | | • | • | • | | |
| SUBSCAPULARIS | | | | | • | • | • | • | |
| PECTORALIS MAJOR | | | | | • | • | • | • | • |
| PECTORALIS MINOR | | | | | | • | • | • | |
| CORACOBRACHIALIS | | | | | | • | • | | |
| LATISSIMUS DORSI | | | | | | • | • | • | |
| ANCONEUS | | | | | | | • | • | |
| TRICEPS | | | | | | • | • | • | |
| BRACHIORADIALIS | | | | | • | • | | | |
| SUPINATOR | | | | | • | • | | | |
| PRONATOR TERES | | | | | | • | • | | |
| EXT. CARPI RADIALIS LONG. & BREV. | | | | | | • | • | • | |
| FLEXOR CARPI ULNARIS | | | | | | • | • | • | |
| FLEXOR CARPI RADIALIS | | | | | | • | • | • | |
| EXTENSOR DIGITORUM | | | | | | | • | • | |
| EXTENSOR CARPI ULNARIS | | | | | | | • | • | |
| EXTENSOR INDICES | | | | | | | • | • | |
| EXT. DIGITI QUINTI | | | | | | | • | • | |
| EXT. POLLICIS LONGUS | | | | | | | • | • | |
| EXT. POLLICIS BREVIS | | | | | | | • | • | |
| ABDUCTOR POLLICIS LONGUS | | | | | | | • | • | |
| PALMARIS LONGUS | | | | | | | • | • | • |
| PRONATOR QUADRATUS | | | | | | | • | • | • |
| FLEXOR DIGITORUM SUBLIMIS | | | | | | | • | • | • |
| FLEXOR DIGITORUM PROFUNDUS | | | | | | | • | • | • |
| FLEXOR POLLICIS LONGUS | | | | | | | • | • | • |
| OPPONENS POLLICIS | | | | | | | | • | • |
| ABDUCTOR POLLICIS BREVIS | | | | | | | | • | • |
| FLEXOR POLLICIS BREVIS | | | | | | | | • | • |
| PALMARIS BREVIS | | | | | | | | • | • |
| ADDUCTOR POLLICIS | | | | | | | | • | • |
| FLEXOR DIGITI QUINTI | | | | | | | | • | • |
| ABDUCTOR DIGITI QUINTI | | | | | | | | • | • |
| OPPONENS DIGITI QUINTI | | | | | | | | • | • |
| INTEROSSEI | | | | | | | | • | • |
| LUMBRICALES | | | | | | | • | • | • |

in the thecal sac, a lesion at this level by sparing some roots while involving others may be manifested clinically by an erratic anatomic distribution.[18]

With regard to sensory innervation (Fig. 1), the shoulder and upper arm are supplied by C5 and C6, the radial side of the arm and hand by C6, the index and middle fingers by C7, and the ulnar portion of the hand by C8.

## TABLE 2.
## SEGMENTAL INNERVATION OF MUSCLES (L1–S2)

| | L1 | L2 | L3 | L4 | L5 | S1 | S2 |
|---|---|---|---|---|---|---|---|
| ILIOPSOAS | • | • | • | • | | | |
| GRACILIS | | • | • | • | | | |
| SARTORIUS | | • | • | • | | | |
| PECTINEUS | | • | • | • | | | |
| ADDUCTOR LONGUS | | • | • | • | | | |
| ADDUCTOR BREVIS | | • | • | • | | | |
| ADDUCTOR MINIMUS | | • | • | • | | | |
| QUADRATUS FEMORIS | | • | • | • | | | |
| ADDUCTOR MAGNUS | | • | • | • | | | |
| OBDURATOR EXTERNUS | | | • | • | • | • | |
| TENSOR FASCIAE LATAE | | | • | • | • | | |
| GLUTEUS MEDIUS | | | | • | • | • | |
| GLUTEUS MINIMUS | | | | • | • | • | |
| QUADRICEPS FEMORIS | | | | • | • | • | |
| GEMELLI | | | | • | • | • | • |
| SEMITENDINOSUS | | | | • | • | • | • |
| SEMIMEMBRANOSUS | | | | • | • | • | • |
| PIRIFORMIS | | | | • | • | • | • |
| OBDURATOR INTERNIS | | | | | • | • | • |
| BICEPS FEMORIS | | | | | • | • | • |
| GLUTEUS MAXIMUS | | | | | • | • | • |
| TIBIALIS ANTERIOR | | | | | • | • | • |
| POPLITEUS | | | | • | • | • | |
| PLANTARIS | | | | • | • | • | |
| PERONEUS TERTIUS | | | | • | • | • | |
| EXTENSOR DIGITORUM LONGUS | | | | • | • | • | |
| ABDUCTOR HALLUCIS | | | | • | • | • | • |
| FLEXOR DIGITORUM BREVIS | | | | | • | • | |
| FLEXOR HALLUCIS BREVIS | | | | | • | • | |
| EXTENSOR HALLUCIS BREVIS | | | | | • | • | |
| FLEXOR DIGITORUM LONGUS | | | | | • | • | |
| PERONEUS LONGUS | | | | | • | • | • |
| PERONEUS BREVIS | | | | | • | • | • |
| TIBIALIS POSTERIOR | | | | | • | • | • |
| FLEXOR HALLUCIS LONGUS | | | | | • | • | • |
| EXTENSOR HALLUCIS LONGUS | | | | | • | • | • |
| SOLEUS | | | | | • | • | • |
| GASTROCNEMIUS | | | | | • | • | • |
| EXTENSOR DIGITORUM BREVIS | | | | | | • | • |
| FLEXOR DIGITORUM ACCESSORIUS | | | | | | • | • |
| ADDUCTOR HALLUCIS | | | | | | • | • |
| ABDUCTOR DIGITI QUINTI | | | | | | • | • |
| FLEXOR DIGITI QUINTI BREVIS | | | | | | • | • |
| INTEROSSEI | | | | | | • | • |
| LUMBRICALES | | | | • | • | • | • |

The medial aspect of the upper limb above the hand is innervated distally by the T1 segment and proximally (including the axilla) by T1 and T2. It is important to remember that the C5 dermatome is not represented on the chest and that the C4 dermatome forms a collar around the lower neck and upper thorax. The second rib is a useful landmark, corresponding approximately to the line of demarcation between the fourth cervical segment and the second thoracic dermatome. The intervening dermatomes supply the upper limb exclusively. Boundaries between dermatomes are not as sharp or as constant as suggested by the schematic drawings in most neuroanatomy textbooks.[18] There is considerable overlap of innervation, but dermatomal charts (Fig. 1) are nevertheless quite useful, as they do represent a certain measure of consistency and provide a reasonably accurate guide as to the level of spinal cord (segmental) involvement.

Dermatomal sensory patterns (Fig. 1) in the thoracic and lumbosacral areas are as follows: T5 is at the nipple line; the lower rib borders correspond to T7, 8. The T10 level is at the umbilicus, and the line of demarcation between the T12 and L1 dermatomes is represented by the inguinal ligament. The lower lumbar segments run obliquely so that L4 crosses the patella and continues medially to the great toe, and L5 proceeds obliquely down the lateral side of the calf into the middle three toes. S1 supplies the lateral border of the foot. The posterior innervation of the leg is provided by S1 distally and S2 proximally; the back of the thigh is also innervated by S2. S3–S5 supply sensation to the perianal region.

The motor innervation of the deep tendon reflexes commonly elicited is as follows: biceps—C5, C6; triceps—C6, C7; knee—L2, L3, L4; and ankle—S1, S2.

## EMBRYOLOGY

Development of the spine begins early in embryonic life and ends in the third decade of life. The origin of malformations of the vertebral column and spinal cord can be explained embryologically, but malformations seldom play a role in spinal injury, although the spinal cord is more vulnerable to injury under certain circumstances, such as in the case of a persistent os odontoideum.

### The Vertebral Column

The mesenchyme of the soon-to-be-developed vertebral column comes from bilateral serially arranged pairs of mesodermal somites alongside the embryonic notochord, which is the early embryonic supporting structure in all vertebrates. During the fourth week of development, each somite liberates a mass composed of diffuse cells, the sclerotome, which migrates toward and surrounds the notochord. The notochord becomes part of the nucleus pulposus, and sclerotomes form vertebrae and ribs. Intersegmental arteries develop, and each sclerotome is separated from those caudal and cephalad to it by these arteries. The caudal half of each sclerotome thickens and combines with the looser cranial half of the sclerotome just caudal to it. Hence, the adult vertebrae do not correspond to primitive somites or sclerotomes but rather to combinations of two halves. The sclerotome grows and establishes the vertebral body ventrally, and the lamina and other bony structures dorsally.

The intervertebral discs develop during this period. A remnant of the notochord within each disc persists as a nucleus pulposus. Adjacent mesenchyme develops into the various vertebral ligaments. The neural arch remains open until the third month, and if it remains open, results in spina bifida. By the sixth week, centers of chondrification appear in the area of the vertebral column; by three months, these centers appear lateral to the notochord and fuse around it to complete the chondrous centrum. At nine weeks, ossification within the cartilage begins, and by the fifth month, bony replacement of the early cartilage is occurring in almost all the cervical, thoracic, and lumbar vertebrae. Complete union of primary bone components is not achieved until several years after birth.

During development, the vertebra of the atlas is taken over by the axis and becomes the dens or odontoid of the axis. By about the sixteenth year, most of the vertebral column is ossified, but in some cases as long as 25 years is required for the cartilaginous early structures of the sacrum and coccyx to become ossified.

## The Spinal Cord

In the human embryo, the first sign of a nervous system is the appearance of the neural plate, an oval thickened area on the upper surface of the two-layered embryo. Surrounding it is the prospective epidermis. The neural plate develops into the neural tube, from which the entire neuraxis eventually develops. As edges of the neural plate elevate, boundary cells become roughened and acquire pigment. These are the cells of the future neural crest. The major sectors of the neural tube, the alar and basal plates, are being formed. The neural crest, formerly flattened, develops a paired and segmental structure. While doing so, it forms parasympathetic and sympathetic ganglia, adrenal medulla, and melanocytes for later skin pigmentation. On about the seventh day of gestation, cells at the center of the dorsal layer of the bilaminar embryonic disk invaginate to form what is called the primitive pit. The cells around this opening form the primitive knot and also form ectoderm and endoderm as well as the notochord. The mesoderm is to become the musculature, and forms laterally in a paraxial manner.

Schwann cells, which produce the sheaths of peripheral nerves, also develop from the neural crest. As the developing spinal cord grows, its vertical lumen becomes taller, and the sulcus limitans appears on both sides. The basal plate enlarges to form the ventral horns of the spinal cord. Three concentric zones develop, including the ependymal layer; the mantle layer, consisting of spongioblastic nuclei and their distal processes, forms the marginal layer. Later, axonal sprouting occurs, and various tracts are formed. There is progressive movement by axons but there is also resorption. Unknown directing forces seem to prevail.

By 10 weeks, motor neurons in the basal plate are beginning to connect with muscle structures. Sensory neurons in the posterior root ganglia are growing in, and establishing connections with, alar plate interneurons. Dorsal root ganglion cells appear to differentiate later than motor neurons in the basal plate. Continued development of the alar plate continues as spinal cord nuclei and laminae aggregate to bring about the actual adult butterfly configuration of spinal gray matter. The central canal is reduced in size, and its dorsal margins fuse to form the posterior portions of the spinal cord. Basal plates become larger on either side of the floor plate and account for the ventral median fissure.

In embryonic life, the spinal cord tapers gradually. In the fourth month of embryonic life, cervical and lumbosacral enlargements appear. After the third month, the vertebral column grows faster than the spinal cord, and longer. Subsequently, the spinal cord is shortened in relation to the vertebral column. Finally, the tip of the conus medullaris usually ends between T12 and L1 because of the growth disparity.

## THE VERTEBRAL COLUMN

The vertebral column is composed usually of 33 vertebrae consisting of 7 cervical (Fig. 2), 12 thoracic, 5 lumbar, 5 (fused) sacral, and 3, 4, or 5 (fused) coccygeal vertebrae (Fig. 3). Bodies of the vertebrae are separated from each

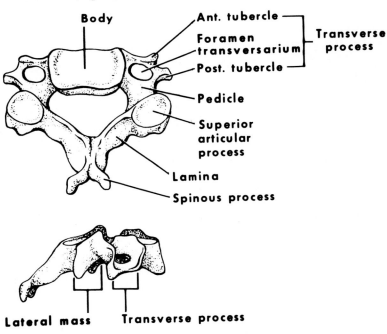

Body

Ant. tubercle ┐
Foramen transversarium ├ Transverse process
Post. tubercle ┘

Pedicle

Superior articular process

Lamina

Spinous process

Lateral mass    Transverse process

*Fig. 2.* Anatomy of cervical vertebra.

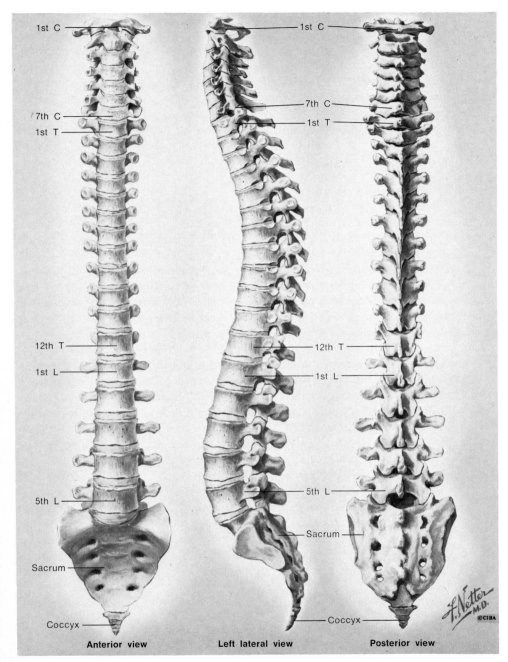

1st C

7th C
1st T

12th T

1st L

5th L

Sacrum

Coccyx

**Anterior view**

1st C

7th C
1st T

12th T

1st L

5th L

Sacrum

Coccyx

**Left lateral view**

**Posterior view**

*Fig. 3.* General configuration of vertebral column.[14] Copyright © 1953, 1972 CIBA Pharmaceutical Company, Division of CIBA-GEIGY Corporation. Reproduced, with permission, from *The CIBA Collection of Medical Illustrations* by Frank H. Netter, M.D. All rights reserved.

other by intervertebral discs, except the first and second vertebrae and the fused sacral and coccygeal regions. These discs provide a large portion, about one-fourth, of the length of the vertebral column above the sacrum. Shrinkage of the discs accounts for loss of height in the order of one-half to three-fourths of an inch during a day of standing, or in old age. Occasionally, there is an extra lumbar vertebra which may be compensated for by one less thoracic vertebra.

A typical vertebra consists of a body and an arch, called either a vertebral or neural arch. The spinal cord lies within the vertebral foramen. The arch itself consists of three parts: the lateral pedicles form its sides and unite it to the body; the roof or lamina spans the pedicles and provides dorsal protection; the spinous process protrudes from the lamina, and the transverse processes protrude from the junction of the pedicles and lamina. All these structures serve for muscular attachments. The superior articular process projects forward on each side from the pedicles with its cartilaginous surface superior. It makes contact with the inferior articulating facet from the vertebral body above it. The inferior articulating facet lies atop the superior articulating facet, and its cartilaginous surface is inferior. Adjacent vertebrae except for C1 and C2 are connected by an intervertebral disc. The vertebra contains no central medullary cavity, as is true of the long skeletal bones. It is composed of spongy bone throughout. A layer of more compact cortical bone covers the spongy bone.

Cervical vertebrae are all small and, in addition to the vertebral foramen, contain a so-called transverse foramen in which the vertebral artery is carried. The atlas, or first cervical vertebra, lacks a body and consists of an anterior and posterior arch. The dens articulates at the anterior arch on its inner surface. The second cervical vertebra is also known as the axis or epistropheus. It has a body from which the dens projects into the arch of C1 (Fig. 4). The seventh cervical vertebra is also different from the third, fourth, fifth, and sixth in that the spinous process is usually unbifurcated, whereas between C2 and C6 there is bifurcation of the spinous process terminally. The bifid spinous processes are sometimes helpful in vertebral identification at posterior surgery. Bifid processes are visualized on anteroposterior radiographs. C7 can be felt easily through the skin on palpation of the back at the base of the neck. Its spinous processes give it the name vertebra prominens. The spinous process is not bifid. The transverse foramen of C7 does not transmit the vertebral artery (Fig. 5).

Typically, nerve roots arise between adjacent vertebral bodies. For example, in the cervical spine the C4 nerve root arises between C3 and C4, the C5 between C4 and C5, the C6 between C5 and C6, and the C7 between C6 and C7. The C8 nerve root arises between C7 and T1, and the T1 nerve root arises between T1 and T2. The level of origin of the nerve root is important in assessing the extent of injury. The thoracic vertebrae increase in size as they proceed caudally. Their basic structure is similar to that of cervical vertebrae. In addition, they bear facets on their lateral anterior surfaces for articulation

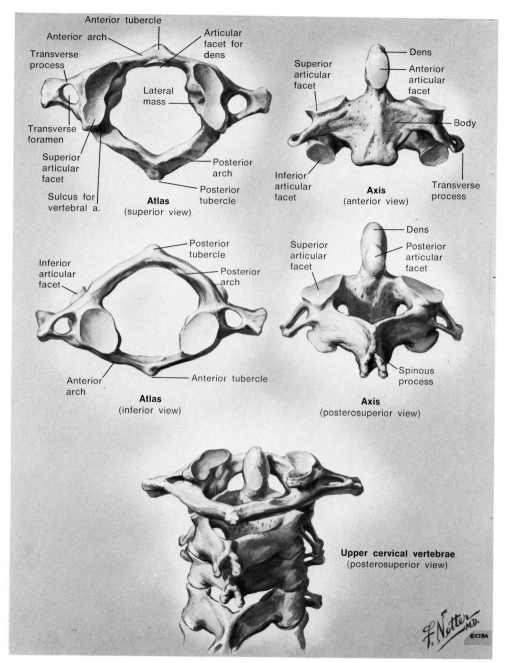

*Fig. 4.* Atlas and axis.[14] Copyright © 1953, 1972 CIBA Pharmaceutical Company, Division of CIBA-GEIGY Corporation. Reproduced, with permission, from *The CIBA Collection of Medical Illustrations* by Frank H. Netter, M.D. All rights reserved.

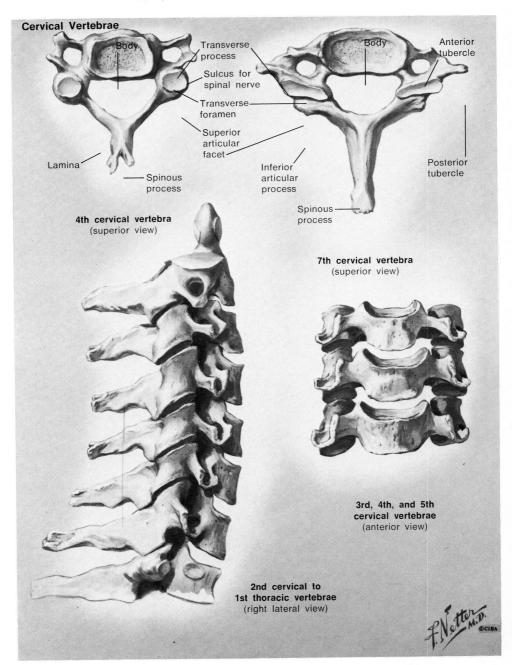

Cervical Vertebrae

Body — Transverse process

Sulcus for spinal nerve

Transverse foramen

Superior articular facet

Lamina

Spinous process

Body — Anterior tubercle

Inferior articular process

Posterior tubercle

Spinous process

**4th cervical vertebra**
(superior view)

**7th cervical vertebra**
(superior view)

**3rd, 4th, and 5th cervical vertebrae**
(anterior view)

**2nd cervical to 1st thoracic vertebrae**
(right lateral view)

*Fig. 5.* Cervical vertebrae.[14] Copyright © 1953, 1972 CIBA Pharmaceutical Company, Division of CIBA-GEIGY Corporation. Reproduced, with permission, from *The CIBA Collection of Medical Illustrations* by Frank H. Netter, M.D. All rights reserved.

with the tubercles of the ribs. The lumbar vertebrae are largest and have square spinous processes in contrast to the pointed spinous processes in thoracic and cervical areas (Figs. 6, 7). The sacrum is composed of five fused sacral vertebrae. It is curved on lateral view from ventral to dorsal as one proceeds caudally. To identify the intervertebral disc, palpation of the interlaminar space between L5 and S1 is an excellent landmark for proceeding cephalad to identify lower lumbar disc spaces.

## Ligaments

Certain ligaments must be considered in the assessment of spinal cord injury, but many ligaments will not be mentioned here, and standard anatomy volumes should be consulted for complete information.[16]

The anterior longitudinal ligament is a broad band on the anterior surface of the vertebral bodies extending from the axis and the skull itself all the way down to the sacrum. The posterior longitudinal ligament lies on the posterior surface of the vertebral bodies and on the anterior surface of the spinal canal, and extends from the axis and the base of the skull to the sacrum. It is continuous with the tectorial membrane which passes from the axis to the occipital bone. The anterior longitudinal ligament limits extension of the vertebral column; the posterior longitudinal ligament prevents hyperflexion of the vertebral column.

In addition, capsular ligaments surround the synovial joints between adjacent articular processes, and intertransverse ligaments and the ligamentum flavum are placed posteriorly atop the dura-invested spinal cord and beneath the laminar surface. The latter is elastic tissue and allows a certain degree of movement. Its function is probably protective. This so-called yellow ligament may bulge and contribute to damage in central cord injury with cervical spondylosis. Hypertrophy may occur and contribute to damage sustained in spinal injury in a narrowed canal. Supraspinous ligaments connect each spinous process inferiorly at its base.

## Intervertebral Discs

The intervertebral disc is frequently involved in spinal injury.[19] The outer portion, composed of fibrocartilage, is the so-called anulus fibrosus, and the soft mucoid inner portion is the nucleus pulposus. Although the chief element of the nucleus pulposus has been described as a mucoid material, in our opinion it is more solid and would best be described as a substance more or less resembling crabmeat. The nucleus pulposus has a very high water content, said to be over 80 percent. Under chronic pressure with the body in the erect position, the disc is said to lose water content, and this apparently accounts for height loss during the day.

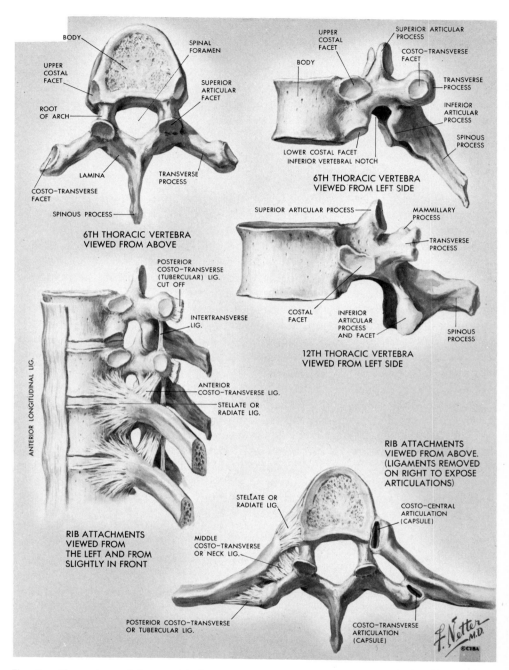

*Fig. 6.* Thoracic vertebrae with ligamentous attachments.[14] Copyright © 1953, 1972 CIBA Pharmaceutical Company, Division of CIBA-GEIGY Corporation. Reproduced, with permission, from *The CIBA Collection of Medical Illustrations* by Frank H. Netter, M.D. All rights reserved.

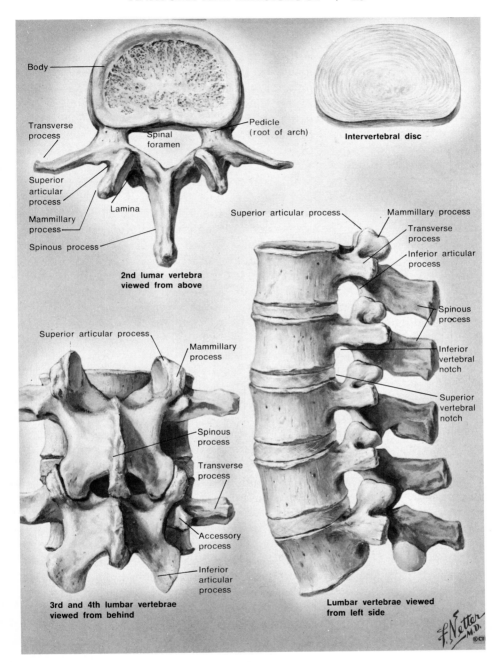

Body

Transverse
process

Spinal
foramen

Pedicle
(root of arch)

Intervertebral disc

Superior
articular
process

Lamina

Mammillary
process

Spinous process

**2nd lumar vertebra
viewed from above**

Superior articular process

Mammillary process

Transverse
process

Inferior articular
process

Spinous
process

Inferior
vertebral
notch

Superior
vertebral
notch

Superior articular process

Mammillary
process

Spinous
process

Transverse
process

Accessory
process

Inferior
articular
process

**3rd and 4th lumbar vertebrae
viewed from behind**

**Lumbar vertebrae viewed
from left side**

*Fig. 7.* Lumbar vertebrae.[14] Copyright © 1953, 1972 CIBA Pharmaceutical Company, Division of CIBA-GEIGY Corporation. Reproduced, with permission, from *The CIBA Collection of Medical Illustrations* by Frank H. Netter, M.D. All rights reserved.

## THE SPINAL CORD AND NERVE ROOTS

The spinal cord lies in the vertebral canal surrounded by the meninges, consisting of the tough, leather-like dura, the arachnoid, and the pia attached to the cord itself (Fig. 8). The epidural space contains blood vessels and adipose tissue. Vertebral venous plexuses and veins form part of Batson's veins, which are notable because of the absence or incompetence of valvular structures and the fact that they can receive blood from the pelvis and abdomen and conduct infection or metastases to the cranial area without circulation through the pulmonary system.

Spinal arteries are tributaries of the vertebral arteries in the neck, of the posterior branches of the intercostal lumbar arteries in the chest and abdomen, and of the lateral sacral arteries in the pelvis. They divide into three branches as they enter the intervertebral foramen. One artery passes toward the lamina dorsally, one passes ventrally toward the vertebral body, and the more important middle branch runs along the nerve root and supplies the spinal cord. On the sides of the cord, the pia and the arachnoid, as well as the dura, are attached by bilateral bands of connective tissue called the denticulate (dentate) ligaments.[17] They pass from the spinal cord to the dura, the first dentate ligament attached at the C1 area, and the last at the level of T12. In most patients, the spinal cord ends at about L1, but sometimes the termination is between L1 and L2. There is considerable variation. The conus medullaris, or the tapered lower end of the spinal cord, continues in the filum terminale, a nonnervous structure. There are 31 pairs of spinal nerve roots arising from the spinal cord, divided into anterior and posterior roots: 8 cervical, 12 thoracic, 5 lumbar, 5 sacral, and 1 coccygeal.

Numerous tracts are involved in the white matter, and the reader is urged to consult a standard neuroanatomic text for the identification. The structures, previously thought simple, are now recognized to be more complicated, but, by and large, various tracts have retained their classic descriptions for the purpose of identifying damage in spinal cord injury.

The caudal spinal cord (conus medullaris) tapers to end usually opposite the L1 vertebral body. It may terminate normally as high as the middle of the twelfth thoracic vertebral body or as low as the inferior border of the second lumbar vertebra. Descending from the tapered end of the conus medullaris is the filum terminale. This fibrous nonneural structure attaches to the dorsum of the coccyx after penetrating the dura. The anterior and posterior roots of the cauda equina are derived from the conus and lie loosely in the thecal sac.

The relation of the spinal cord segments to the vertebral bodies is of practical importance. The eighth cervical cord segment is located between the bodies of C6 and C7. The T12 spinal segment is usually located at a level corresponding approximately to the body of the tenth thoracic vertebra. In the thoracic spine, a given spinal cord segment is generally located one and one-half to two vertebral bodies higher than its numerically equivalent vertebral bony counterpart. In the clinical diagnosis of a thoracic lesion, this

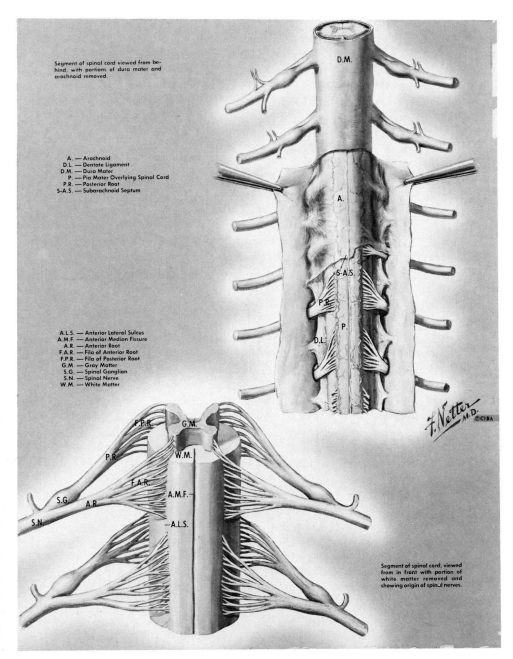

Segment of spinal cord viewed from behind, with portions of dura mater and arachnoid removed.

A. — Arachnoid
D.L. — Dentate Ligament
D.M. — Dura Mater
P. — Pia Mater Overlying Spinal Cord
P.R. — Posterior Root
S-A.S. — Subarachnoid Septum

A.L.S. — Anterior Lateral Sulcus
A.M.F. — Anterior Median Fissure
A.R. — Anterior Root
F.A.R. — Fila of Anterior Root
F.P.R. — Fila of Posterior Root
G.M. — Gray Matter
S.G. — Spinal Ganglion
S.N. — Spinal Nerve
W.M. — White Matter

D.M.

A.

S-A.S.

P.R.

P.

D.L.

F.P.R.   G.M.

P.R.       W.M.

F.A.R.

S.G.    A.R.    A.M.F.—

S.N.

—A.L.S.

Segment of spinal cord, viewed from in front with portion of white matter removed and showing origin of spinal nerves.

*Fig. 8.* Spinal membranes and roots.[14] Copyright © 1953, 1972 CIBA Pharmaceutical Company, Division of CIBA-GEIGY Corporation. Reproduced, with permission, from *The CIBA Collection of Medical Illustrations* by Frank H. Netter, M.D. All rights reserved.

should be taken into account for anatomic localization. Below L1 the spinal segments of the conus are in close apposition, and it is impractical to attempt to relate them to their corresponding vertebral levels. The L1 vertebra can be differentiated from that of T12 by the sharp tip of the spinous process of the latter opposed to the blunt spinous process of the former.

Regarding sensory transmission within the spinal cord, the anterolateral tracts convey pain and temperature sensation and, to a lesser extent, impulses perceived as pressure and touch. The posterior columns transmit gnostic sensation—touch, pressure, vibration, and muscle, tendon, and joint sensibility (position sense).

Serious disturbances in respiration result from lesions of segments C3–C5 that involve the motor cells of the phrenic nerves. Destruction of these cells or their outgoing fibers leads to paralysis of the diaphragm, while irritation induced by nearby lesions results in hiccough, dyspnea, and coughing. Affection of reticulospinal fibers from the medullary respiratory center is another cause of respiratory distress. These fibers constitute the major component of the respiratory pathway and are concerned with automatic respiration. Voluntary respiration is mediated by the lateral pyramidal tract. The reticulospinal pathway is probably a diffuse one, medial in location to the lateral spinothalamic and lateral corticospinal tracts.

In our experience, earliest return of sensation is signaled by the interpretation as touch of stimuli that ordinarily cause deep pain. For example, pressure on the Achilles tendon, great toe, or tibia of a degree that would ordinarily cause disagreeable deep pain is experienced by the cord-injured patient as a feeling of touch or pressure, which he tolerates well. Tugging on a Foley catheter inserted into the bladder causes deep pain, or at least a sensation of touch, and, on occasion, is the only sign of sensory function that remains following injury. Early motor functional return is revealed by barely discernible muscle contractions best palpated rather than observed. Electromyographic evidence of function in volitional motor units verifies this impression.

The Brown-Sequard syndrome is caused by a lesion that involves the lateral half of the spinal cord over one or more segments. In cases of trauma it occurs following hemisection of the cord—most commonly as a result of a knife wound.[13] At the level of the lesion, there is an ipsilateral segmental lower motor neuron paralysis as well as complete sensory loss in the corresponding dermatomic area. Below the level of the lesion, on the same side, destruction of the descending motor fibers causes a variable loss of voluntary motion, increased tone, increase of the deep reflexes, absence of superficial reflexes, and a positive Babinski toe sign. With regard to sensory signs, analgesia and thermoanesthesia are demonstrable a few segments below the lesion on the opposite side. The discrepancy in levels corresponds to the distance that fibers transmitting sensations of pain and temperature ascend on the same side of the cord prior to crossing, which is usually two to four segments. Tactile sensibility is usually, but not always, intact, because of the many crossed as well as uncrossed fibers subserving this modality. Perception of vibration and muscle and joint sensibility are impaired on the ipsilateral

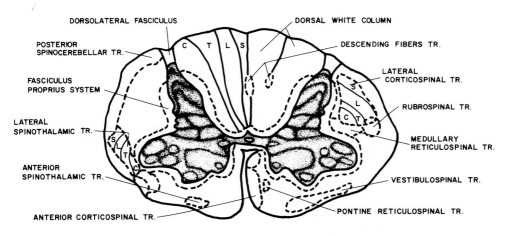

DORSOLATERAL FASCICULUS

DORSAL WHITE COLUMN

POSTERIOR
SPINOCEREBELLAR TR.

DESCENDING FIBERS TR.

FASCICULUS
PROPRIUS SYSTEM

LATERAL
CORTICOSPINAL TR.

RUBROSPINAL TR.

LATERAL
SPINOTHALAMIC TR.

MEDULLARY
RETICULOSPINAL TR.

ANTERIOR
SPINOTHALAMIC TR.

VESTIBULOSPINAL TR.

ANTERIOR CORTICOSPINAL TR.

PONTINE RETICULOSPINAL TR.

*Fig. 9.* Neuroanatomy of the spinal cord.

side below the lesion. The classic picture of hemisection is rare but partial syndromes are common (Fig. 9).

Fibers comprising the corticospinal tract originate in the cerebral cortex, most of them from the precentral area.[10] The fibers course downward through the brain and brain stem and upon reaching the lower end of the medulla oblongata, 80 percent cross the midline forming the pyramidal tract. At each spinal segmental level, almost to the very end of the spinal cord, fibers from the tract synapse either with interneurons at the base of the posterior horn or with motor neurons of the anterior horn. About 20 percent of corticospinal fibers do not cross in the pyramidal decussation. Instead, they proceed directly down the cord ipsilateral to their site of origin. Some of these fibers course downward in the anterior column of the cord and others descend in the lateral column of the cord. These fibers then cross at approximately the level of the segments they innervate and synapse either with interneurons or anterior horn cells.

In order to distinguish between radicular paralysis of a segmental nature and peripheral nerve paralysis, it is necessary to keep in mind the pattern of peripheral nerve innervation as well as segmental innervation (Tables 1, 2). If muscles supplied by the same peripheral nerve are affected, the site of the lesion must be peripheral in the nerve. On the other hand, if there is partial or complete paralysis of a group of muscles each with the same radicular innervation, the lesion must then be located at the anterior root level or in the spinal cord. The same kind of reasoning applies when diagnosing the level of brachial plexus injuries.

## Blood Supply

The anterior spinal artery originates by fusion of two inferiorly directed branches arising from the vertebral arteries, and is a single artery running in

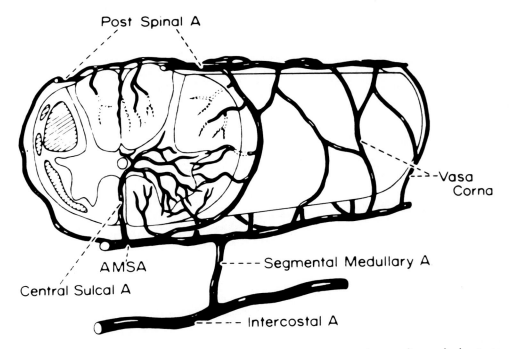

Post Spinal A

Vasa Corna

AMSA

Segmental Medullary A

Central Sulcal A

Intercostal A

Fig. 10. Arterial circulation of the spinal cord; AMSA = anterior median sulcal artery. (Courtesy of Ahmann et al, Neurology 25:301, 1975)

the anterior median fissure[1] (Fig. 10). The posterior spinal arteries originate from the posterior inferior cerebellar arteries or the vertebral arteries themselves. These three arteries proceed throughout the length of the cord and are small at their origins but are reinforced at various intervals by branches of radicular arteries. Typically, the anterior spinal artery distributes to the ventral two-thirds of the spinal cord, and the dorsal one-third of the spinal cord is supplied by the lesser or posterior spinal arteries, although variations exist. Two watershed areas where perfusion is thought to be less are the upper thoracic spine and the middle to lower thoracic spine. The venous drainage of the spinal cord is irregular but resembles the arterial supply.

The anterior spinal artery, which supplies the anterior two-thirds of the cord, originates from intracranial branches of both vertebral arteries and is fed by anterior radicular branches emanating from the vertebral, subclavian, intercostal, and lumbar arteries as one proceeds caudally. The first four thoracic segments are most vulnerable to ischemic change as a result of damage to either the anterior spinal artery or its tributaries. This is due to poor collateral circulation in this area. The communicating branches that enter the vertebral canal with the anterior spinal roots contribute significantly to the circulation of the spinal cord, especially the artery of Adamkiewicz which accompanies one of the lower thoracic or upper lumbar anterior roots, most often on the left side. The paired posterior spinal arteries, which are actually one plexiform channel, generally supply the posterior (dorsal) one-third of the cord, and communicate with the anterior spinal artery by way of numerous arterial coronae. In the cervical cord, the posterior spinal arteries are formed by inconstant branches of the posterior inferior cerebellar or vertebral arteries. In the thoracic cord, compromise of the spinal arterial supply may give rise to clinical evidence of a level above the actual site of the lesion due to proximal (cephalic) ischemia, particularly in the watershed between T1 andT4.

## PHYSIOLOGY

Spinal transection suddenly interrupts all descending pathways that influence spinal reflexes either by facilitation or inhibition. Monosynaptic segmental reflexes are normally influenced to a considerable extent by descending suprasegmental impulses, and undergo an abrupt change in reactivity when deprived of these influences. In lower animals, the vestibulospinal and reticulospinal tracts are thought to convey "shock-preventing" impulses; in man, corticospinal connections play a more important role in this respect.

In addition to paralysis and loss of the deep tendon and superficial reflexes, perception of sensation and autonomic function are abolished below the site of transection (Fig. 11). The bladder and bowel are paralyzed with resultant urinary retention, ileus, and meteorism. Owing to lack of vasomotor

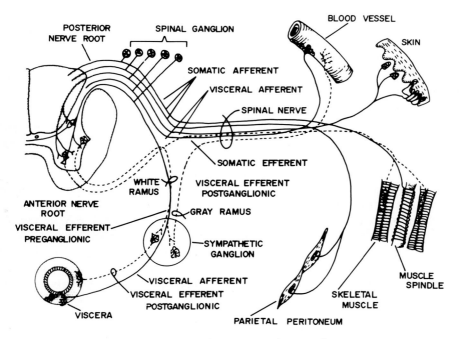

*Fig. 11.* Innervation of somatic and visceral structures.

control, the blood pressure falls temporarily. Sweat secretion is absent below the lesion. In man the period of spinal shock varies from days to weeks. It is generally agreed that the intensity and duration of spinal shock increase as one ascends the evolutionary scale, especially in primates. The state of spinal shock may be prolonged as a result of toxic and septic conditions.

The first movements to return following a period of areflexia are withdrawal movements in response to plantar stimulation, dorsiflexion of the big toe (the sign of Babinski), and anal and bulbocavernosus reflexes. In the later stages the withdrawal response becomes more vigorous and can be elicited by a minimal stimulus applied to the lower extremities. In spinal cord transection above T5, both abdominal and cremasteric reflexes are almost always lost. Occasionally in cases of complete lesions, these reflexes, although diminished and readily exhaustible, may be elicited during the subacute and chronic stages.

It was formerly believed that extensor hypertonus (paraplegia in extension) as opposed to increased flexor tone (paraplegia in flexion), beginning soon after transection, indicated that the spinal cord was not completely severed and that some degree of functional recovery might occur. This was not borne out by experience gained in World War II, when it was found that paraplegia in extension may occur following complete transection. The order of recovery of the spinal reflexes following trauma varies and, in cases of complete transection, extensor movements of the paraplegic limbs may be observed following a period of flexor activity.[8,12] Generally, increased tone appears sooner in incomplete than in complete lesions. In the chronic phase of spinal injury, crossed reflexes occur as a result of heightened reflex activity of the isolated spinal cord. Such crossed reflexes may also occur in cases of incomplete lesions. The most common crossed reflex resulting from plantar stimulation of the foot is the extensor thrust of the contralateral leg involving contraction of the adductors, quadriceps, and hip extensors, together with plantar flexion of the foot and toes (Philippson's reflex).[15]

In addition to hyperreflexia and extensor plantar responses, clonus and other signs indicative of pyramidal tract dysfunction are demonstrable when increased reflex activity supervenes following spinal transection.

Stretch reflexes even at the segmental level are highly complex in their organization. The concept of muscular hypertonus as a release phenomenon from descending inhibition must also take into account the altered function of the gamma efferent (fusimotor) system. There is evidence that, in large measure, the brain stem influences alpha motor neurons indirectly by altering the rate of discharge of the gamma motor neurons. Spasticity appears to be associated with hyperactivity of the gamma motor neurons of antigravity muscles, which presumably occurs as a result of being released from inhibitory influences. Withdrawal of facilitating effects by interference with cerebellar connections concerned with the integration of the gamma and alpha systems may lead to a suppression of gamma motor activity.

Cephalad effects attributed to interference with ascending impulses acting upon antagonistic reflex arcs have also been demonstrated following spinal transection.

Patients with complete spinal cord transection lose sympathetic reflex responses that depend on efferent pathways from medullary centers to the thoracic cord. Disturbances of vasomotor control result in postural hypotension. There is no vasoconstriction in response to cold, nor is there sweating in response to heat following injury. Later, adaptation takes place. Quadriplegic patients are unable to control their body temperature. It is also generally observed that the heart rate of quadriplegics is not increased in response to a variety of systemic pathologic factors as occurs in the non-spinally injured. Thus the vital signs may not reflect the true pathophysiologic systemic status of the patient. Of interest in this connection are the observations of Jennett,[11] who found that following cervical spinal cord transection, the response of the heart rate to hypoxia (breathing 10 percent oxygen for three minutes) was not markedly different from that of a group of normal controls. Jennett concluded that an intact sympathetic pathway from medulla to spinal cord is not essential for the development of tachycardia subsequent to hypoxia.

The vasomotor reflex or reflex erythema may, in some cases, be utilized to help determine the level of a spinal lesion. It is of localizing value only when absent in the region of the radicular field corresponding to a spinal cord lesion and present above and below this segmental field. The absence of a pilomotor reflex in such a radicular field has the same significance.

## SPINAL SHOCK

The term "spinal shock" was coined by Marshall Hall in 1850 and is still used despite its inappropriateness. Spinal shock bears no relation to surgical shock. It merely signifies absence of reflexes following a severe spinal injury. Absence of reflexes occurs when the spinal cord is suddenly sectioned experimentally or accidentally. Disconnection may be anatomic or physiologic, which occurs when anatomic continuity is preserved. Spinal shock also occurs when the spinal cord is cooled or when a local anesthetic is injected into it. The result of an acute transection of the spinal cord by any of these means causes absence of reflexes. Such an areflexive state in man may last for several weeks. The lower the animal species, the sooner do the reflexes return following cord transection. It has been observed clinically that a patient with an incomplete transection will have return of deep tendon reflexes within a few days following injury. The return of reflexes means that the cord has not been sectioned completely and that there is some remaining function below the site of injury. Functional recovery can then theoretically occur, although recovery is very uncommon in severe injuries with complete loss of voluntary function.

Spinal transection represents a sudden withdrawal of the many excitatory and inhibitory influences that occur within the spinal cord, which finally act in some way upon muscles. It can be reasoned that the basic activity of a section of spinal cord detached from higher control is one of hypoactivity, flaccidity, or areflexia.

Several weeks following injury, reflexes do return, and hyperreflexia may occur. Following recovery from spinal shock, reflex activity returns and, eventually, in many cases withdrawal movements accompanied by excessive visceral autonomic discharge appear. In such cases, plantar stimulation of the foot may evoke violent withdrawal of the lower extremities, profuse sweating, and evacuation of the bladder and bowel. This reaction is termed a mass reflex, and is indicative of automatic activity of the isolated segment of spinal cord. The Babinski sign may be elicited, and withdrawal and spontaneous nonvoluntary movements can occur in response to stimulation. Anal and genital reflexes recur, and in some cases mass reflexes begin to appear (see Chapter 23). With a relatively minor sensory stimulus of the skin or a full bladder or rectum, the patient may begin to sweat profusely, the bladder and rectum may empty, and the lower extremities may withdraw violently. This is frequently distressing to the patient. In addition to the hyperactive reflexes, clonus may occur.

In spinal shock, sudden withdrawal of facilitation decreases excitability of spinal motor neurons and interneurons. The function of higher control, therefore, at least at the time of injury and in the several weeks thereafter, is to reduce excitability. Later, circuits within the spinal cord recover and cause increase of reflexes. Spinal shock is also accompanied by other autonomic deviations from normal. Blood pressure usually drops, owing to loss of sympathetic control and tone. There is an ileus because of loss of autonomic control. Hypothermia and bradycardia occur.

A mechanism that might explain the increase in excitability of the reflex arc below a spinal transection is hyperactivity of the reflex arc, thus accounting for the spasticity which occurs weeks to months following spinal injury. There is some evidence both anatomically and electrophysiologically that following spinal transection, posterior root fibers in the area of injury sprout new collaterals and produce more synaptic connections with motor neurons and interneurons. Such an increase in connections might increase the magnitude of reflex response to peripheral stimulation.

## REFERENCES

1. Ahmann PA, Smith SA, Schwartz JF, Clark DB: Spinal cord infarction due to minor trauma in children. Neurology 25:301–307, 1975
2. Angevine JB, Jr: Clinically Relevant Embryology of the Vertebral Column and Spinal Cord. In Clinical Neurosurgery, Proc Cong Neurol Surg, Denver, Colorado, 1972. Baltimore, Williams & Wilkins, 1973, chap 7, pp 95–113
3. Arey LB: Developmental Anatomy. A Textbook and Laboartory Manual of Embryology. Philadelphia, WB Saunders, 1965, p 695
4. Burrington JD, Brown C, Wayne ER, Odom J: Anterior approach to the thoracolumbar spine. Technical considerations. Arch Surg 111:456–460, 1976
5. DiChiro G, Fried LC: Blood flow currents in spinal cord arteries. Neurology 21:1088–1096, 1971
6. Dommisse GF: Morphological aspects of the lumbar spine and lumbosacral region. Ortho Clin North Am 6:163–175, 1975
7. Dommisse GF, Grobler L: Arteries and veins of the lumbar nerve roots and cauda equina. Clin Orthop 115:22–29, 1976

8. Guttmann L: Clinical Symptomatology of Spinal Cord Lesions. In Vinken PJ, Bruyn GW, Biemond A (eds): Handbook of Clinical Neurology, vol I. Localization in Clinical Neurology. Amsterdam, North Holland Pub, 1969, pp 176–216

9. Hollinshead WH: Anatomy for Surgeons, vol III. The Back and Limbs. New York, Hoeber-Harper, 1958, pp 82–200

10. Jane JA, Yashon D, DeMyer WE, Bucy PC: The contribution of the precentral gyrus to the corticospinal tract of man. J Neurosurg 26:244, 1967

11. Jennett S: The response of heart rate to hypoxia in man after cervical spinal cord transection. Paraplegia 8:1, 1970

12. Kuhn RA: Functional capacity of the isolated human spinal cord. Brain 73:1, 1950

13. Lipschitz R: Associated injuries and complications of stab wounds in the spinal cord. Paraplegia 5:75, 1967

14. Netter FH: The Ciba Collection of Medical Illustrations, vol I. The Nervous System. Summit, NJ, Ciba, 1953, p 168

15. Ruch TC: Transection of the Human Spinal Cord: The Nature of Higher Control. In Ruch TC, Patton HD, Woodbury JW, Rowe AL (eds): Neurophysiology, 2nd ed. Philadephia, WB Saunders, 1965, pp 207–214

16. Schneider RC, Cherry G, Pantek H: The syndrome of acute central cervical spinal cord injury. J Neurosurg 11:546, 1954

17. Teng P: Ligamentum denticulatum: An anatomical review and its role in various neurosurgical problems of the spinal cord. J Mount Sinai Hosp (New York) 32: 567–577, 1965

18. Truex RC: Functional neuroanatomy of the spinal cord: Clinical implications. Clin Neurosurg 20:29–55, 1973

19. Walker AE: Anatomical factors related to pathogenesis of acute spine injuries. J Bone Joint Surg 46-A:1806–1810, 1964

20. Yashon D, White RJ: Injuries of the Vertebral Column and Spinal Cord. In Feiring EH (ed): Brock's Injuries of the Brain and Spinal Cord, 5th ed. New York, Springer, 1974, p 962

# 4

## Etiology and Predisposing Factors

### INTRODUCTION

The commonest cause of vertebral and spinal cord injury is vehicular accident,[100] automobile or motorcycle. Possibly diving accidents and missile injuries follow, in that order. Key and Retief[62] found of 300 spinal cord injuries admitted to the spinal cord injury center in Capetown, South Africa, one-third were due to motor vehicle accidents and 23 percent were due to stabs. Other accidents as well as fights and falls accounted for 30 percent; sports injuries accounted for 5.3 percent; medical accidents accounted for 3 percent; and gunshot, train accidents, and rock falls accounted for the remainder.

Many less common causes and several predisposing diseases will be reviewed as well as iatrogenic, congenital, vascular, degenerative, infectious, and neoplastic conditions not ordinarily thought of as causing spinal injury per se (Table 1). These conditions have in common an external source of compressive forces on a basically normal spinal cord and cauda equina. They are discussed briefly since they are not the main province of this volume but in the literal sense are responsible for spinal "injury."

### STAB WOUNDS

Stab wounds of the spinal cord are a common cause of spinal injury in certain parts of the world where firearms are not readily available. Occasionally they are encountered in Western countries. Lipschitz and Block[71] described a large series, and the reader is referred to the chapter on stab wounds. Buczynski and Makowsa[15] described a case of traumatic transection of the cervical spinal

## TABLE 1.
## ETIOLOGY OF VERTEBRAL INJURY AND SPINAL CORD COMPRESSION

**ACCIDENTS**

Vehicles
Diving
Missiles and blasts
Knife wounds
Athletics
Suicide
Birth injury
"Clay-shoveler's" fracture
Electrical accidents
Herniated disc
Seat-belt injuries
Gas bubbles (decompression)

**PREDISPOSING AND DEGENERATIVE CONDITIONS**

Rheumatoid arthritis
Ankylosing
Paget's disease
Arachnoiditis
Pseudohypoparathyroidism
Spondylitis

**NEOPLASMS**

Hodgkin's disease
Multiple myeloma
Metastatic carcinoma
Others

**TOXINS**

Triorthocresyl phosphate
Chlordane
Others

**VASCULAR DISEASE**

Spontaneous spinal hematoma (Usually epidural)
Following temporary aortic occlusion
Following cardiac arrest
Dissecting aortic aneurysm
Spinal artery occlusion
Sickle cell disease

**IATROGENIC DISEASE**

Following spinal puncture
Following spinal cord arteriography
Radiation myelitis
Accidents following laminectomy
In conjunction with use of anticoagulants
Spinal anesthesia
Arachnoiditis
Hypokalemia (As in ureteric transplants)

**INFECTIOUS DISEASE**

Abscess (Usually epidural)
Atlantoaxial dislocation with pharyngeal infections
Sarcoidosis
Tuberculoma
Syphilis
Schistosomiasis
Cysticercosis
Herpes zoster

**CONGENITAL DISEASE**

Mongolism
Achondroplasia

cord by glass caused by a splinter when a patient fell through a glass door. The glass was lodged at C4–C5 within the canal. The patient expired after operation.

## CLAY SHOVELER'S FRACTURE

Fracture of one or more spinous processes in the lower cervical spine or upper thoracic vertebra has been called "clay-shoveler's fracture"[41] (Fig. 1). It was so named because it was a frequent occupational injury among untrained

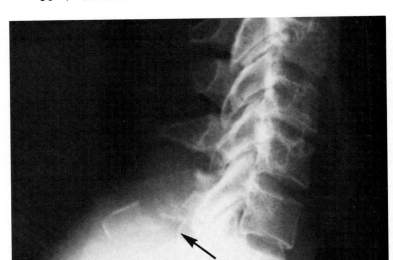

*Fig. 1.* Clay shoveler's fracture of spinous process of C7.

workers digging through clay soil to drain swampy areas in southwestern Australia. The injury resulted from tossing clay up 10 to 15 feet with a long-handled shovel. This fracture had also been noted among industrial metal dippers and other workers, but recently its incidence has been reduced owing to automation and mechanization. This condition also occurs among football players and been termed "root-puller's fracture," stress fracture of the spinous process, and Schmitt's disease.[41]

The usual presenting symptom is sudden pain in the midline of the lower neck or between the shoulder blades while shoveling or lifting a heavy object. Physical examination reveals tenderness and sometimes swelling over the fractured spinous process. The diagnosis is confirmed by radiographic examination in both the anteroposterior (AP) and lateral planes. The AP view may show a double shadow of the spinous process due to displacement (usually downward) of the avulsed bone fragment. Sometimes lateral films are inadequate because of overlying soft tissue so that the fracture may go unrecognized unless visualized on the AP projection. Swimmer's view may be helpful in diagnosis. Management of this fracture is nonsurgical, consisting of simple analgesia and rest.

## SPINAL HEMATOMA

Kirkpatrick and Goodman[64] reported a subarachnoid and subdural spinal hematoma following spinal puncture. This complication has been reported frequently in the past.[95] Spinal hematomas typically present with severe well-localized back pain, and rapidly progressive myelopathy. Prognosis for functional recovery is poor unless immediate decompression is carried out. Anticoagulant therapy enhances the possibility of such a hematoma. Occasionally such hematomas occur spontaneously with no history of trauma.[4] In several reported cases primary bleeding diatheses have been implicated. Epidural hematoma is most common. If the hematoma is in the high lumbar area, a lumbar puncture may be unsuccessful because of collapse of the subarachnoid space. A cisternal myelogram may be required to demonstrate the site of the block.

## INFECTION

Infection in vertebral bodies is uncommon but may cause spinal cord damage by compression. Epidural abscesses may occur spontaneously, may be metastatic following a distant infection,[117] or may be due to tuberculosis. Several other infections have been implicated in spinal injury. Treatment is generally directed to the underlying etiologic agent.

Keuter[60] described nontraumatic atlantoaxial dislocation associated with nasopharyngeal infections. He reviewed the literature and suggested that this was not uncommon. Martin[79] reported atlantoaxial dislocation following cervical infection. The eponym, Grisel's disease (after the 1930 description), has been generally accepted. Apparently there is metastatic infection or infection by direct contiguity of the odontoid with an infected pharynx followed by osteomyelitis. Healing is generally brought about by antibiotics, and fusion is almost never required.

Singh et al.[110] reported a patient with paraplegia due to spinal cysticercosis and Bird[11] reported a case of spinal cord injury due to schistosomiasis, both patients presenting with transverse myelitis. Herpes zoster has occasionally produced transverse myelitis, perhaps due to local vasculitis and consequent ischemia. Ramani and Sengupta[92] described cauda equina compression due to tabetic arthropathy of the spine. All are low-grade infectious processes rather than actual trauma. Alergant[6] reported root compression from tabetic spinal arthropathy and Campbell and Doyle[18] reported eight cases. In these patients proliferation of facet joint tissues encroaches on vital neural structures.

Ahn[3] described treatment for Pott's paraplegia. Tuberculous involvement of the vertebral column, usually in the thoracic area, almost certainly results in spinal cord dysfunction due to direct pressure by the infectious mass. Hodgson and Stock[47] reported an anterior spinal fusion on 100 patients with tuberculosis of the spine. Many advocate costotransversectomy and drainage of the cold abscess followed by immobilization to enhance spontaneous fusion.

## ARACHNOIDITIS

Spinal cord and cauda equina dysfunction may be due to arachnoiditis caused by remote trauma, which results in scarring of the covering membranes of the spinal cord and cauda equina causing pain and other symptoms and signs. Chemical, viral, and bacteriologic causes have been suggested. Chemical causes have been implicated most frequently, but usually the exact etiology is obscure. We have seen patients with severe spinal cord injury following intra-thecal streptomycin injection for TB meningitis. We have also seen severe arachnoiditis in patients who have had multiple myelograms or injections of steroids for low back pain and herniated disc disease. It should be stressed that the etiology is usually unclear. One would expect a certain amount of subarachnoid hemorrhage to accompany severe spinal injury. This can lead to or contribute to arachnoiditis. Clinical symptoms and signs may vary greatly. Usually extreme pain is a prominent complaint. Radiolographic manifestations will be discussed further in the section on Radiology.

## ANKYLOSING SPONDYLITIS

Ankylosing spondylitis is a disease affecting the spinal column in which even relatively minor trauma[65,77] may result in a severe vertebral fracture and spinal injury.[9] Spontaneous dislocations have been reported.[108] This condition is also known as rheumatoid spondylitis and Marie-Strumpell disease. The spine has the radiographic appearance of bamboo, hence the designation "bamboo spine" (Fig. 2). Calcification and ossification of the ligaments, synovial joints, and other vertebral soft tissue converts the spine into a long tube of rigid bone.[40] Associated osteoporosis also predisposes to severe injury.[78] Cervical injuries are most common (Fig. 2).[46,93,127]

Janda et al.[55] reported a patient with ankylosing spondylitis and a fracture dislocation of the cervical spinal column who had considerable neurologic recovery after treatment with the halo traction apparatus. Although their patient had severe neurologic deficit, myelopathy was incomplete. Freeman[32] presented a patient with severe cervical deformity in which correction was also accomplished by halo traction. Hollin et al.[49] described four rheumatoid spondylitis patients with fractures of the cervical spine. They stressed the high mortality.

Yau and Chan[128] reported stress fractures in the lumbodorsal spine in patients with ankylosing spondylitis pointing out that the destructive lesions in ankylosing spondylitis might be a response to delayed union or nonunion of a fracture. They believe that the fractures and destructive lesions seen in ankylosing spondylitis are not truly destructive but rather a failure to reconstruct bone. Most authors, however, believe that the ankylosed spine breaks like a long bone in a transverse plane as a result of bending force. In fractures in the cervical spine it is difficult to ascertain which theory is correct. Fracture of the thoracolumbar spine in ankylosing spondylitis is relatively uncommon, whereas destructive lesions in the nonfractured thoracolumbar spine are relatively frequent. The reader is referred to discussions by Yau and Chan,[128] as well as other discussions listed in the references.

Osgood et al.[88,89] emphasized that concomitant cervical and thoracic

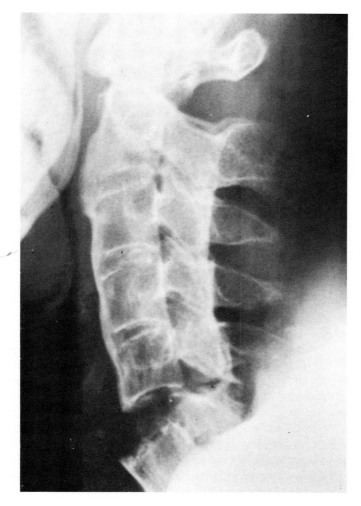

*Fig. 2.* Fracture-dislocation of C5–C6 in ankylosing spondylitis.

spine fractures can occur in patients with advanced ankylosing spondylitis and, although uncommon, the possibility should be considered. Grisolia et al.[38] reported six patients with fractures and dislocations of the spine complicating ankylosing spondylitis and stressed that any type of neurologic deficit or even no deficit may result. Rosenberg and Horowitz[98] also reported a patient with fracture dislocation of the cervical spine in rheumatoid spondylitis.

Hansen et al.[43] discussed fracture dislocations of the ankylosed thoracic spine in rheumatoid spondylitis. They believe that fractures of the thoracic and lumbar spine have not received the attention given cervical spine fractures. The ankylosed spine is comparable to a long bone. There is no motion and no give, hence fractures are somewhat atypical in appearance. Because of

the predisposition to fracture and a relatively high incidence of lack of neurologic signs initially, it is important to warn the patient and be cognizant of a
subclinical but potentially dangerous spinal fracture. Sometimes muscle
spasm, stiff neck or back, and pain in the fractured area may be the only
complaints.

## RADIATION MYELITIS

Radiation injury of the spinal cord is due to excessive radiation dosage or improper ports of administration or is an idiosyncratic reaction in a patient receiving low dosage. The neurologic deficit is almost always progressive[94] but
may not be so. Transient radiation myelitis has been reported,[58] as has improvement in neurologic deficit in this condition. Solheim[114] described five
cases of late radiation myelopathy in which pareses and sensory disturbances
progressed for some time after latent periods of 5 to 19 months. Four of the
five patients then improved considerably and he suggested that the clinical
course of late radiation myelopathy is not always chronic or progressive. In
the absence of a history of spinal injury, myelography may be required to
rule out a compressive lesion.

The interval between termination of radiation and onset of neurologic
symptoms varies from five months up to three years. Myelograms are normal. The neurologic findings are predominantly sensory but almost any neurologic picture can be seen. On occasion a Brown-Sequard syndrome may be
present. The differential diagnosis concerns mainly tumor metastases and remote carcinomatoid myelopathy.[94]

Radiation myelitis may show itself initially by numbness or paresthesia
(pins and needles sensations) affecting the hands, feet, or trunk, which may
be brought on or aggravated by flexion or extension of the neck. These symptoms may be evanescent without further progression or may herald the onset
of severe myelitis. Lhermitte's sign is occasionally seen.[58] The patient will occasionally complain of vibrating or electric shocklike sensations. Neck flexion
is usually the trigger for this phenomenon and in addition to Lhermitte's
sign, it is sometimes referred to as the "barber's chair sign." Patients having
received radiation for neoplasms of the upper respiratory tract, chest, thyroid,
and metastatic tumors are most commonly affected. Doses may be relatively
low (3000 rad). Long periods of radiation in small individual dosages may
lessen the incidence of radiation myelitis.

Pathologic studies of progressive radiation myelopathy in every instance
reveal gross cord degeneration. Myelomalacia is associated with extensive loss
of myelin. Large zones of necrosis show a predilection for the white matter,
and extensive change in blood vessels, mainly in the form of arteriolar degeneration, exists. There is some necrosis of vascular tissue. It has been suggested that systemic hypertension may be an important factor in determining the
incidence of severe progressive radiation myelopathy in man.

## COMPRESSION FRACTURE

The commonest cause of compression fracture is trauma, usually in a vertical or near vertical plane (Table 2). In a fall from a height, the patient may also suffer calcaneal or other fracture of the feet and legs.

Buhr[16] reported compression fracture common in elderly patients with osteoporotic spines, most occuring spontaneously or with minor trauma. Attempted reduction by hyperextension is not likely to succeed, so treatment should be kept simple. Paralytic ileus may accompany the fracture, particularly if hyperextension is attempted. Because these fractures are almost always stable, the patient with osteoporosis and compression fracture should be mobilized as the severity of pain permits. The treatment of compression fracture with regard to bracing, immobilization, and hospitalization is controversial. External support may help the pain but should be kept to a minimum. Hospitalization, if necessary, should also be kept to a minimum. Many times these fractures are seen incidentally, particularly on lateral chest x-rays. The differential diagnosis should include metastatic carcinoma to a vertebral body, but this is not usually difficult to ascertain. In patients with no related medical or traumatic history, the finding of a compression fracture may be difficult to differentiate from carcinoma.

Harris and Cunningham[44] described stress compression fracture in patients with osteoporosis of the spine. This condition, usually seen in the elderly, may result from trivial stress and can be easily overlooked in an industrial population where the incidence of so-called low back strain is high. Since neurological deficit is minimal, treatment is supportive and nonspecific. Disability is usually due to pain.

### TABLE 2.
### CAUSES OF VERTEBRAL COMPRESSION FRACTURE

Falls from heights

Osteoporosis

Tetanus

Epileptic seizures

Snowmobile injuries

Electroconvulsive therapy

Ejections from aircraft

Parachute jumps

Helicopter accidents

Following chlordane poisoning

Davis and Rowland[24] described upper thoracic vertebral fractures in West Africans suffering from tetanus, finding vertebral fractures in 19 of 33 patients, with a greater degree of compression occurring in children. They observed that vertebral fracture is usually not an important complication of tetanus, since it causes little pain, does not prolong the illness, and gives rise to no permanent disability. It also has no effect on mortality. Mukherjee[85] reported fractures of vertebra in conjunction with tetanus, reviewed the literature, and concluded that this was a relatively rare complication. Colangelo[21] reported tetanus in a 16-year-old boy complicated by multiple compression fractures of the third through ninth thoracic vertebrae. The patient recovered. Most compression fractures in tetanus occur in the thoracic spine. Mechanical factors accompanying seizures are believed to be operant, but a vascular factor such as destruction of the spongiosa cannot be excluded. Major mechanical factors relate to abnormal sustained paravertebral muscle contraction with flexion and hyperextension. It is doubtful that trauma during tetanic spasms accounts for fracture.

Vasconcelos[122] described compression fractures of the vertebrae in about 15 percent of patients having major epileptic seizures. He felt that fractures were caused by sustained muscular contraction. Another cause might be direct trauma sustained during a fall. There is no way of being certain which of these causes of fracture is commonest during seizures.

Lutz[75] reported vertebral fractures occurring during electroconvulsive psychiatric therapy, presenting 33 patients with compression fractures from the third through eighth thoracic vertebra. Most were minimal, but some were moderate. In no case did he describe neurologic deficit and in all cases the fractures took place prior to the fifth shock treatment. He suggested that succinyl choline chloride, the paralytic agent, is an important modification in electroconvulsive therapy and has reduced the incidence of compression fractures. He stated that because the paralytic technique is somewhat inconvenient it may not be widely used. Stranger and Kerridge[116] reported multiple compression fractures of the dorsal spine following chlordane poisoning. The patient ingested a large amount of this material and had convulsive seizures that appeared to be the cause of the fractures.

Roberts et al.[97] drew attention to the high incidence of snowmobile spine injuries, stating that compression fractures of the spine account for a significant number. They presented six patients who had no severe neurologic deficit, but some did have pain and other sequelae. The injuries are caused by the bumping vertical forces to the vertebral column during transit over rough terrain.

Chubb et al.[20] studied 928 aircraft ejections occurring from 1960 through 1964. Of 44 persons sustaining vertebral compression fractures, 28 were believed to have received them during ejection and 16 during parachute landing. Sitting in the erect position with hips and head firmly against the seat was the most significant factor in preventing compression fractures, and increasing age, lack of tower training, use of rocket catapults, and ejection from bombers were possibly contributing interrelated factors.

Ewing[28] analyzed vertebral fracture rates in U.S. Naval aircraft accidents between 1959 and 1963. The highest rates were found in jet aircraft ejections, and he suggested that inadequate sitting height accommodations in certain aircraft cause vertebral fractures with rapid ejection. Of all vertebral fractures, 60 percent[104] occurred in jets and the trend seems upward; 60 percent[62] of vertebral fractures in jet aircraft occurred in conjunction with the ejection maneuver itself.

Italiano[53] surveyed helicopter accidents finding spinal fractures most commonly located in the dorsal lumbar vertebrae, which were compression fractures resulting from forward tilting at the time of the crash. The anterior body is more severely involved because of this biomechanical effect.

## SPONDYLOSIS

Vertebral spondylosis, both cervical and lumbosacral, is another cause of damage to the spinal cord not due to trauma. It is a slow, relentless, osteoarthritic, degenerative process that results from aging. Joffe et al.[57] described several cases and reviewed the literature. Constriction of the canal is caused by hypertrophic laminal arches, pedicles, bony spurs, and articular facets with or without disc herniation. Hypertrophic yellow ligament may add to the problem. Pain and radicular or long tract neurologic deficit can be present.[27] Intermittent ischemia, resulting from compression either by herniated disc or the spondylotic process, may cause intermittent claudication[14] of the legs identical, but more frequently atypical, to that seen in vascular disease. Although both types of claudication[113] are relieved by rest, relief may not be immediate in this type of "narrow spinal canal" syndrome. The lordotic posture may accentuate leg pain in standing. The kyphotic posture relieves the discomfort occasionally. Diagnosis is based on examination and investigative electromyogram and myelogram. Measuring the anterior-posterior diameter or interpedicular distance on plain x-rays may not provide a diagnosis, since these measurements are frequently within normal limits. A constricted dural sac demonstrated by myelography is diagnostic. Appropriate laminectomy may provide relief. Further details are discussed by Joffe et al.,[57] Snyder et al.,[113] and Wilson.[124]

## RHEUMATOID ARTHRITIS

Chronic proliferative inflammatory changes of rheumatoid arthritis may involve almost all nonneural tissue of the cervical spine.[8,111] Radiographs of the upper cervical area can demonstrate erosions of the dens, narrowing of the atlantoaxial and atlanto-occipital joints with erosions of adjacent bone, and abnormal mobility of the atlas on flexion. Distance between the anterior margin of the dens and the posterior border of the anterior arch of the atlas may exceed normal (about 4 mm). Stress films may show abnormal mobility.

Below the axis, the disc spaces may be narrow and bone plate erosion without osteophytosis may result in abnormal mobility and dislocation at multiple levels.[50] In rheumatoid arthritis, hyperemia and inflammatory changes in joints are accompanied by osteoporosis and ligamentous abnormalities. Dislocation may be spontaneous[74,108] and has been reported in juvenile arthritics.[86]

Ferlic et al.[30] described unstable cervical spines in rheumatoid arthritis and those resulting from surgical treatment. They stated that rheumatoid arthritis is not infrequently accompanied by spontaneous subluxation of cervical vertebrae, which can be managed by nonsurgical treatment. Surgery is necessary when neural involvement exists or when conservative therapy fails. The issue as to when surgical fusion should be done because of instability has not been resolved. Each patient is different and that decision requires serious consideration by experienced physicians. If the patient is in good condition, we seriously consider fusion if the spine is unstable even without neurologic deficit. Subluxation may develop even in bedridden individuals.

Meijers et al.[82] described dislocation of the cervical spine with spinal cord compression in rheumatoid arthritis in 14 patients. The neurologic syndromes included almost any variation of symptoms and signs associated with spinal cord compression. Several patients complained of suboccipital pain. Gleason and Urist[36] described a patient with rheumatoid arthritis in which the condition produced erosions, separation, and displacement of the odontoid process into the base of the skull and was finally fatal. Lemmen and Laing[69] reported fractures of the cervical spine in patients with rheumatoid arthritis at the C5–C6 level in two patients, and a C6–C7 fracture in another. They pointed out that even in rheumatoid patients, one should always consider locking of the facets and the impossibility of reducing the fracture by ordinary means.

## SPORTS INJURIES

Serious injuries of the vertebral column and spinal cord occur in almost all sports. Accurate diagnosis is important so that a potential spinal injury is not converted to irreversible paralysis. Leidholt[57,68] described spinal injuries in sports, stressing the fact that the spine is injured very frequently in competitive sports and that injuries to the spine occur in every sport.

Of all sports, football probably accounts for most injuries. In collating serious and fatal neurosurgical football injuries, Schneider[103–105] found most occurred in players well equipped with armor. Only 11.8 percent of the group were sandlot players who had not worn equipment. Spearing, in which the head is directly utilized to impale a runner or block a tackler, is dangerous because of possible hyperflexion or hyperextension. In Schneider's lab, Gosch et al.[37] showed that in experimental head injuries cervical spine cord hemorrhages are not only possible but common. It appears that a head injury enhances the possibility of masked spinal injury under certain circumstances. Funk and Wells[34] described football injuries of the cervical spine, reviewing mechanisms that included extension, flexion, impaction, and lateral stretch injuries. They also emphasized that at times the initial presentation of congenital instability of the vertebral column may be falsely attributed to an athletic accident. Lateral flexion neck injuries were emphasized by Chrisman et al.[19] They felt that lateral head and neck movement predisposed to cervical root compression syndromes. Harris et al.[45] emphasized the etiology of cervical intervertebral disc trauma causing paralysis.

Liss[72] described a fatal cervical spinal cord injury in a swimmer. There was no impact against any moving or immobile object and the fatal injury was demonstrated in a thin gray matter segment at the C2–C3 level in the form of acute petechial hemorrhages. To our knowledge no similar case has been reported. Burke[17] described 52 patients admitted to an Australian spinal injury unit because of injuries due to water sport accidents; 48 of these were caused by diving into shallow water and striking their heads on the bottom. Almost all were cervical spine injuries and many had severe neurologic deficit. Kewalramani and Taylor[61] also reported injuries to the cervical spine from diving accidents. Of 126 cases of spinal injury admitted to their facility in California, 18 percent were secondary to diving accidents over a 46-month period. Males ranging from 15 to 47 years of age composed 91 percent of the group; 90 percent occurred in the summer months. Chronic recurrent cervical vertebral (and spinal) trauma occurs in repetitive high diving. Papo and Alvarez[90] described the effects in Acapulco's divers.

Ellis et al.[26] described five patients who sustained serious neurologic injuries tumbling on the trampoline. One of these resulted from a backward somersault imperfectly executed by a person unskilled in gymnastics.

## VASCULAR INJURY

Vascular injury to the spinal cord is caused by many etiologic factors, most commonly an ischemic injury due to vascular occlusion with perfusion deficit. The midthoracic and upper thoracic spinal cord is subject to ischemia because of poor circulation from radicular arteries and spinal arteries (see Chap. 2). Consequently lesions interrupting radicular flow may cause paraplegia.

Ahmann et al.[2] described spinal cord infarctions in children due to minor trauma. They described two children, ages 22 months and four years, who after slight trauma developed flaccid weakness of both arms and flaccid quadriplegia with involved sphincters. No fracture or dislocation was found. Myelograms were negative and diagnosis was made only after the full clinical syndrome evolved. Pathologic studies revealed ischemic infarction involving the cervical cord and central gray matter without hematomyelia or external compressive lesions. They felt that the infarction might be related to spasm of distal branches of the central sulcal arteries in a terminal arterial bed. Pathogenesis of myelomalacia due to vascular involvement following trauma contributes to spinal cord damage. Bischof and Nittner[12] detailed this type of injury.

Condon and Rose[22] and Kepes[59] described spinal cord injury due to a dissecting aneurysm of the aorta. Paraplegia was undoubtedly due to ischemia following interruption of the intercostal and radicular arterial supply of the spinal cord.[63] Paraplegia can occur in conjunction with seemingly uneventful aortic surgery.[1,48] Severe spinal neurologic deficit has been reported secondary to hypotension and cardiac arrest.[5]

Spinal cord damage has been recorded after abdominal aortic angiography.[76] This is a rare but tragic complication when the procedure involves arteries that have communications with the spinal cord circulation. High concentrations of contrast media are neurotoxic and if an undiluted bolus is inadvertently introduced directly into the vasculature of the cord, massive spinal cord parenchymal necrosis may result. A still rarer cause of spinal cord damage during percutaneous vertebral angiography or translumbar aortography may result from accidental misplacement of the needle into the spinal theca. If the mistake is not recognized, angiographic contrast medium injected into the subarachnoid space may cause severe spinal damage and respiratory distress, and may in fact prove fatal.[81]

When spinal cord damage has occurred, basically little can be done to prevent its progress. Steroids and other supportive measures are indicated. Mishkin et al.[83] and McCleery and Lewtas[81] used a scheme in which the spinal fluid is washed out in aliquots of 19 ml, the patient being placed in a head-up posture so that the hyperbaric contrast medium gravitates downward away from the brain. Rapid reduction of cerebrospinal fluid (CSF) iodine level can be achieved, and they reported concomitant improvement of the neurologic status in these patients. Curare with artificial ventilation may be required to control extensor spasms. The rationale for the washout treatment is that Mishkin et al.[83] noted that the iodine content of CSF was elevated after this rare neurologic complication of angiography.

Schneider et al.[102] described spinal cord lesions following temporary circulatory arrest. Gilles and Nag[35] demonstrated vulnerability of the human spinal cord in transient cardiac arrest. They described six young children who had neuronal necrosis within the gray matter of the spinal cord after transient cardiac arrest. Similar lesions follow Stokes-Adams attacks and clamping of the aorta. Mozingo and Denton[84] suggested that the neurologic deficit seen with aortic occlusion resulted from acute peripheral nerve ischemia and not from spinal cord ischemia as had been assumed previously. They stated that the final neurologic deficit due to acute peripheral nerve ischemia may masquerade as that seen with a transverse spinal cord lesion. This, of course, is controversial, since any postmortem examination done soon after such an insult might show little in the way of changes in the spinal cord.

Blaisdell and Cooley[13] described paraplegia after temporary occlusion of the thoracic aorta. In this case, the loss of spinal function is probably due to ischemia. The spinal cord tolerates ischemia poorly as does the brain.

Wolman and Hardy[126] described spinal cord infarction associated with the sickle cell trait. Progressive paraplegia with an ascending level occurred in a 60-year-old woman who was found to have sickle cell trait. Death resulted from respiratory failure and autopsy revealed several small infarcts of varying age confined to the central nervous system. There were infarcts throughout the nervous system, but these were most numerous and extensive in the spinal cord.

Hallenbeck et al.[42] studied mechanisms underlying spinal cord damage and decompression sickness in dogs and suggested that spinal cord infarction in decompression sickness is caused by obstruction of spinal cord venous drainage at the level of the epidural vertebral venous system. Hughes[52] reported a patient who suffered venous infarction of the spinal cord. The patient had a thrombotic diathesis perhaps due to a carcinoma of the pancreas.

## SEAT-BELT INJURIES

Seat belts may prevent serious injury due to ejection or buffeting during automobile accidents, but care must be taken in application and positioning. Seat belts are said to reduce serious injuries by 35 percent. However, some injuries may be due to the seat belt itself (Fig. 3). When only lap belts were worn, it was felt that the addition of "bandolier" or shoulder-type seat belts would reduce the number of seat-belt-related accidents. That may be true, but bandolier-type seat belts themselves may be responsible for neck, chest, and other injuries.

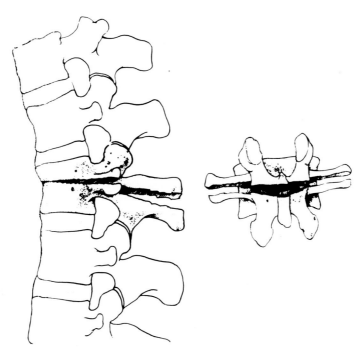

*Fig. 3.* Seat-belt injury of lumbar spine (from Smith, Kaufer: J Bone Joint Surg 51A: 239, 1969).

Smith and Kaufer[112] reported that among 24 lumbar spine fractures in lap seat-belt wearers, 20 showed an unusual and consistent pattern of injury characterized by separation of posterior elements without the usually expected decrease in height of the anterior portion of the vertebral bodies. They suggested that tension stress is primarily responsible for the unusual patterns in seat-belt injuries. Although the seat belt was instrumental in producing the lesion described, they did not indict lap-type seat belts because it was their opinion that more people were helped than hurt by this device. Friedman et al.[33] also described a case of seat-belt lumbar fracture. Howland et al.[51] reported a patient with a transverse fracture induced by an improperly highly placed seat belt, which acted as a central fulcrum.

Saldeen[101] ascribed fatal neck injuries to the use of diagonal safety belts. He stated that this belt configuration did reduce the number of injuries generally at least 50 percent and was particularly effective in preventing head and trunk injuries, but he described three cases of fatal neck injury in persons wearing the diagonal safety belt that were probably caused by the lower jaw being temporarily impaled in the belt when the person slipped out of the belt and was ejected from the car. Fletcher and Brogdon[31] presented a "fulcrum" fracture of the lumbar spine, presumably due to a lap seat belt and a sternum fracture due to the diagonal safety belt. We feel that safety belts certainly contribute to vertebral injuries but generally prevent more serious injuries.

## MISCELLANEOUS

Many other conditions that predispose to vertebral and spinal injuries are by and large uncommon but should be considered in the evaluation of a patient with a spinal injury.

Livingston[73] observed several cases over a three-year period in which spinal manipulation caused injury. He classified seven patients as "direct" injuries, which included joint or soft tissue injury, spinal cord or nerve injury, vascular injury, or bony injury. He defined "indirect injuries" as injury by omission. There were four patients in this category in whom the proper diagnosis of spinal disease was delayed because of manipulation.

Levine et al.[70] reported that spinal cord injury by electrical current had been identified in only 2 of 111 victims of electrical accidents seen in a 21-year period. In one patient, the injury was fatal and postmortem examination of the spinal cord documented the extent of injury. They suggested that electrical injury to the spinal cord may be either transient or permanent.[109] In transient injuries, the neurologic symptoms appear immediately and usually clear within 24 hours. Permanent injuries may not be apparent until days following the accident and may be associated with minimal visible structural injury to the skin and underlying organs. Extent of such injury ranges from localized paresis to quadriplegia. Motor deficits occur more frequently than sensory loss. Clinical presentation may be characterized by either complete or partial paralysis. Jackson et al.[54] presented a patient who developed delayed quadriplegia following an electrical burn. Necrosis of the spinal cord may occur.[66]

Schwarz and Bevilacqua[106] described spinal cord injury following spinal anesthesia. This has been reported with a number of currently used anesthetic agents and it may result in immediate paraplegia or the insidious onset of paraplegia weeks later. Demyelination, necrosis, arachnoiditis, and vasculitis were shown at postmortem.

Taylor et al.[118] and Richter and Behnke[96] described a spinal injury in deep sea divers following a scuba dive. They suggested that many decompression injuries in deep sea divers and caisson workers cause symptoms and signs referable to the presence of intravascular or extravascular nascent gas bubbles. Although the most common type of injury is the peripheral cramp-like muscular pain known as the bends, occasionally the nervous system is involved. Richter and Behnke[96] warned against diving to unwarranted depths unless adequate compression chamber facilities are available. Richter and Behnke's patient improved considerably following recompression but still had considerable residual weakness, spasticity, and sensory loss in the lower extremities after a long follow-up period.

Wolman[125] described a patient with a blast injury of the spinal cord who survived for 43 years. Although both legs were paralyzed initially, a good recovery occurred after 18 months. No evidence of any fracture of the spine was found, but in the lower cervical spinal cord there was a transverse elongated slit surrounded by dense gliosis in the ventral part of the posterior columns. Wolman[125] concluded that the lesion, together with small scattered foci of gliosis in the adjacent posterior and lateral columns, was more consistent with an old contusion from being thrown to the ground than attributable to the direct blast effect of sudden change in air pressure.

Paget's disease can occur in the spine and result in neurologic symptoms and signs.[56,107,120] Feldman and Seaman[29] stated that the cervical spine is rarely affected by Paget's disease but when it is, the x-ray appearance frequently differs from that seen in other parts of the skeleton. A striking frequency of clinical neurologic symptoms and signs in the four patients they described was related to encroachment of the spinal cord or intervertebral foramina as a consequence of the disease process. Symptoms and signs, they felt, might also arise from interference with the blood supply to the spinal cord. Whalley[123] and Ramamurthi and Visvanathan[91] reported a patient with Paget's disease of the axis causing quadriplegia. Teng et al.[119] presented patients with compression of the spinal cord caused by Paget's disease, giant cell tumor, and Albright's syndrome (polyostotic fibrous dysplasia).

Spinal cord injury with paraplegia has occurred secondary to triothocresyl phosphate poisoning. This so called "Jamaica ginger palsy" was first encountered in the 1920s during the prohibition era. Apparently these patients show direct spinal damage, but also may have peripheral neuropathy. Vitamin B-12 and folate deficiency causes subacute combined (posterior and lateral spinal tracts) degeneration of the cord.

Cullen and Pearce[23] presented a case of pseudohypoparathyroidism presenting with spastic paraplegia. The spinal condition was caused by an abnormal overgrowth of bone from a vertebral lamina. Although ectopic bone is characteristic of pseudohypoparathyroidism, usually in the subcutaneous tissues or basal ganglia, theirs was the first report of affliction of the spinal cord. Rosencrantz[99] reported a case of fibrous dysplasia (Jaffe-Lichtenstein disease) with vertebral fracture and compression of the spinal cord. The patient was paraplegic.

Angeloni and Scott[7] described a patient who developed flaccid quadriplegia following ureteric transplant. They ascribed this to hypokalemia developing nine years after ureterosigmoidostomy. Paralysis was first thought to be acute poliomyelitis but responded dramatically to correction of the metabolic abnormalities. Paralysis due to hypokalemia has been reported several times usually due to ureterosigmoidostomy. Treatment with potassium is usually dramatic. Matheson[80] described a case of paraplegia due to severe flexion of the spine from the high lithotomy position.

Norrell and Llewellyn[87] reported a patient with migration of a threaded Steinman pin from the acromioclavicular joint into the spinal canal, which occurred 10 years after internal fixation of an acromioclavicular separation. This is quite an unusual case. The patient suffered only severe pain, and the relation of the position of the pin to symptoms went undiagnosed for some time. The pain was relieved by removal of the pin from the spinal canal.

Spencer[115] described a nail-gun fatality in which the nail was fired anteriorly into the upper neck resulting in a complete block to myelography at the level of the second cervical vertebra. Surgical exploration revealed severe damage of the spinal cord.

Dzenitis[25] reported the first case of spontaneous atlantoaxial dislocation spinal cord compression in a Mongoloid child. He observed that nontraumatic or spontaneous atlantoaxial dislocation is common in Mongolism and may be due to congenital laxity of ligaments and joints in these patients.

Gulati and Rout[39] described atlantoaxial dislocation with quadriparesis in an achondroplastic patient who was successfully treated with skeletal traction and cervical fusion. Spondylosis at thoracic and lumbar levels is frequent in these individuals.

## COMPRESSION BY NEOPLASTIC LESIONS

Any cause of compression or distortion or lack of blood supply to the spinal cord might literally be considered a traumatic event. This can result from neoplasms, arteriovenous malformations, as well as infectious diseases like tuberculosis. Venous infarction of the spinal cord usually occurs in conjunction with a congenital blood vessel abnormality, but may occur spontaneously and be confused with a neoplastic or other nontraumatic cause of spinal damage. Low-grade neoplasms such as giant cell tumor as well as processes possibly neoplastic, like aneurysmal bone cyst, can cause spinal cord compression. Van Beusekom[121] described spinal cord compression in patients with Hodgkin's disease in whom spinal cord dysfunction was due to direct pressure from the tumor. Bhagwati and McKissoch[10] reviewed 10 cases. Although any such externally compressive lesion is traumatic, this volume is concerned with true trauma and its sequelae.

## REFERENCES

1. Adams HD, van Geertruyden HH: Neurologic complications of aortic surgery. Ann Surg 144:574–610, 1956
2. Ahmann PA, Smith SA, Schwartz JF, Clark DB: Spinal cord infarction due to minor trauma in children. Neurology (Minneapolis) 25:301–307, 1975
3. Ahn BH: Treatment for Pott's paraplegia. Acta Ortho Scand 39:145–160, 1968
4. Ainslie J: Paraplegia due to spontaneous extradural or subdural hemorrhage. Brit J Surg 45:565–567, 1958
5. Albert MS, Greer WER, Kantrowitz W: Paraplegia secondary to hypotension and cardiac arrest in a patient who has had previous thoracic surgery. Neurology (Minneapolis) 19:915–918, 1969
6. Alergant CD: Tabetic spinal arthropathy. Two cases with motor symptoms due to root compression. Brit J Venereal Dis 36:261–265, 1960
7. Angeloni JM, Scott GW: Flaccid quadriplegia following ureteric transplant. Lancet 1:1005–1006, 1960
8. Ball J, Sharp J: Rheumatoid arthritis of the cervical spine. Mod Trends Rheumat 2:117–138, 1971
9. Bergmann EW: Fractures of the ankylosed spine. J Bone Joint Surg 31A:669–671, 1949
10. Bhagwati SN, McKissock W: Spinal cord compression in Hodgkin's disease. A review of 10 cases. Brit J Surg 48:672–677, 1961
11. Bird A: Acute spinal schistosomiasis. Neurology 14:647–656, 1964
12. Bischof W, Nittner K: Zur Klinik und Pathgenese der Vaskular Bedingten Myelomalazien. Neurochirug (Stuttgart) 8:215–231, 1965
13. Blaisdell F, Cooley D: Paraplegia after temporary thoracic aortic occlusion. Surgery 51:351–355, 1962
14. Blau JN, Logue V: Intermittent claudication of the cauda equina. Lancet 1:1081–1086, 1961
15. Bucynski AZ, Makowski J: A case of traumatic transection of cervical spinal cord by glass. Paraplegia 12:167–169, 1974
16. Buhr AJ: The aging spine, fractures and osteoporosis. Nova Scotia Med Bull 45:317–321, 1966
17. Burke DC: Spinal cord injuries from water sports. Med J Aust 2:1190–1194, 1972
18. Campbell DJ, Doyle JO: Tabetic Charcot's spine: report of eight cases. Brit Med J 1:1018–1020, 1954
19. Chrisman OD, Snook GA, Stanitis JM, Keedy VA: Lateral-flexion neck injuries in athletic competition. JAMA 192:117–119, 1965
20. Chubb RM, Detrick WR, Shannon RH: Compression fractures of the spine during USAF ejections. Aerospace Med 36:968–972, 1965
21. Colangelo C: Compression fractures of the thoracic vertebrae in a patient with tetanus. JAMA 170:455–457, 1959
22. Condon JR, Rose FC: Neurological manifestations of dissecting aneurysm of aorta. Postgrad Med J 45:419–422, 1969
23. Cullen DR, Pearce JMS: Spinal cord compression in pseudohypoparathyroidism. J Neurol Neurosurg Psychiatry 27:459–462, 1964

24. Davis PR, Rowland HAK: Vertebral fractures in West Africans suffering from tetanus: a clinical and osteological study. J Bone Joint Surg 47B:61–71, 1965

25. Dzenitis AJ: Spontaneous atlanto axial dislocation in a mongoloid child with spinal cord compression. Case report. J Neurosurg 25:458–460, 1966

26. Ellis WG, Green D, Holzaepfel NR, Sahs AL: The trampoline and serious neurological injuries. A report of five cases. JAMA 174:1673–1676, 1960

27. Epstein JA, Epstein BS, Lavine L: Nerve root compression associated with narrowing of the lumbar spinal canal. J Neurol Neurosurg Psychiatry 25:165–176, 1962

28. Ewing CL: Vertebral fracture in jet aircraft accidents: a statistical analysis for the period 1959 through 1963, U.S. Navy. Aerospace Med 37:505–508, 1966

29. Feldman F, Seaman WB: The neurologic complications of Paget's disease in the cervical spine. Am J Roentgenol Radium Ther Nuc Med 105:375–382, 1969

30. Ferlic DC, Clayton ML, Leidholt JD, Gamble WE: Surgical treatment of the symptomatic unstable cervical spine in rheumatoid arthritis. J Bone Joint Surg 57A:349–354, 1975

31. Fletcher BD, Brogdon BG: Seat-belt fractures of the spine and sternum. JAMA 200:167–168, 1967

32. Freeman GE, Jr: Correction of severe deformity of the cervical spine in ankylosing spondylitis with the halo device. J Bone Joint Surg 43A:547–552, 1961

33. Friedman MM, Becker L, Reichmister JP, Neviaser JS: Seat belt spinal fractures. Am Surg 35:617–618, 1969

34. Funk F, Jr, Wells RE: Injuries of the cervical spine in football. Clin Orthop 109:50–58, 1975

35. Gilles FH, Nag D: Vulnerability of human spinal cord in transient cardiac arrest. Neurology (Minneapolis) 21:833–839, 1971

36. Gleason IO, Urist MR: Atlanto-axial dislocation with odontoid separation in rheumatoid disease. Clin Orthop 42:121–129, 1965

37. Gosch HH, Gooding E, Schneider RC: Cervical spinal cord hemorrhages in experimental head injuries. J Neurosurg 33:640–645, 1970

38. Grisolia A, Bell RL, Peltier LF: Fractures and dislocations of the spine complicating ankylosing spondylitis. J Bone Joint Surg 49A:339–344, 1967

39. Gulati DR, Rout D: Atlanto-axial dislocation with quadriparesis in achondroplasia. J Neurosurg 40:394–396, 1974

40. Guttmann L: Traumatic paraplegia and tetraplegia in ankylosing spondylitis. Paraplegia 4:189–203, 1966

41. Hakkal HG: Clay shoveler's fracture. Am Fam Phys 8:104–106, 1973

42. Hallenbeck JM, Bove AA, Elliott DH: Mechanisms underlying spinal cord damage in decompression sickness. Neurology (Minneapolis) 25:308–316, 1975

43. Hansen ST, Jr, Taylor TKF, Honet JC, Lewis FR: Fracture dislocation of the ankylosed thoracic spine in rheumatoid spondylitis, ankylosing spondylitis, Marie-Strumpell disease. J Trauma 7:827–837, 1967

44. Harris JL, Cunningham EB: Stress fractures of the lumbar vertebrae. J Occup Med 7:255–256, 1965

45. Harris WH, Hamblen DL, Ojemann RG: Traumatic disruption of cervical intervertebral disk from hyperextension injury. Clin Orthop 60:163–167, 1968

46. Hinck VC: Cervical fracture dislocation in rheumatoid spondylitis. Am J Roentgenol Radium Ther Nucl Med 82:257–258, 1959

47. Hodgson AR, Stock FE: Anterior spinal fusion for the treatment of tuberculosis of the spine. The operative findings and results of treatment in the first one hundred cases. J Bone Joint Surg 42A:295–310, 1960

48. Hogan EL, Romanul FCA: Spinal cord infarction occurring during insertion of aortic graft. Neurology (Minneapolis) 16:67–74, 1966

49. Hollin SA, Gross SW, Levin P: Fracture of the cervical spine in patients with rheumatoid spondylitis. Am Surg 31:532–536, 1965

50. Hopkins JS: Lower cervical rheumatoid subluxation with tetraplegia. J Bone Joint Surg 49B:46–51, 1967
51. Howland WJ, Curry JL, Buffington CB: Fulcrum fractures of the lumbar spine. Transverse fracture injured by an improperly placed seat belt. JAMA 193:240–241, 1965
52. Hughes JT: Venous infarction of the spinal cord. Neurology (Minneapolis) 21:794–800, 1971
53. Italiano P: Le fratture vertebrali del piloti negli incidenti da elicuttero. Riv Med Aero 29:577–602, 1966
54. Jackson FE, Marin R, Davis R: Delayed quadriplegia following electrical burn. Milit Med 130:601–605, 1965
55. Janda WE, Kelly PJ, Rhoton AL, Jr, Layton DD, Jr: Fracture-dislocation of the cervical part of the spinal column in patients with ankylosing spondylitis. Mayo Clin Proc 43:714–721, 1968
56. Janetos GP: Paget's disease in cervical spine. Am J Roentgenol Radium Ther Nuc Med 97:655–657, 1966
57. Joffe R, Appleby A, Arjona V: 'Intermittent ischaemia' of the cauda equina due to stenosis of the lumbar canal. J Neurol Neurosurg Psychiatry 29:315–318, 1966
58. Jones A: Transient radiation myelopathy. Brit J Radiol 37:727–744, 1964
59. Kepes JJ: Selective necrosis of spinal gray matter. A complication of dissecting aneurysm of the aorta. Acta Neuropath (Berlin) 4:293–298, 1965
60. Keuter EJW: Non-traumatic atlanto-axial dislocation associated with nasopharyngeal infections (Grisel's disease). Acta Neurochir 21:11–22, 1969
61. Kewalramani LS, Taylor RG: Injuries to the cervical spine from diving accidents. J Trauma 15:130–142, 1975
62. Key AG, Retief PJM: Spinal cord injuries, an analysis of 300 new lesions. Paraplegia 7:243–249, 1972
63. Killen DA: Paraplegia in the dog following mobilization of the abdominal and lower thoracic aorta from the posterior parietes. Surgery 57:542–548, 1965
64. Kirkpatrick D, Goodman SJ: Combined subarachnoid and subdural spinal hematoma following lumbar puncture. Surg Neurol 3:109–111, 1975
65. Kornblum D, Clayton ML, Nash HH: Nontraumatic cervical dislocations in rheumatoid spondylitis. JAMA 149:431–435, 1952
66. Langworthy OR: Necrosis of the spinal cord produced by electrical injuries. Bull Johns Hopkins Hosp 51:210–216, 1932
67. Leidholt JD: Spinal injuries in sports. Surg Clin North Am 43:351–361, 1963
68. Leidholt JD: Spinal injuries in athletes: be prepared. Orthop Clin North Am 4:691–707, 1973
69. Lemmen LJ, Laing PG: Fracture of the cervical spine in patients with rheumatoid arthritis. J Neurosurg 16:542–550, 1959
70. Levine NS, Arnold A, McKeel DW, Peck SD, Pruitt BA: Spinal cord injury following electrical accidents: Case reports. J Trauma 15:459–463, 1975
71. Lipschitz R, Block J: Stab wounds of the spinal cord. Lancet 2:169–172, 1962
72. Liss L: Fatal cervical cord injury in swimmers. Neurology (Minneapolis) 15:675–677, 1965
73. Livingston MC: Spinal manipulation causing injury. A three year study. Clin Orthop 81:82–86, 1971
74. Lourie H, Stewart WA: Spontaneous atlantoaxial dislocation. A complication of rheumatoid disease. N Engl J Med 265:677–681, 1961
75. Lutz EG: Electroconvulsive therapy and cerebral inhibition changes of susceptibility to fractures during electroconvulsive therapy. Int J Neuropsychiatry 3:125–130, 1967
76. Margolis G, Tarazi AK, Grimson KS: Contrast medium injury to the spinal cord produced by aortography. J Neurosurg 13:349–365, 1956
77. Margulies ME, Katz I, Rosenberg M: Spontaneous dislocation of the atlanto-axial

joint in rheumatoid spondylitis. Recovery from quadriplegia following surgical decompression. Neurology (Minneapolis) 5:290–294, 1955

78. Martel W, Page JW: Cervical vertebral erosions and subluxations in rheumatoid arthritis and ankylosing spondylitis. Arthrit Rheumat 3:546–556, 1960
79. Martin RC: Atlas-axis dislocation following cervical infection. JAMA 118:874–875, 1942
80. Matheson AT: Paraplegia from flexion injury of the spine: danger of the high lithotomy position. J Ob-Gyn Brit Comm 68:656–657, 1961
81. McCleery WNC, Lewtas NA: Subarachnoid injection of contrast medium. A complication of vertebral angiography. Br J Radiol 39:112–114, 1966
82. Meijers KAE, van Beusekom GTh, Luyendijk W, Duijfjes F: Dislocation of the cervical spine with cord compression in rheumatoid arthritis. J Bone Joint Surg 56B:668–680, 1974
83. Mishkin MM, Baum S, Chiro G: Emergency treatment of angiography induced paraplegia and tetraplegia. N Engl J Med 288:1184–1185, 1973
84. Mozingo JR, Denton IC: The neurological deficit associated with sudden occlusion of abdominal aorta due to blunt trauma. Surgery 77:118–125, 1975
85. Mukherjee SK: Fracture vertebra following tetanus. J Indian Med Assoc 63:158–160, 1974
86. Nathan FF, Bickel WH: Spontaneous axial subluxation in a child as the first sign of juvenile rheumatoid arthritis. J Bone Joint Surg 50A:1675–1678, 1968
87. Norrell H, Jr, Llewellyn RC: Migration of a threaded Steinmann pin from an acromioclavicular joint into the spinal canal, a case report. J Bone Joint Surg 47A:1024–1026, 1965
88. Osgood CP, Abbasy M, Mathews T: Multiple spine fractures in ankylosing spondylitis. J Trauma 15:163–166, 1975
89. Osgood CP, Ackerman E, Martin LG: Fractures of the cervical spine in rheumatoid spondylitis. J Neurosurg 39:764–769, 1973
90. Papo M, Alvarez CS: The effects of chronic recurrent spinal trauma in high-diving. A study of Acapulco's divers. J Bone Joint Surg 44A:648–658, 1962
91. Ramamurthi B, Visvanathan GS: Paget's disease of axis causing quadriplegia. J Neurosurg 14:580–583, 1957
92. Ramani PS, Sengupta RP: Cauda equina compression due to tabetic arthropathy of the spine. J Neurol Neurosurg Psychiatry 36:260–264, 1973
93. Rand RW, Stern WE: Cervical fractures of the ankylosed rheumatoid spine. Neurochirurgia 4:137–148, 1961
94. Reagan ThJ, Thomas JE, Colby MY: Chronic progressive radiation myelopathy. JAMA 203:106–110, 1968
95. Rengachary S, Nurphy D: Subarachnoid hematoma following lumbar puncture causing compression of the cauda equina. J Neurosurg 41:252–254, 1974
96. Richter RW, Behnke AR: Spinal cord injury following a scuba dive to a depth of 350 feet. U.S. Armed Forces Med J 10:1227–1234, 1959
97. Roberts VL, Noyes FR, Hubbard RP, McCabe J: Biomechanics of snowmobile spine injuries. J Biomech 4:569–577, 1971
98. Rosenberg MA, Horowitz I: Fractured dislocation of the cervical spine with rheumatoid spondylitis: case report and review of literature. J Can Assoc Radiol 16:241–243, 1965
99. Rosencrantz M: A case of fibrous dysphasia (Jaffe-Lichtenstein) with vertebra fracture and compression of the spinal cord. Acta Orthop Scand 36:435–440, 1965
100. Ruge D: Spinal Cord Injuries. Springfield, Charles C Thomas, 1969
101. Saldeen T: Fatal neck injuries caused by use of diagonal safety belts. J Trauma 7:856–862, 1967
102. Schneider D, Dralle J, Ebhardt G: Lasionen des Ruckenmarks nach temporarem Kreislaufstillstand. Z Neurol 204:165–178, 1973

103. Schneider RC: Serious and fatal neurosurgical football injuries. Clin Neurosurg 12:226–236, 1964
104. Schneider RC, Gosch HH, Norrell H, et al: Vascular insufficiency and differential distortion of brain and cord caused by cervicomedullary football injuries. J Neurosurg 33:363–375, 1970
105. Schneider RC, Reifel E, Chrisler HO, Oosterbaan BG: Serious and fatal football injuries involving the head and spinal cord. JAMA 177:362–367, 1961
106. Schwarz F, Bevilacqua J: Paraplegia following spinal anesthesia. Arch Neurol 10:308–321, 1964
107. Schwarz G, Reback S: Compression of spinal cord in osteitis deformans (Paget's disease) of vertebrae. Am J Roentgenol Radium Ther Nucl Med 42:345–366, 1939
108. Sharp J, Purser DW: Spontaneous atlanto-axial dislocation in ankylosing spondylitis and rheumatoid arthritis. Ann Rheumat Dis 20:47–77, 1961
109. Silversides J: The neurologic sequelae of electrical injury. Can Med Assoc J 91:195–204, 1964
110. Singh A, Aggarwal ND, Malhotra KC, Puri DS: Paraplegia in cysticercosis: Case of spinal cysticercosis with paraplegia (India). Brit Med J 2:685–686, 1966
111. Smith PH, Benn RT, Sharp J: Natural history of rheumatoid cervical luxations. Ann Rheumat Dis 31:431–439, 1972
112. Smith WS, Kaufer H: Patterns and mechanisms of lumbar injuries associated with lap seat belts. J Bone Joint Surg (Am) 51:239–254, 1969
113. Snyder EN, Jr, Mulfinger GC, Lambert RW: Claudication caused by compression of the cauda equina. Am J Surg 130:172–177, 1975
114. Solheim OP: Radiation injury of the spinal cord. Acta Radiol 10:474–480, 1971
115. Spencer GT: Nail-gun accident. Br Med J 1:181, 1968
116. Stranger J, Kerridge G: Multiple fracture of the dorsal part of the spine following chlordane poisoning. Med J Aust 1:267–268, 1968
117. Sullivan AW: Subluxation of the atlanto-axial joint; sequel to inflammatory processes of the neck. J Pediatr 35:451–464, 1949
118. Taylor WL, Santos GW, Behnke AR: Localization of spinal cord injury in a deep sea diver. U.S. Armed Forces Med J 10:1223–1226, 1959
119. Teng P, Gross SW, Newman CM: Compression of spinal cord by osteitis deformans (Paget's disease), giant-cell tumor and polyostotic fibrous dysplasia (Albright's syndrome) of vertebrae: report of four cases. J Neurosurg 8:482–493, 1951
120. Turner JWA: Spinal complications of Paget's disease (osteitis deformans). Brain 63:321–349, 1940
121. Van Beusekom GTh: Spinal cord compression in patients with Hodgkin's disease. Psychiatr Neurol Neurochir 72:17–22, 1969
122. Vasconcelos D: Compression fractures of the vertebrae during major epileptic seizures. Epilepsia 14:323–328, 1973
123. Whalley N: Paget's disease of atlas and axis. J Neurol Neurosurg Psychiatr 9:84–86, 1946
124. Wilson CB: Significance of the small lumbar spinal canal: Cauda equina compression syndrome due to spondylitis. J Neurosurg 31:499–506, 1969
125. Wolman L: Blast injury of the spinal cord. Paraplegia 5:83–88, 1967
126. Wolman L, Hardy AG: Spinal cord infarction associated with the sickle cell trait. Paraplegia 7:282–291, 1970
127. Woodruff FP, Dewing SB: Fracture of the cervical spine in patients with ankylosing spondylitis. Radiology 80:17–21, 1963
128. Yau CMC, Chan RNW: Stress fracture of the fused lumbodorsal spine in ankylosing spondylitis. A report of three cases. J Bone Joint Surg 56B:681–687, 1974

# 5

## Emergency Management

### ACCIDENT SITE

Proper care of a person sustaining a spinal cord injury must begin at the accident site.[17] Early assessment is essential to avoid undue movement of the patient. Since many such patients are conscious, careful questioning concerning extremity movement, absence of feeling, and presence and location of pain will indicate to the informed layman the existence of spinal cord damage.[9] Unless the patient is in shock from obvious bleeding or is in serious respiratory distress, the principle of nonmovement of the patient should always be observed until suitable assistance and proper equipment are available. The patient may be rolled onto a firmly supported stretcher, or better, a broad piece of plywood, for transportation to the hospital (Fig. 1). The spine must not be allowed to angulate, thus the patient should be moved en-bloc. It is wrong for two people to attempt to lift a spine-damaged patient, one lifting under the armpits and another lifting the dangling legs. In the presence of suspected cervical spine injury, efforts should be directed toward stabilizing the patient's head and neck with available items (e.g., cushions, sandbags, clothing). While longitudinal hand traction to the head can be applied during movement of the patient, we believe that securing of head and trunk to a solid flat surface prior to and during movement of the patient is superior. Trained personnel should be with the patient during the trip to the hospital to provide respiratory assistance. Relief for respiratory distress or vomiting takes precedence over body positioning, and the patient may have to be placed on his side, with the proper vertebral support, for adequate drainage and naso-oral suction. Vogl[14] reported on experiences treating spine fractures in emergency vehicles in Germany, including use of x-ray and alignment-reduction.

Bucy[1] summarized emergency treatment at the accident site stating that:

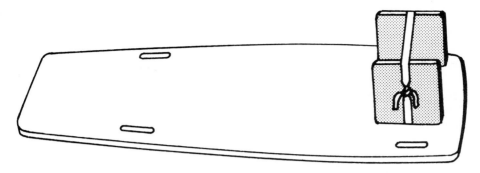

*Fig. 1.* Depiction of spine board with cervical support for transportation of patient with vertebral injury.

(1) the patient should not be moved, flexed, or rotated if he has a potentially fractured spine (he should be moved only as indicated above). (2) The patient should be immobilized without any attempt at correction of the position and the spine should be kept immobile. (3) Intramuscular injection of 10 to 20 mg of dexamethasone should be given immediately if the patient is paralyzed even slightly. (4) The patient should be transferred promptly to the care of an expert who understands such injuries and is prepared to treat them. In that regard Giesler et al.[4] reported 26 vertebral injuries possibly made worse by well-intentioned but faulty first aid care and Gillingham[5] emphasized prevention of further damage by well-intentioned lay or professional people following head and spinal injuries.

Many roadside cervical spine splinting devices have been described. They are basically constructed of thick nonpliable plastic with Velcro fasteners. They are slipped carefully into position so as to immobilize the fractured cervical spine without movement. Unfortunately most emergency squads are not equipped with such devices.

## EMERGENCY ROOM

All persons suspected of having sustained serious spinal trauma should be transported to properly equipped and staffed centers. Such facilities should be well known to emergency personnel and geographically located to serve areas recognized as potential sites of trauma. Examination should be carried out before the patient is transferred from ambulance stretcher to hospital examining table or spinal cart.

When a patient is suspected of having sustained a cervical spine injury, immediate but momentary attention must be directed to demonstrating adequacy of respiratory exchange and the presence or absence of associated trauma to other organ systems, particularly those that can lead to circulatory compromise. The most frequent location of vertebral fracture dislocations is in regions of greatest mobility, between C5–T1 and T11–L2. While the documentation of a clear airway, adequate excursion of the thorax, normal color of the nail beds and skin, and the near-normal mental responsiveness of the patient, together with a normal blood pressure and pulse, sustains the clinical impression of excellent pulmonary performance and circulatory adequacy, far greater concern is due those patients in whom one or all of these clinical criteria are abnormal.[2] In the face of respiratory distress that does not clear with judicious toilet of the nasal-oral pharyngeal pathways, we recommend awake nasotracheal intubation or tracheostomy. Great care should be exercized not to overextend the neck for orotracheal intubation. It must always be kept in mind that cervical cord transections are invariably accompanied by mild hypotension and bradycardia as well as lowered body core temperatures and that such a state is not indicative of hemorrhagic shock. Morphine should never be given to patients with spinal injuries when respiration, either phrenic or intercostal, is affected. In the presence of lumbar lesions, opiates may be administered since respiration is seldom significantly altered.

Assurance that the respiratory and circulatory states are secure permits rapid neurologic examination of the patient following efforts to externally stabilize the head-neck-body axis. For this purpose either halter traction or sandbag splinting is adequate for temporarily minimizing motion during examination. Careful interrogation of the patient concerning extremity movement, lack of feeling, presence of pain, parasthesias, bladder and bowel function, and circumstances of the accident should be recorded. Fracture of the cervical spine should be suspected whenever the patient complains of severe pain or stiffness in his neck.[2] Fracture of the thoracic and lumbar spines should be suspected whenever an injured person complains of pain and stiffness in those areas. Root compression causing radiation of pain in accordance with the distribution of the particular roots suggests fracture.

It is recommended that examination be implemented in these patients in the emergency room, with recording of detailed observations according to the following flow sheet.

   1. An initial thorough neurologic examination must be performed to serve not only as an estimate of cord involvement, but also as a base line for future examinations. Of particular importance is to document the level of cord or root injury, the demonstration of extent and level of sensory and motor dysfunction. In cervical cord injuries considered to represent complete transection, considerable effort must be expended to uncover any area of sensory alterations, e.g., sacral dermatomes, presence of sensation on catheter tug, deep pain interpreted as touch or pressure, and evidence of residual muscle activity.

   2. Search must be made to uncover any associated injury, particularly to the abdominal and thoracic cavities, which may have escaped initial cursory examination.

3. Base-line laboratory studies, including hematocrit, blood sugar, urea, electrolytes, blood gases, and urinalysis should be rapidly carried out when indicated. Intravenous fluids should be started both to increase circulating volume and to provide an avenue for necessary medications and other intravenous treatment. Dexamethasone in high dosage should be administered. Indwelling catheterization should be placed in patients with severe spinal injury to prevent bladder distention and to record output of urine. Guttman[7] suggests that catheterization be delayed for 24 hours so that a program of intermittent catheterization can be begun under relaxed, sterile circumstances. Some authors believe that nasogastric intubation is necessary to decompress gastric contents and increase ventilation. We believe that use of this measure should depend on individual circumstances. If surgery is to be performed, blood grouping should be ascertained.

Advisability of performing lumbar puncture for diagnostic purposes in spinal cord injuries remains controversial. We feel that results of the Queckenstedt test performed during lumbar puncture should not appreciably influence selection of cases for laminectomy. After all, only a patency equal to an 18-gauge needle need be present for the test to be normal, in spite of the presence of considerable spinal cord compression.

## RADIOLOGIC EXAMINATION

On a flat, firm frame in halter traction or with adequate skeletal support the patient is transported to the x-ray department with a physician in attendance, if possible. There is little danger in a straight longitudinal pull on the head for cervical traction in cervical spine injury. It will not damage the cord and, in our view, it will not produce further displacement of vertebral fragments. Under careful manual control every reasonable effort is made to demonstrate the extent of bony involvement. Standard lateral and anteroposterior (AP) projections of the appropriate spinal area are sometimes insufficient, particularly in fractures of lower cervical vertebrae; consequently special views, e.g., lateral projections taken with countertraction on the arms or with the arms in the position of a swimmer (swimmer's view) may be necessary. In upper cervical or craniocervical trauma, the odontoid should be seen. To accomplish this, open mouth views are extremely valuable. Polytomography may be required for adequate visualization of the bony lesion. In all cases of serious injury, additional films of the skull, chest, and abdomen are advised. In most head injuries it is important to obtain cervical spine films to rule out fracture of the spine, since almost any injury causing cerebral damage can cause a cervical vertebral lesion. Myelography with introduction of the contrast material laterally at C1–C2 in cervical injuries is recommended in selected cases.

The advantage of this introduction site is that it may be accomplished with the patient in the supine position, but in most cases myelography with introduction of radiopaque material into the lumbar theca will suffice. Rarely cisternal introduction is advisable, particularly in lumbar injuries. The presence of swelling and hemorrhage into lumbar theca causes inaccuracies of contrast material injection in lumbar injuries, with attendant danger of misinterpretation. Patients with cervical cord injuries have problems with postural hypotension and we have seen patients, particularly in the acute and subacute phase both during myelography or on circular beds, who could not be placed in the standing vertical position due to severe cerebral ischemic symptoms. Likewise, some with partial respiratory paralysis cannot be placed in the standing-on-head position because of inhibition of diaphragmatic breathing by abdominal organs. It should be stressed that myelography is not always required.

Any patient with a severe spinal cord injury and/or a severe vertebral column injury should be radiographed on the original stretcher or board on admission to the emergency room. After determination of the type of fracture and severity, the patient may be transferred to a turning frame from which other x-rays, surgery, and subacute to chronic care may be carried out without further movement. We advocate the Stryker wedge turning frame. In the past, various frames have been somewhat dangerous because when the patient was turned his weight would cause him to slide out in a downward direction during the turn. Modern frames are wedges or V-shaped, and the patient is turned into the wedge thereby obviating any chance of slipping while being turned. We do not advocate turning until at least 24 hours or even longer after the injury, although depending on the circumstances, turning can be begun earlier. Others have advocated immediate turning but we feel that the patient's condition should be stabilized prior to turning since many patients cannot tolerate the prone position because respiration is inhibited. We feel that until the fracture is definitely healed, either by surgical or nonsurgical means, a circular electric turning bed should not be utilized. Smith et al.[12] and Roberts and Curtiss[10] have advised against the use of the circular electric turning frame in spinal injuries because of complications caused by the vertical position during the turning maneuver. In addition to systemic effects of hypotension that can occur in the paralyzed sympathetic system, there may be movement of the fracture itself and this could be dangerous. Surgery and chronic care can be carried out on the Stryker wedge frame without these problems.[13]

## TYPES OF INJURIES

### Subluxation Without Obvious Fracture

Subluxation of one vertebra upon another may occur without evidence of fracture on x-ray.[11] When this happens, a fracture of an articulating facet not seen on x-ray is likely. In some cases the vertebra may have returned to normal position by the time the roentgenogram is taken and instability may not be evident on lateral x-ray views made in the neutral position, even if other fractures are visualized. If it is deemed necessary, the unstable, subluxed vertebra may be demonstrated by forward flexion of the neck or by gentle extension (these procedures are potentially dangerous and must be carried out under a physician's direction) in the emergency room. Allowing the patient himself to determine the tolerable extent of flexion and extension reduces danger to a possibly unstable spine. The attending physician should stop the procedure immediately if symptoms or signs are produced by these maneuvers. On our service these stress films of the cervical spine are deemed necessary only when alignment is excellent and generally need not be done during the emergency phase of care. If an overt fracture dislocation exists, nothing is gained by demonstrating assumed instability at this early stage.

Subluxations of mild degree may not be associated with neurologic abnormalities, but subluxations of severe degree are usually, though not always, accompanied by severe neurologic change. Transient subluxation may occasionally occur causing severe cord injury that persists even though the vertebral bodies return to normal position and the patient has neurologic loss without evident bony abnormality. When this happens, flexion and extension may establish the presence of dislocation. When severe degrees of subluxation and neurologic deficit exist, immobilization, skeletal traction, and reduction are indicated. Laminectomy should be considered in the acute phase if profound neurologic loss is present. Early fusion should also be considered in these cases as well as in all patients demonstrating persistent bony instability. The most appropriate treatment may vary depending on the actual situation, and choices will be discussed under appropriate headings.

### Fracture-Dislocation

Dislocation with obvious fracture is the most dire of spinal injuries. In these cases facets or intra-articular joints are subluxed and usually pedicles and pars intra-articularis fractured. Other vertebral elements, such as bodies and laminae, may also be fractured. Vertebral bodies are displaced and displacement is usually greatest at the moment of impact, with some degree of spontaneous reduction. Initial treatment in cervical injuries, usually on an emergency basis, is skeletal tong traction and an attempt should be made to reduce (realign) the fracture-dislocation. We do this rapidly, employing up to 75 pounds of weight (see Chap. 9). With adequate spinal column realignment and minimal or no neurologic dysfunction, early fusion has been recommended to significantly reduce the lengthy period of immobility required by the use of the classical method of prolonged skeletal traction.[15,16] Posterior fusion can be used to provide internal stabilization to the spine. This type of fusion is of particular value when multiple vertebral levels are involved, when facets are locked and must be operatively reduced (sometimes during the early phase), when the architecture of deformity would mitigate against anterior fusion, or when a laminectomy has been performed and a decision is made to undertake a fusion procedure at the same time.[11] Anterior fusion, also performed early, is a valuable procedure for permanent and rapid spinal stabilization when only one cervical level (e.g., C5–C6) is involved. To prevent subsequent dislocation and damage, our regimen following both posterior and anterior fusion is to keep patients in tongs for three to six weeks, in bed without tongs for three to six weeks longer, and then to permit the patient to be up in a four-post brace for three to six months. Stress films are obtained four to six months following fusion to evaluate results. Lately, use of halo traction devices have made earlier ambulation possible in some types of injuries.

### Compression Fracture

Fractures may occur with or without dislocation or subluxation.[11] Compression fracture of the vertebral body without subluxation is commonest. Generally one vertebra alone is involved, but occasionally more than one may be crushed. Such fractures are usually considered stable because the posterior bony elements, the laminae, facets, and pedicles, are intact. Also contributing to stability are the posterior and anterior longitudinal ligaments and related musculotendinous structures. Treatment is generally conservative in the absence of neurologic signs or instability. Uncommonly, however, disc material moval of the offending disc material via an anterior approach that can be foling in neurologic signs and symptoms. Under these circumstances myelography is indicated. Failure to demonstrate an obstructive or deforming lesion usually eliminates the necessity of surgical decompression by laminectomy. If the myelogram indicates such a lesion, an alternative to laminectomy is removal of the offending disk material via an anterior approach that can be followed by anterior fusion.

## OTHER LESIONS

It should be kept in mind that other lesions resulting from traumatic spinal cord injury do occur. Compound injuries inflicted by knife and gunshot are *stable* but may require surgical debridement.[8] Spinal damage may result from minor injury in rheumatoid arthritis and ankylosing spondylitis,[6] and on occasions, subdural and epidural hematoma have been reported.

## OTHER COMPLICATIONS

In patients with no sensory and motor function below the level of a high thoracic or cervical cord lesion, symptoms reflecting surgically significant abdominal trauma may be absent. These patients complain only of nausea and may have referred pain of diaphragmatic origin in the supraclavicular area.

Because of the spinal injury and its sequelae many of the signs and symptoms of abdominal injuries are absent.

## REFERENCES

1. Bucy PD: Editorial: Emergency treatment of spinal cord injury. Surg Neurol 1:216, 1973
2. Cave EF: Immediate treatment of specific fractures. Surg Clin North Am 46:771–788, 1966
3. Cooke DA, Littler EN, Williams HO: A simple 'plastazote' splint for the treatment of cervical and high dorsal injuries at the roadside. Practitioner 213:65–68, 1974
4. Giesler WO, Wynne-Jones M, Jousse AT: Early management of the patient with trauma to the spinal cord. Med Serv J Can 22:512–523, 1966
5. Gillingham J: The problem of head and spinal injuries—prevention of the second accident. Med Sci Law 10:104–109, 1970
6. Grisolia A, Bell RL, Peltier LF: Fractures and dislocations of the spine complicating ankylosing spondylitis. J Bone Joint Surg 49A:339–344, 1967
7. Guttman L: Spinal Cord Injuries: Comprehensive Management and Research. Oxford, Blackwell Sci Publ, 1973, p 124
8. Lipschitz R: Associated injuries and complications of stab wounds of the spinal cord. Paraplegia 5:75–82, 1967
9. Melvin WJ: The emergency treatment of diving accidents. Appl Ther 7:459–462, 1965
10. Roberts JB, Curtiss PH, Jr: Stability of the thoracic and lumbar spine in traumatic paraplegia following fracture of fracture-dislocation. J Bone Joint Surg 52A:1115–1130, 1970
11. Schneider RC: Trauma to the spine and spinal cord. In Kahn EA, Crosby EC, Schneider RC, Taren JA (eds): Correlative Neurosurgery, 2d ed. Springfield, Ill., Charles C Thomas, 1969, pp 597–648
12. Smith TK, Whitaker J, Stauffer ES: Complications associated with the use of the circular electrical turning frame. J Bone Joint Surg 57A:711–713, 1975
13. Stryker H: A device for turning the frame patient. JAMA 113:1731–1732, 1939
14. Vogl A: Zur mobile behandlung Von Wirbelbruchen. Zbl Chir 93:439–444, 1968
15. White RJ, Yashon D: General care of cervical spine injuries. In Youmans JR (ed): Neurological Surgery. Philadephia, Saunders, 1973, pp 1049–1066
16. White RJ, Yashon D: Dorsal and lumbar spine injuries. In Youmans JR (ed): Neurological Surgery. Philadelphia, Saunders, 1973, pp 1085–1088
17. Yashon D, White RJ: Injuries of the vertebral column and spinal cord. In Feiring EH (ed): Brock's Injuries of the Brain and Spinal Cord and Their Coverings, 5th ed. New York, Springer, 1974, pp 668–743

# 6

# Radiology

## RADIOLOGIC DIAGNOSIS

Radiographic examination is of utmost importance in the diagnosis of bony vertebral injury in spinal cord or root trauma. High-quality radiography begins in the emergency room. Although the patient is usually on a litter, it is possible to obtain diagnostic films without significantly altering the position of the patient. His safety must not be compromised during the examination. With the patient supine on the table, lateral and anteroposterior films are made of the vertebral area. For examination of the cervical spine, an open-mouth view of the dens is taken with the central ray passing through the center of the open mouth along the midsagittal plane of the skull. It is important to project the maxillary teeth away from the base of the dens, so it may be helpful to use a prolonged exposure with the patient repeatedly opening and closing his mouth so the maxilla can be obscured. McRae[23] considers stereoscopic lateral films of the cervical spine essential, but we disagree and do not in fact obtain these films.

Positions for x-ray examination of the spine depend on the specific areas to be visualized. In addition to the primary views mentioned, another, although not routine, includes a basilar view in which the first cervical vertebrae may be visualized through the skull in a vertico-submental projection. The patient lies prone with the neck hyperextended, and the chin must be firmly supported several inches above the tabletop so that the base line of the skull (the line between the outer canthus of the eye and the external auditory meatus) is parallel to the tabletop. The x-ray beam is focused just behind the ear to project the atlas in the center of the field. This view is not to be used when instability is in question because of the necessity to hyperextend the head. If the patient is unable to lie prone, a reverse view with the patient supine can be utilized. Open-mouth views are generally more satisfactory.

In addition to ordinary anteroposterior views, an anteroposterior view angled 20° cephalad gives a better view of the uncinate processes and joints of Luschka in the lateral mass region.

If there is no question about acute instability, flexion and extension views may be carried out. This provides additional information concerning stability and abnormal movement of one vertebral body upon another. During flexion, placing the chin upon the chest does not suffice; the entire cervical spine must be rolled forward. Dynamic films utilizing cinefluoroscopy are of value in judging C1–C2 stability in the lateral projection. Cine films can also assist in diagnosing instability in the lateral view during flexion and extension in the lower cervical spine.

Oblique views are sometimes helpful, and are made with the patient prone in the right and left anterior oblique cervical positions. The purpose of these views is to visualize the articular processes, apophyseal joints, facet surfaces, intervertebral foramina, pedicles (pillars), laminae, and joints of Luschka on the downside. One side must be contrasted against the other. Generally, oblique views are employed to diagnose minor fractures or ancient effects of trauma. In the cervical spine, occult small fractures of minor importance may occur in many areas.[1] These include the interarticular isthmus, facets, linear fractures through the lamina, fractures about the joints of Luschka, fractures of transverse processes, and fractures of spinous processes.

Vines[29] stressed the diagnosis of occult fractures in the cervical spine. He emphasized that the lateral masses (articular pillars) should be visualized by means of bilateral oblique views. Figure 1 shows changes in the lateral masses that can be detected on ordinary anteroposterior films as the result of ancient

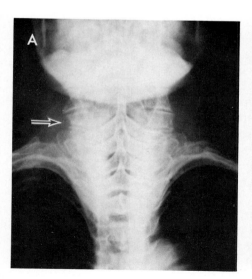 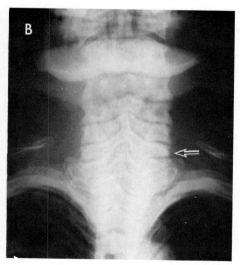

*Fig. 1.* Remote spinal injury. A. Compare change in right pillar (arrow) with opposite (normal) side. B. Compare change in left pillar with opposite (normal) side.

trauma. Compare the traumatized side with the opposite side. Vines emphasized that standard anteroposterior and lateral films are not adequate to evaluate the lateral masses. Boylstron[3] also suggested that occult fractures and dislocations could be diagnosed radiographically by oblique views in flexion and extension. Chiroff and Sachs[5] stressed discontinuity of the spinous processes on anteroposterior and lateral views as an aid in the diagnosis of unstable fractures of the spine; a fracture severe enough to cause discontinuity should be considered unstable until proved otherwise.

Weir[31] emphasized the importance of subtle signs of cervical spine injury, such as prevertebral soft tissue swelling observed on lateral cervical spine films. The normal width of the prevertebral soft tissue space measures 2.6 to 4.8 mm from the normal tracheal air shadow to the anterior border of the vertebral body; a soft tissue thickness of 5 mm or more is indirect evidence of cervical vertebral injury. Loss of the normal lordotic curve in the neutral position is another suspicious sign.

Shapiro et al.[25] warned against overdiagnosis of pseudofractures. Superimposed shadows may project over the odontoid or other bony structure to create the illusion of a radiolucent line which may be confused with a linear fracture. In the area of the dens, the two most common examples of pseudofracture are visualization of the maxillary central incisor teeth and the posterior arch of the atlas. A slight change in angulation of the x-ray beam or the use of stereoscopy may clarify the problem.

Janda et al.[17] emphasized the need for polytomography of the cervical spine if a suspected fracture is not visualized on routine radiographs. This is especially true in the C1–C2 area where fractures are sometimes difficult to visualize.[19,33] Russin and Guinto[24] compared tomographs with ordinary radiographs in cervical spine injuries, and found that in a significant number of patients the extent of the fracture was not appreciated on ordinary x-rays. They advised the use of tomography when a fracture is not revealed by plain radiographs. An additional advantage of the use of tomography is aid in evaluation of fractures that would require oblique views or angled views, such as a pillar view for evaluation of the lateral masses. Polytomes can be performed without unnecessary manipulation of the head and neck, which would otherwise be necessary. Gargano et al.[11] advised transverse axial tomography for axial viewing of the vertebral column. Axial tomography gives an accurate cross-section view of the spinal cord, and the size and shape of the canal can be demonstrated exactly in only that projection. Whether this new technic will have value in acute spinal cord trauma remains to be proved.

Myelography is frequently performed for evaluation of a spinal cord lesion. Indications remain controversial, and the decision is left to the judgment of the physician caring for the acutely injured patient. In chronic spinally injured patients, myelography can help assess cyst formation, osteophyte formation causing pain, and blockage to the flow of contrast material. Myelography is ordinarily carried out with a non-water-soluble oily material called Pantopaque (iophendylate). We have found this to be satisfactory for trauma patients, despite the theoretical objection that the cerebrospinal fluid is bloody in many cases of spinal cord trauma. It has been said that arachnoiditis can be accentuated or caused by a combination of Pantopaque and blood in the cerebrospinal fluid.

The use of a water-soluble contrast medium (metrizamide) described by Skalpe and Amundsen[28] results in good quality myelograms, and adverse affects are minor. Some water-soluble contrast materials cause convulsions and pain. Another advantage of water-soluble radiopaque solution is that it does not require removal. However, in most spinal injury patients only a small amount of Pantopaque (3 to 4 cc) is used and removal is also not necessary. The major problem with water-soluble contrast material is rapid dilution of the contrast medium with cerebrospinal fluid, so that examination must be performed quickly while contrast is adequate. For a cervical myelogram, if lumbar injection is made, the contrast medium may diffuse with cerebrospinal fluid too rapidly, so C1–C2 lateral spinal puncture can be used for injection of water-soluble (or oily) contrast. Another advantage to C1–C2 lateral puncture over lumbar and cisternal taps is that the patient does not have to be moved. Iophendylate myelography can be performed via a C1–C2 puncture with the patient in the supine position and then tilted to a reverse Trendelenburg position so that the dye may run down to the area of blocked spinal fluid flow.

Gas myelography was developed by Dandy[7] in the early 1920s and has been utilized in spinal cord lesions but seldom in trauma. Air or other gas can be injected into the lumbar spine, and lumbar x-rays can be obtained if the air is trapped in the lumber area by elevating the buttocks and legs of the patient. Heinz and Goldman[16] advocated C1–C2 puncture with the body in an upward-slanting position so that gas is trapped below the level of the foramen magnum. By this method, they could evaluate the entire spinal canal, including the cervical medullary junction. In our experience, this technique does not supply adequate definition for making a decision regarding surgery in most cases. Sicard and Lavarde[26,27] advocated gas myelography in traumatic tetraplegia. They felt that its usefulness was primarily in patients with tetraplegia but without evidence of bony disruption. The problem with gas myelography, in our opinion, is that usually one cannot see enough detail. The advantage of gas myelography in cervical trauma is that the procedure may be performed with the patient in the supine position without the necessity for movement.

The disc space itself can be injected with saline or water-soluble or non-soluble contrast. Discography has been utilized in vertebral injury, but has not been considered helpful, although it has some usefulness in the diagnosis of ruptured disc. Interosseous venography has also been utilized without much value in spinal trauma.[18,30]

Arteriography of the spinal cord has been employed in post-traumatic paraplegia. Gargour et al.[12] selectively catheterized intercostal and lumbar arteries for consistent demonstration of vessels of the thoracolumbar segment. Selective catheterization of vertebral arteries and costal cervical trunks was also used in the diagnosis of cervical and high thoracic spinal cord injuries.

Following their demonstration, others employed angiography in injured patients. Wener et al.[32] found little use for angiography in the study of cervical cord injury. Doppman[9] concluded that neither spinal arteries nor epidural veins showed consistent diagnostic changes following experimental trauma due to acute epidural compression in monkeys. Djindjian et al.[8] felt that spinal cord angiography did have some value in compressive lesions. Bussat et al.[4] described spinal cord angiography in dorsolumbar fractures with neurologic involvement. They employed selective angiography of the intercostal and lumbar artery to delineate the origin and course of the great radicular artery. In dorsolumbar spine fractures, selective angiography demonstrated the site and level of origin of the artery of Adamkiewicz. Deviations in the normal course of this artery were felt to provide information concerning whether surgical decompression was required. Spinal cord angiography has not found favor among clinicians for use in diagnosing spinal injury. The information obtained is indirect, and this technique will probably not be utilized extensively in the future.

Spinal cord damage has been reported after angiography.[10] If an undiluted bolus is inadvertently directed into the vasculature of the cord, massive medullary necrosis may result. Any factor that decreases the outflow of contrast medium from the aorta into the peripheral vascular bed will increase the diversion of injected contrast to the spinal cord after aortic injection or after selective intercostal or vertebral injections. In some cases this may be caused by organic blockage of, for example, the iliac or femoral vessels. A similar effect may follow administration of vasopressor drugs, which produce peripheral vasoconstriction with hypertension in the somatic circulation. The spinal cord vasculature does not participate in the general vasoconstriction, so an excessive dose of contrast medium may be diverted from a high-pressure area in the aorta to the low-pressure area in the spinal circulation. Breath holding can have a similar affect. When aortography is performed with the patient in the supine position, the gravitational affect of the heavy contrast medium may also increase flow to the posterior (dorsal) spinal cord. Multiple doses may cause vasodilation in intercostal and spinal vessels, open up the medullary circulation, and alter the endothelial barrier to cause damage. Mishkin et al.[21] observed that the iodine content of the cerebral spinal fluid was raised if paralysis occurred after spinal angiography, so they performed immediate lumbar puncture and withdrew cerebrospinal fluid in 10-ml aliquots with replacement by isotonic saline.

A rarer cause of spinal cord damage during vertebral angiography or translumbar aortography may be accidental misplacement of the needle into the spinal theca and intraspinal injection of contrast. This can cause spasms and seizures that may prove fatal due to respiratory arrest. Such patients may require curare with artificial ventilation until spasms and seizures are diminished. Margolis et al.[19,20] studied the pathologic anatomy of experimental contrast medium injury to the spinal cord produced by aortography, and found severe myelomalacia and a toxic reaction in the spinal cord. They found that water-soluble contrast medium caused a striking acceleration of blood flow.

McCleery and Lewtas[22] presented a patient who had subarachnoid injection of contrast medium as a complication of vertebral angiography. The patient had a severe reaction. Gonzales and Osterholm[13] reported that renografin-76 did not extend the injury in experimentally spinal damaged cases, in spite of a massive dose injected into the upper thoracic aorta.

Alffran and Lindberg[2] used strontium-85 to assess the bone in vertebral fractures. They examined 51 patients with vertebral fractures by external counting over the vertebral spine 14 days after intravenous isotope injections. Increased uptake of strontium-85 was regularly found over fractures not over six months of age. After that, peak values fell, and practically all fractures over 18 months of age displayed values of strontium-85 within normal limits. Griffiths et al.[14] used I-125 photon scanning in the evaluation of bone density in a group of 100 patients with spinal cord injury. Observations were compared to those in normal persons. Cortical bone was found to be normal in the spinal cord injury patients. Hand radiographs demonstrated severe loss of trabecular bone in 52 patients, suggesting that in spinal cord injury, cortical bone is preserved generally, while trabecular bone is lost.

## REFERENCES

1. Abel MS: Occult Traumatic Lesions of the Cervical Vertebrae. St. Louis, Warren H. Green, 1971, p 148
2. Alffran P-A, Lindberg L: External counting of [85]Sr in vertebral fractures. J Bone Joint Surg 50A:563–569, 1968
3. Boylstron BF: Oblique roentgenographic views of the cervical spine in flexion and extension. J Bone Joint Surg 39A:1302–1309, 1957
4. Bussat P, Rossier AB, Djindjian R, Vasey H, Berney J: Spinal cord angiography in dorsolumbar vertebral fractures with neurological involvement. Radiology 109:617–620, 1973
5. Chiroff RT, Sachs BL: Discontinuity of the spinous process on standard roentgenographs as an aid in the diagnosis of unstable fractures of the spine. J Trauma 16:313–316, 1976
6. Cloward RB: Cervical discography. Acta Radiol (Diagn) 1:675–688, 1963
7. Dandy WE: Diagnosis and localization of spinal cord tumors. Bull Johns Hopkins Hosp 33:190, 1922
8. Djindjian R, Houdart R, Hurth M: L'arteriographie dans les compressions medullaires. Rev Neurol (Paris) 118:109–110, 1968
9. Doppman JL: Angiographic changes following acute spinal cord compression: an experimental study in monkeys. Br J Radiol 49:398–406, 1976
10. Editorial: Spinal cord damage after angiography. Lancet 2:1067–1068, 1973
11. Gargano FP, Meyer J, Houdek PV, Charyulu KKN: Transverse axial tomography of the cervical spine. Radiology 113:363–367, 1974
12. Gargour GW, Wener L, DiChiro G: Selective arteriography of the spinal cord in posttraumatic paraplegia. Neurology (Minneapolis) 22:132–134, 1972
13. Gonzales CF, Osterholm JL: The lack of renografin-76 toxicity in acute severe spinal cord injury. Radiology 112:605–608, 1974
14. Griffiths HF, D'Orsi CJ, Zimmerman RE: Use of [125]I photon scanning in the evaluation of bone density in a group of patients with spinal cord injury. Invest Radiol 7:107–111, 1972

15. Guttmann L: Traumatic paraplegia and tetraplegia in ankylosing spondylitis. Paraplegia 4:188–203, 1966
16. Heinz ER, Goldman RL: The role of gas myelography in neuroradiologic diagnosis. Radiology 102:629–634, 1972
17. Janda WE, Kelly PJ, Rhoton AL, Layton DD: Fracture-dislocation of the cervical part of the spinal column in patients with ankylosing spondylitis. Mayo Clin Proc 43:714–721, 1968
18. Lessmann FP, Perese DM: Intraosseous vertebral venography, a new diagnostic method. Neurochirurgia (Stuttgart) 2:175, 1960
19. Margolis G, Tarazi AK, Grimson KS: Contrast medium injury to the spinal cord produced by aortography. Pathologic anatomy of the experimental lesion. J Neurosurg 13:261–267, 1956
20. Margolis G, Griffin AT, Kenan PD, et al: Contrast-medium injury to the spinal cord. The role of altered circulatory dynamics. J Neurosurg 16:390–406, 1959
21. Mishkin MM: Emergency treatment of angiography-induced paraplegia and tetraplegia. N Engl J Med 288:1184–1185, 1973
22. McCleery WNC, Lewtas NA: Subarachnoid injection of contrast medium. A complication of vertebral angiography. Br J Radiol 39:112–114, 1966
23. McRae DL: The cervical spine and neurologic disease. Radiol Clin North Am 4:145–158, 1966
24. Russin LD, Guinto FC: Multidirectional tomography in cervical spine injury. J Neurosurg 45:9–11, 1976
25. Shapiro R, Youngberg AS, Rothman SLG: The differential diagnosis of traumatic lesions of the occipito-atlanto-axial segment. Radiol Clin North Am 11:505–526, 1973
26. Sicard A, Lavarde G: La myelographie gazeuse dans les tetraplegies traumatiques recentes. J Chir (Paris) 96:293–296, 1968
27. Sicard A, Lavarde G: La place de la tomomyelographie gazeuse dans les traumatismes du rachis. Acta Chir Belgica 9:898–905, 1968
28. Skalpe IO, Amundsen P: Thoracic and cervical myeolography with metrizamide. Radiology 116:101–106, 1975
29. Vines FS: The significance of "occult" fractures of the cervical spine. Am J Roentgenol Radium Ther Nucl Med 107:493–504, 1969
30. Vogelsang H: Intraosseous Spinal Venography. Baltimore, Williams & Wilkins, 1970
31. Weir DC: Roentgenographic signs of cervical injury. Orthop Dig 2:17–27, 1974
32. Wener L, DiChiro G, Gargour GW: Angiography of cervical cord injuries. Radiology 112:597–604, 1974
33. Woodruff FP, Dewing SB: Fracture of the cervical spine in patient with ankylosing spondylitis. Radiology 80:17–21, 1963

# 7

# Pathology and Pathogenesis

## LIFE EXPECTANCY

The paralyzed patient's life expectancy is generally less than that of the population at large. Price[69] points out that suicide is not uncommon among traumatic spinal cord injury patients and that many, possibly justifiably, have severe personality problems. In a study of 599 patients, Breithaupt et al.[14] found that for complete quadriplegia, the death rate was 12 times that of the total population; for complete paraplegia, four and three-quarter times; for partial transection of the cord in the cervical area, just over three times; and for partial paraplegia, one and one-third times. Life insurance tables were used to determine statistics. In their study, as well as in all others, genitourinary sepsis remains the single most common cause of death, accounting for 50 percent or more of fatalities. Other causes of death were related to the gastrointestinal tract in about 10 percent and to cardiovascular disease in 10 percent. Pneumonia, infected pressure sores, and cerebrovascular accidents account for others. Intracerebral hemorrhages have been reported due to markedly elevated blood pressure during episodes of autonomic hyperreflexia caused, for example, by distention of the bladder during irrigation or by urinary retention. Amyloidosis is present in many of these patients. Its etiology is not clear, except that it occurs in many chronic diseases. Gastrointestinal deaths have also occurred due to liver failure and perforation of a peptic ulcer. Acute dilation of the stomach has been reported responsible for deaths, but can be prevented if treatment is instituted early.

The autopsy findings of Dietrick and Russi[20] corroborate the foregoing statistics. In addition to cerebral vascular accidents as a result of elevated blood pressure, they also mention myocardial infarction. They found splenomegaly in 40 percent of patients, which was associated in every case with acute infection, liver disease, or amyloidosis. They also found atrophy of the testes to be common. Cooper et al.[16] as well as Cooper and Hoen[17] noted that many paraplegics have testicular atrophy, hypoproteinemia, reversal of the albumin-globulin ratio, and low 17-ketosteroid excretion. Gynecomastia was also noted. Dietrick and Russi[20] suggested that liver failure could account for testicular atrophy and gynecomastia. Approximately 50 percent of their patients had tecticular atrophy, but they also had severe lesions of the liver. Amyloidosis was found in 23.5 percent of their patients at autopsy. In addition, Watkins[92] reported a patient who sustained a ruptured diaphragm as a late cause of death in paraplegia.

Burke et al.[55] compared a series of 5575 paraplegic patients with corresponding age groups in the general population. They reported that during the first year after spinal cord trauma, mortality was 5 to 10 times higher than it was among patients who survived the first year, when life expectancy increased significantly. Freed et al.[28] reported that in a series of 243 patients with traumatic spinal cord impairment, 54 died, and the cause of death was directly related to the spinal injury in 59 percent. They found that the paraplegic patient has a greater probability of survival than the quadriplegic.

Freed et al.[28] as well as Spatz[80] were concerned about cardiac arrest during anesthesia in the second month following injury. This will be discussed in the chapter on anesthesia, but these deaths were most likely due to serum potassium increase and consequent cardiac arrest owing to the action of succinylcholine on the paraplegic's muscle. The mechanism of release of muscular intracellular potassium is unknown. Other causes of early death included pulmonary embolism.

Tribe[83] presents data indicating that in spinal injured patients during World War I, overall mortality was 80 percent, with 47 percent dying within six to eight weeks following injury. Tribe distinguished deaths occurring in acute cases from those in chronic cases; in acute cases, death occurred within two months, and the primary causes were respiratory failure and pneumonitis in high cervical lesions and pulmonary embolus due to deep vein thrombosis. In chronic cases, many deaths were not attributed to the spinal injured state, but to concomitant disease such as carcinoma, tuberculosis, and arteriosclerosis. However, renal failure with attendant hypertension, amyloidosis, and cerebral hemorrhage were the most common causes of death in chronic patients, and this was true in all other reported series.

In a continuation of the study of Breithaupt et al.,[14] Jousse et al.[48] in 1968 reported on 835 patients with traumatic transverse myelitis. The leading cause of death was kidney failure, accounting for 36 percent of deaths. They concluded that mortality in patients with traumatic paraplegia varies with the extent of the disease. In minimal paraplegia, it is almost the same as the expected mortality rate in the general population; in partial quadriplegia, it is almost twice the expected rate; in complete paraplegia it is almost four times the expected rate; and in complete quadriplegia, it is about 12 times the rate expected in the general population.

## GROSS PATHOLOGY

Bedbrook[10] examined 24 autopsy specimens from all stages of the postaccident state varying from one day to 20 years and observed that microscopically, the neural lesion is always over one or more segments and that cysts are
frequent. The cord is crushed in certain injuries, and root damage and arachnoiditis, as well as dense scar tissue, is observed. He felt that epidural scar is
worsened by operative interference. Edema of the spinal cord was also observed, and based on his autopsy observations, Bedbrook felt that operative
laminectomy was rarely justified (Figs. 1–14).

In chronic cases we have examined, there is considerable scarring with
obliteration of all anatomic structures. Old fractures are evident with adherent
scar tissue, cystic pockets of cerebrospinal fluid, and vascular structures resembling venous lakes. In acute cases (Figs. 1–8) there is subarachnoid hemorrhage, contusion of the spinal cord, and swelling so severe that at surgery
the dura frequently cannot be closed. On occasion, at exploratory early surgery the spinal cord has appeared normal in spite of total paralysis (Figs.
15–18).

Rosencrantz[71] described a case of fibrous dysplasia (Jaffe-Lichtenstein)
with vertebral fracture and secondary compression of the spinal cord. The patient had lesions in thoracic vertebrae and became paraplegic. Lesions in the

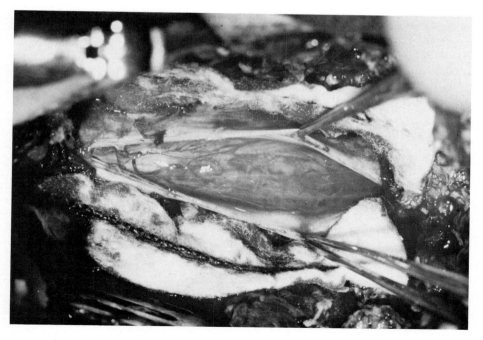

*Fig. 1.* Contused swollen spinal cord at surgery, 6 hours after injury. Permanent
quadriplegia.

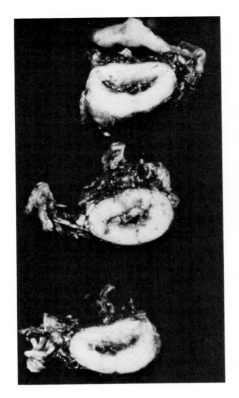

*Fig. 2.* Sections of spinal cord. Acute injury demonstrating central gray hemorrhage over several segments.

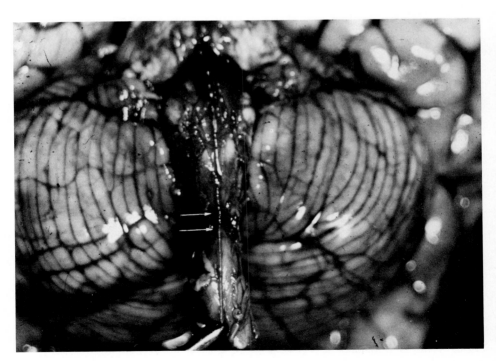

*Fig. 3.* Sudden death due to contusion-laceration cervicomedullary junction (arrows).

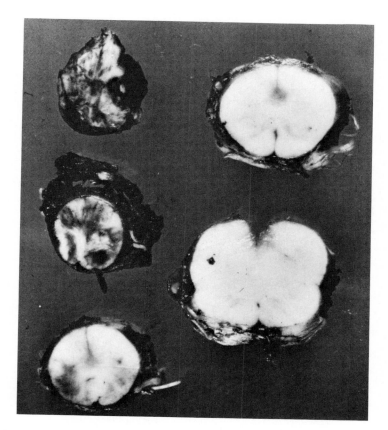

*Fig. 4.* Same case as Figure 3, showing cervical and medullary contusion and hemorrhage.

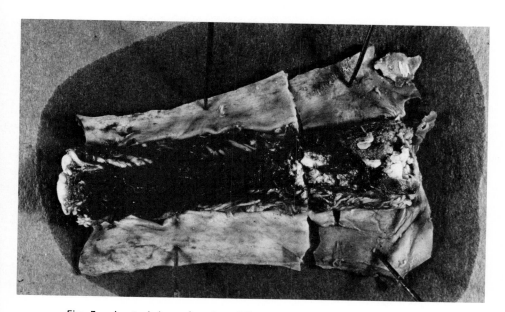

*Fig. 5.* Acute injury showing diffuse clotted subdural hematoma.

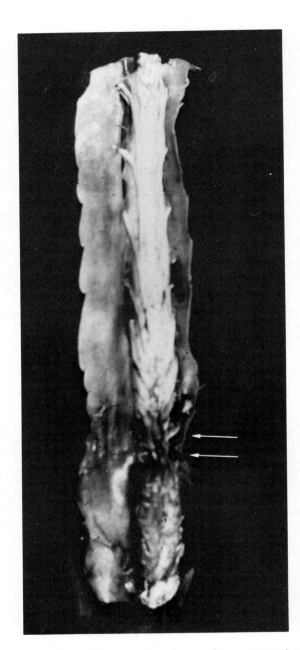

*Fig. 6.* Acute injury with laceration, hemorrhage, contusion (arrows).

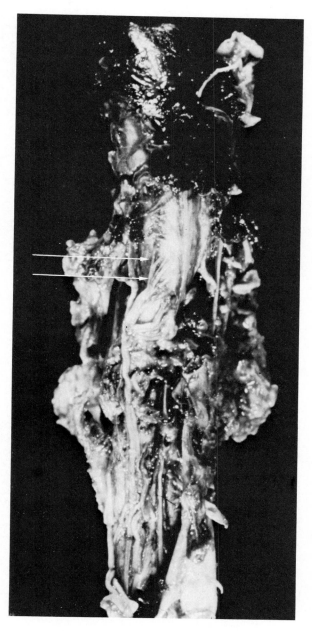

*Fig. 7.* Acute injury to lower spinal cord and cauda equina showing laceration, contusion, hemorrhage. Conus medullaris (arrows).

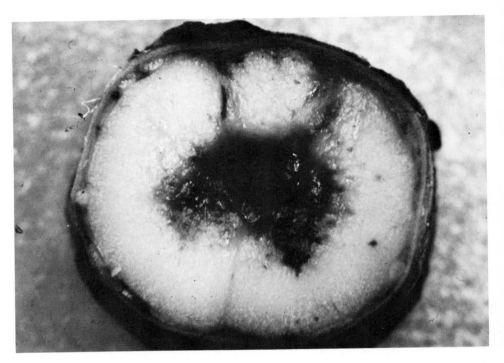

Fig. 8.  Acute injury showing central gray hemorrhage and dorsal epidural and sub-dural hemorrhage.

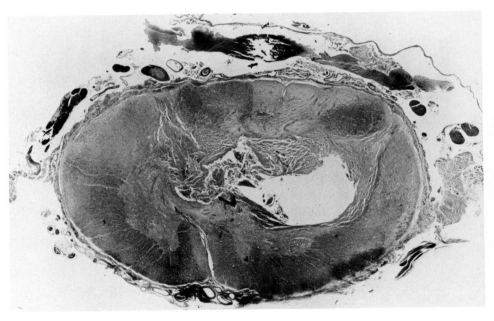

Fig. 9.  Cavitation in central gray in chronic injury. Distortion of normal internal anatomy.

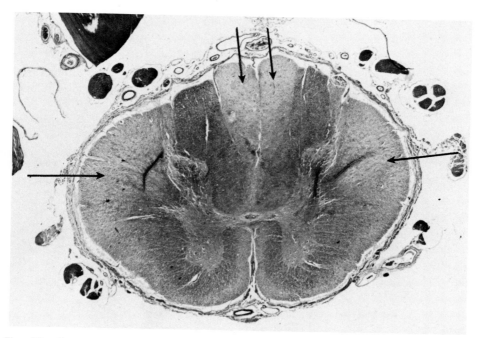

*Fig. 10.* Same case as Figure 9. Demyelination (arrows) at a distance from actual trauma.

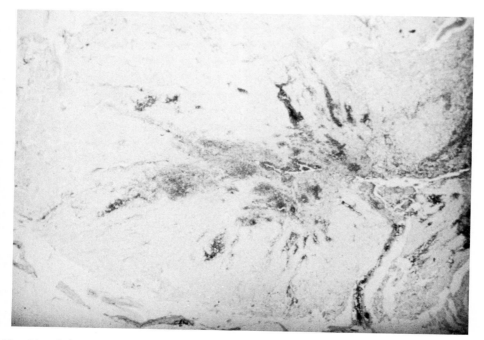

*Fig. 11.* Subacute injury. Gray matter hemorrhage, demyelination, and distortion of internal anatomy.

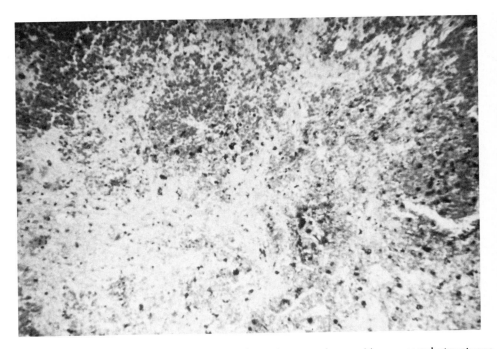

Fig. 12.  Same case as Figure 11. Hemorrhage in central gray. No neuronal structures apparent.

Fig. 13.  Chronic injury. Severe demyelination and distortion of internal anatomy. Central gray hemorrhage resolving (arrow).

*Fig. 14.* Same case as Figure 13. Lacunar spaces, macrophages, demyelination are apparent.

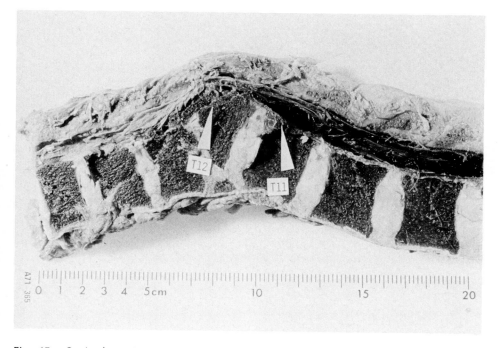

*Fig. 15.* Sagittal section ancient thoracic vertebral injury with cavitation and severe cord injury. Marked constriction of spinal canal. (Courtesy of Dr. G. M. Bedbrook)

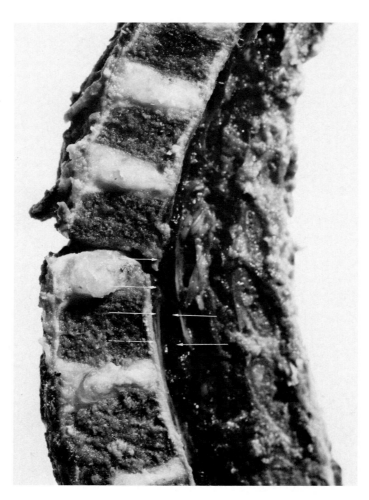

*Fig. 16.* Cervical fracture C4–5. Death 7 hours after injury. Anterior extradural hemorrhage below site of injury (arrows). (Courtesy Dr. G. M. Bedbrook)

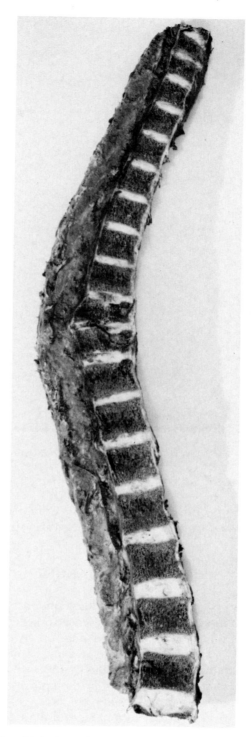

*Fig. 17.*   Sagittal section high thoracic compression fracture with rupture of the posterior longitudinal ligament and cord compression. Anterior longitudinal ligament intact. (Courtesy Dr. G. M. Bedbrook)

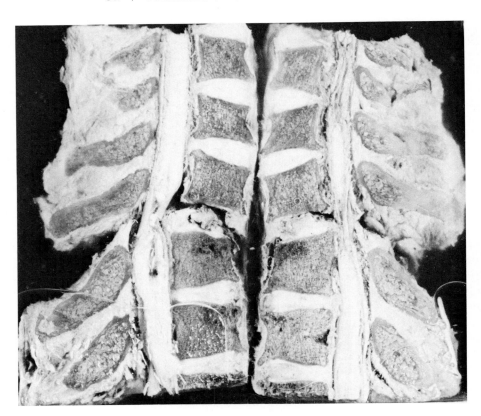

*Fig. 18.* Fracture-dislocation with severe cord compression. (Courtesy Dr. G. M. Bedbrook)

vertebral column are uncommon in this disease. Compressive lesions occur in many other bone diseases with propensity to fracture.

## HISTOLOGIC CHANGES

Bailey,[2-4] in a series of papers, reported alterations in neurons, nerve fibers, and neuroglia in the injured human spinal cord in seven acute and subacute cases. The interval from date of injury to date of death varied from seven hours to 60 days. Chromatolysis and acute swelling of nerve cells appeared at seven hours, and tigroid material loss in the perinuclear zone was noted prior to 30 hours. It appeared that the process in the spinal cord was slower than in injured human cerebral neurons. After 60 days, cells were ghost-like in appearance, thus he reasoned that loss of tigroid material was a direct effect of injury. Intracellular neurofibrils underwent fragmentation in patients who survived over seven hours. From seven hours to 18 days after injury, varicosities and fusiform enlargements were observed, leading to segmentation and granulation of neurons. Granulation appeared to be an immediate effect of the shock of injury, whereas varicosities and fusiform enlargements were effects of less severe trauma. In the region of direct injury there was evidence of disturbance of tissue fluid balance, because injured nerve cells appeared shrunken and irregular and nuclei were degenerated. In the area of contusion, nerve cells were enlarged and irregular with pale nuclei displaced peripherally. These cells had cytoplasmic vacuoles and their nuclei were swollen. Nerve cells in various stages of injury had both nuclear and cell membrane ruptures, and the nucleoplasm and cytoplasm were of gelatinous consistency.

Light microscopy investigation of changes in the nerve fibers and myelin sheaths yielded findings consistent with contusion or laceration interrupting function of the spinal cord below the level of destruction. Formation of end bulbs on both proximal and distal segments was evident, regardless of the point of interruption. After 18 days, the end bulbs on the distal ends of the proximal segment were more intensely impregnable with silver and were simpler in structure. By seven hours, the end bulbs developed on fine, medium, and large nerve fibers, and were at the height of development within four days. Those on the proximal end of the distal segment were detached by nine days, and by 18 days they had been absorbed or were engulfed by compound granular corpuscles. The distal segment underwent granular fragmentary or vacuolar degeneration, ultimately leading to disappearance of axis cylinders (Figs. 9–14).

Bailey also studied alterations in classical neuroglia utilizing Cajal's gold chloride method for astrocytes, and hematoxylin and eosin for nucleolar detail. In response to local compression, the atrocytes had not reacted by the end of 60 days. After contusion, astrocytes showed regressive changes to form amoeboid astrocytes within 30 hours. Active proliferation with double nucleated forms and cells in juxtaposition having single nuclei indicated that amitotic cell division had taken place. Apolar, bipolar, and unipolar forms were found. Jellinger[46] described lesions at some distance from the main lesion, as well as cystic degeneration in human cervical cord injuries.

From an historical perspective, Wolman[95] discussed factors significant in the neuropathology and histopathology of traumatic paraplegia, including compression, traumatic hemorrhage, upper cervical injuries, war injuries, stab wounds, compression, contusion, relationship to bone injury, cord lesions, vascular lesions, the role of the dentate ligaments, compression by prolapsed intervertebral disc, whiplash injuries, birth injuries, repair, and regeneration. He pointed out that the term "concussion" has been used in many ways with different meanings.[100] For example, the functional disturbance of the spinal cord following injury usually resulting in recovery within a period varying from a few hours to a few weeks has been described as "concussion," but the term has also been applied to the force that produces the spinal injury occurring in falls, jolts, shootings, skull fractures, and blast injuries.[100]

The role of the dentate ligament attachment in producing lesions of the cord due to its tethering affect is controversial. Surgical division of the dentate ligaments following trauma to the spinal cord has, in large measure, been abandoned, but several surgeons still persist in sectioning the ligaments to provide yet greater freedom for the entrapped spinal cord. For further details, the reading of Wolman's paper[95] is suggested. In experimental animals, Ducker et al.[25] studied the pathologic evidence of acute spinal cord trauma, using light microscopy. They showed that initially the development of demonstrable spinal cord injury does not parallel the clinical neurologic condition. Although clinical signs may improve, pathologic changes may progress in severity for about one week. Second, spinal cord changes are initially more prominent in the center of the spinal cord, even when the traumatic blow is delivered to the posterior surface. Generally the lesion begins as small gray matter hemorrhages with edema and progresses to central necrosis, adjacent white matter edema, and demyelinization, to finally involve the entire cord in very severe cases. Third, the location and progression of the injured area of the spinal cord is dependent on the force of the trauma. After minimal trauma, after which the animal recovers, alterations are apparent only in gray matter. After moderate trauma accompanied by paresis, changes engulf the central area and involve adjacent white matter. After severe trauma resulting in complete paralysis, changes include the entire spinal cord substance. The location of the histologic changes are important. For example, in a patient who had a fatal cervical cord injury while swimming and who had no apparent trauma, Liss[60] found only degeneration of neurons in the upper cervical cord. A similar lesion in the thoracic cord may have caused little noticeable neurologic loss.

## VASCULAR DAMAGE

Wagner et al.[86,87] described the histologic appearance of the primate spinal cord within four hours following delivery of a force sufficient to produce only transitory paraplegia. The resulting hemorrhagic lesion involved primarily central gray matter and was attributed to the direct effect of trauma on vessels in gray matter with consequent impairment of blood supply to the injured area. Chromatolysis, vacuolation, and alterations in cytoplasmic density and stainability were observed within neurons. Edematous changes in white matter, more marked in the internal layers than in the external layers, appeared minimal and explain, in part, why the paraplegia was considered transient.

In 95 autopsies performed during the period of 1952 to 1963, Wolman[96] found that pathologic disturbances of circulation in the spinal cord during the acute stage commonly consisted of hemorrhage in both cord substance and covering membranes. Gray matter was more frequently involved than white matter, but occasionally there was extensive spread into adjacent white matter. Contusion was also frequent, the contused segment appearing darker macroscopically and bluish red soon after injury. Microscopically, in contusion, white matter was edematous, vacuolated, and pale staining with a honeycombed appearance. Axis cylinders were irregularly swollen, tortuous, and fragmented. The earliest hemorrhages appeared as small collections of red cells often found in congested capillaries and extending into surrounding tissue. They were situated in gray matter, usually in the ventral part of the posterior horn. Compression of the cord appeared more often in fracture-dislocations than in other types of injuries. It also resulted from prolapse of intervertebral disc. The cord appeared narrow and constricted with marked swelling due to edema above and below the site of compression. Thrombosis also occurred, and involvement of vertebral arteries was noted in some cervical injuries, after manipulation of the neck, and after birth injuries. There was occasional occlusion of major spinal arteries and thrombosis of smaller pial and subpial arteries. Pial veins were also occluded.

In late stages following spinal injury there was hemorrhage and resolution of hemorrhage with phagocytosis, hemosiderin pigment, and compound granular corpuscles, as well as proliferation of glia. The eventual chronic picture was one of patchy gliosis that extended longitudinally owing to secondary degeneration of fiber tracts. Hematomyelia occurred with intramedullary cavitation. Arterial changes in chronic cases were constituted of fibrin thrombi within vessels with organization and recanalization of vessels. Wolman[96] also described alterations caused by intrathecal alcohol given to relieve spasticity. In these cases, there was severe intimal proliferation and loss of elastica and replacement of fibrous tissue in pial vessels, as well as hyalinization in spinal vessels.

Parker[67] applied external trauma to the lumbar spinal columns of dogs and used postmortem contrast radiography to identify damage to segmental spinal branches of the aorta. He observed thrombotic occlusion of some aortic branches in every dog. Ahmann et al.[1] and Keith[49] reported on spinal cord infarction due to minor trauma in children. Although infarction of the spinal cord may be an occasional complication of thoracic and aortic surgery and dissection aneurysm, it has also been observed in children who suffered relatively minor trauma followed by permanent spinal cord injury. In the patients described by Ahmann, signs were delayed, beginning with flaccid weakness of both arms and progressing to flaccid quadriparesis with sphincter involvement. No vertebral fracture or dislocation was present. Pathologic examination showed ischemic cord infarction limited to anterior gray matter in the low cervical cord in one child and to the high cervical cord and low medulla in another. Myelography was negative in both patients.

Goodkin and Campbell[33] observed sequential pathologic changes after dropping a weight on the dura-invested spinal cord of the cat. They described early gross involvement of gray matter with a delay in white matter destruction. Both gray and white matter edema were evident. They suggested that there is a period of time during which portions of white matter may be salvaged and long tract function preserved through various methods of treatment. White et al.[93] showed chronic histologic changes occurring after impact injury in subhuman primates. They suggested that the expanding central gray lesion produces centrifugal pressure on circumferential white matter within limiting leptomeninges. They observed that damage to long tracts was delayed beyond that to gray matter. Direct hypothermia to the spinal cord apparently stabilizes the pathologic changes consisting of hemorrhage, edema, and necrosis. Balentine[5] induced central necrosis of the spinal cord by hyperbaric oxygen exposure in rats. Based on their observations, they warned that the therapeutic use of hyperbaric oxygen in patients with spinal cord injury may potentially cause central spinal necrosis.

White[94] reported light microscopy studies on experimentally injured spinal cords. He reviewed alterations in microarchitecture and other pathologic changes after experimental injury and pointed out the progressive nature of the central lesions. He emphasized that small hemorrhages in the central gray matter 30 minutes after severe injury resulted from delayed rupture of thin-walled vessels and erythrocyte leakage into perivascular spaces. Small petechial hemorrhages at this time are often restricted to central gray matter. Within two hours after trauma, central petechiae enlarge while polymorphonuclear and microglial reactions become evident. Neuronal alterations occur, which include ghost cells, eosinophilic nerve cells with indistinct nuclei and cytoplasm, and loss of Nissl bodies. By four hours, the process is advanced to coagulation necrosis of much of the central gray and subadjacent white matter. By 24 hours after injury, the spinal cord is composed of amorphous necrotic tissue and aggregated red blood cells with only a small rim of identifiable white matter.

Wolman[97] studied post-traumatic regeneration of nerve fibers in the human spinal cord and its relation to intramedullary neuroma. He examined spinal cords of 76 patients with traumatic paraplegia surviving from six hours to 43 years after injury. Well-developed axon regeneration was found in 12 cases in or adjacent to the spinal segments sustaining maximal damage. The shortest interval elapsing between injury and death in which regeneration was observed was 12 months, and in cases with longer survival, regenerated processes could be traced.

## DELAYED CYSTIC DEGENERATION

Delayed cystic degeneration of the spinal cord following spinal cord injury has been reported (Figs. 19, 20).[6,52,57,66] Syringomyelic cavities are a late complication of spinal cord injury and consist of a cyst extending from the site of injury cephalad into the cervical cord, but usually not into the medulla. Rossier et al.[72] place the incidence at between 1.0 and 1.5 percent. Usually, clinical evidence of such a cavity is pain and temperature sensory loss, as in classic syringomyelia. The syringomyelia syndrome differs from classic syringomyelia in that there is a history of severe spinal trauma with paralysis. The disorder begins insidiously in segments of the cord adjoining the level of injury and descends and ascends progressively over many years. In classic syringomyelia there are cervicomedullary junction abnormalities, the commonest being downward displacement and elongation of the cerebellar ton-

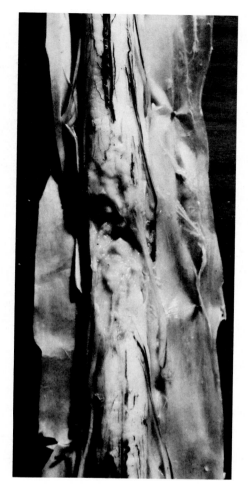

*Fig. 19.* Laceration and cavitation of spinal cord. (Courtesy Dr. G. M. Bedbrook)

sils. In post-traumatic syringomyelia this does not occur. Cysts may be demonstrated by gas myelography. Changing the tilt of the patient from supine to upright demonstrates the expanding lesion. Positive contrast myelography usually shows a normal-sized cord.

McLean et al.[64] documented a case of post-traumatic syringomyelia in which the interior of the cyst was outlined by both positive contrast and gas myelography. The cyst was found to communicate with the fourth ventricle. They suggest that the cyst is originally formed from a central spinal cord hematomyelia and propagated by continued intermittent pressure caused by neck movements, particularly flexion. The authors felt that the cyst should be treated by surgical drainage into the subarachnoid space.

Barnett and Jousse[7] reported a patient with a cavity from the site of in-

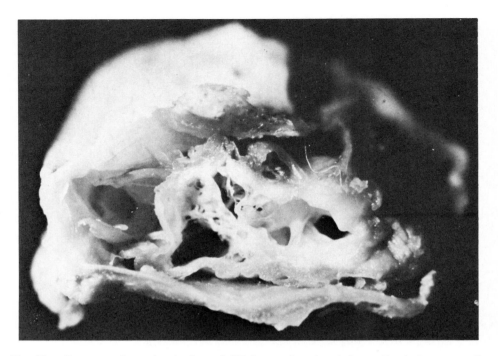

*Fig. 20.* Cross section of spinal cord C7 6 months after injury. Cord almost totally replaced by cavities and glial trabeculae.

jury (L1 segment) into the cervical canal. Barnett[8] suggests that such cavities may result from minor to moderate trauma. Barnett et al.[9] state that such cavities may convert a paraplegic into a tetraplegic. We have not seen any such cases. They also reported a patient in whom clinically significant post-traumatic syringomyelia developed as early as four months following trauma.

Surgical treatment has been attempted to reduce the neurologic deficit by incision of pia to drain the cavity in injured spinal cord. We insert a 3 to 5 cm silastic catheter from the subarachnoid space into the cavity for permanent drainage. Whether this procedure is valuable cannot be proved. Pathogenesis of the cyst is uncertain, but the hemorrhage and necrotic material inside the spinal cord following injury may be forced upward forming a central or paracentral cord cyst and usually extending a number of segments from the site of trauma. Hemorrhage tracking upward from the injury site may also be a possibility. Infarction may occur at a distance because of related arterial occlusion and may be related to formative mechanisms. Barnett et al.[9] emphasized that formation of the syringomyelic cavity is characterized by pain at the onset, and found evidence that the cavity may extend into the brain stem in some instances. Credit for first reports of these cavities is given to Holmes,[43] who, in 1915, found lesions very similar to those described in more recent literature.

Horenstein[44] suggests that diagnostic criteria for intramedullary cyst might include (1) development of a sensorimotor deficit with areflexia and dissociated sensory loss in segments adjacent to the level of injury after an interval of months to years; (2) molding of posterior vertebral bodies to conform to the configuration of the expanded spinal cord with myelographic verification of intramedullary enlargement; and (3) a focus of arachnoiditis by which the spinal cord may be tethered. He suggests that tethering might be remediable by surgery, thus sparing the patient additional loss of function.

## SPINAL HEMATOMA

In the brain, extracerebral hematomas, both subdural and extradural, usually are associated with trauma. Such hematomas are commonly encountered in neurosurgical practice. On the other hand, similar hematomas in the spinal cord are distinctly uncommon and are less often related to trauma. Hematomas in the spinal cord show a distinct predilection for the epidural space. Spinal subdural hematomas are rare, although incidence appears to be increasing as a direct complication of anticoagulant therapy. Owing to the diluting affect of cerebral spinal fluid, localized spinal subarachnoid hematomas occur extremely rarely.

Kirkpatrick and Goodman[51] report a patient who had a combined subarachnoid and subdural spinal hematoma following lumbar puncture. Most intraspinal hematomas of all varieties share a common symptom of severe back pain and rapidly progressive myelopathy, and once paraplegia develops, poor prognosis for recovery. Besides trauma, other causes of spinal epidural hematoma are spinal surgery, a spontaneous bleeding diathesis, spinal puncture, certain medications such as aspirin-like drugs and anticoagulants, and vascular anomalies. A certain number are associated with apparently minor mechanical manuevers such as coughing, straining, and lifting. Many are spontaneous without recognizable cause. The sooner the hematoma can be evacuated by decompressive laminectomy, the better the prognosis. Unfortunately, spinal hematomas are difficult to recognize, and diagnosis is frequently delayed. In the diagnosis of extraspinal hematoma in the lumbar area, a lumbar puncture may be unsuccessful or bloody due to penetration of the needle into the hematoma itself. Also, the return of spinal fluid may be minimal because of compression of the thecal sac by a hematoma immediately above the spinal puncture site. Improvement in a patient's neurologic status may occur following a long period of compression in the cauda equina area, which has greater propensity for recovery.

Since the original report of spinal apoplexy by Jackson[45] in 1869, over 100 cases of spontaneous epidural hematoma have been reported in both adults and children. A minority occurred in the cervical and cervicothoracic region. Hematomas within the lumbar area are sometimes chronic and may simulate a herniated nucleus pulposus both clinically and on myelogram. Most spinal epidural hematomas occur in the thoracic region. The differential diagnosis between spinal epidural hematoma and abscess is frequently difficult without exploratory surgery. A Brown-Sequard syndrome is unusual, but has been reported.[73] Most spinal epidural hematomas occupy a dorsal or dorsolateral position within the spinal canal. Because of this, the patient may have to be placed in the supine as well as lateral position for the diagnosis to be made by myelography. The latter positioning is only necessary when complete block is absent. Frequently these hematomas occupy several segments and because the diagnosis is obscured preoperatively, both lumbar and upper cervical myelography may have to be carried out to establish the full extent of the lesion. Of 33 patients reviewed by Markham et al.,[63] only 16 were restored to normal or near normal condition, 9 had moderate disability, and 6 were paraplegic. Scott et al.[75] reported two patients and emphasized the requirement for upper cervical myelography. Grollmus and Hoff[40] emphasized the radicular pain that may precede onset of paralysis by days or weeks.

By contrast, hematomyelia is not uncommon following spinal trauma. It is infrequently associated with arteriovenous malformations, anticoagulant drugs, systemic or intrathecal chemotherapy and is rarely spontaneous. The treatment of intramedullary spinal hematoma is controversial, but most agree that if the diagnosis is made, the hematoma should be evacuated surgically with a careful myelotomy incision made through the posterior column. The area chosen should have a paucity of blood vessels and is usually slightly off the midline in a vertical cephalocaudal direction.

Locke et al.[62] described a patient who developed an acute spinal epidural hematoma presumably secondary to aspirin-prolonged bleeding. Patients treated with antiplatelet-aggregating drugs such as aspirin should be watched for the above-described signs and symptoms of hematoma. Senelick et al.[76] described a patient on anticoagulant therapy who developed painless spinal epidural hematoma, which is less common.

## RADIATION INJURY

Radiation injury of the spinal cord is an uncommon complication in modern radiation therapy of malignant tumors because of new technics of shielding. There is an exceptionally wide variation in individual tolerance, as well as in radiosensitivity of the cord. This, of course, cannot be ascertained in advance with accuracy in the individual patient, so there is risk of cord injury in irradiation of even extraspinal tumors. Speaking simply, the greater the tumor dose, the greater the chance of radionecrosis of the spinal cord. However, concrete proof that radiation is in fact the cause of myelopathy is difficult. Most reports emphasize that prognosis is poor once irradiation myelopathy is established and the clinical course is chronic and progressive. Solheim[81] suggests, on the other hand, that the clinical course is not always so, and that considerable spinal cord function may be regained.

Most patients with suspected radiation-induced myelopathy have had radiation not for a spinal cord lesion but for carcinomas around the head and neck, particularly the nasopharynx, tonsils, larynx, thyroid, and esophagus. Hodgkin's disease is another in which radiation is delivered to the thoracic cavity with possible consequent myelopathy. Radiation myelopathy is less common now than in the past because of the increased awareness of sequelae by the radiotherapist. Preventive techniques include utilization of ports other than the spinal canal whenever possible, reduced dosage to the spinal canal itself in treatment of spinal cord tumor, and the withholding of radiation in some cases in which it is recognized that irradiation will be of low benefit.

The first signs of neural injury usually appear between six months and two years after exposure to radiation. Symptoms and signs have been grouped into various syndromes: (1) transient radiation myelopathy,[47] (2) acute radiation myelopathy with progression within a few hours or days from the asymptomatic state to the completion of neurologic deficit, (3) chronic progressive radiation myelopathy,[70] and (4) patients who show progression, but then improvement.[81] Steroids have been used in the treatment of radiation myelopathy. The diagnosis may only be presumed after negative myelography; postmortem evaluation is the most precise means of making an exact diagnosis, but sometimes even this is difficult.

A dose even as low as 1000 rads may be dangerous, depending upon the tolerance of the patient. Besides the total dose, the occurrence of radiation myelopathy is dependent on the rate of delivery, the overall time of administration, the size of the individual fraction, the field size, the volume of the area irradiated, the type of irradiation, and the use of hyperbaric oxygen or other special adjuncts during radiation. Concepts of the pathogenesis of radiation myelopathy differ as to whether the effect is primarily on connective tissue and blood vessels, or on nerve cells and axons, or a combination of both. Whether an autoimmune response is involved has also been considered.[30] Pathologic changes observed include thrombosis of vessels, hyalinization of blood vessel walls, necrosis of tissue, and giant cell formation. Gilmore[31] comments on the development of elongated spindle-shaped cells that produce prodigious amounts of fibers demonstrated by reticular stain, and also emphasizes the extensive proliferation of connective tissue-forming cells and the development of connective tissue in experimentally irradiated rat spinal cord.

## ULTRASONIC DAMAGE

Experimental ultrasonic damage to the spinal cord producing paraplegia has been ascribed to heat and cavitation.[82] There has been no clinical situation in which ultrasound damage has occurred in human spinal cord. Past work on the effects of ultrasound on nervous tissue has involved the use of focused sound in such a manner that high rises in temperature caused thermal lesions. Tissue heating caused by absorption of ultrasound is proportional to the frequency utilized, thus thermal damage increases with frequency. The thermal damage theory is controversial, and the possibility of a nonthermal mechanism has been suggested. Taylor[82] found that hypoxia has a synergistic effect on ultrasonic damage to spinal cord in experimental animals.

## MAJOR VESSEL OCCLUSION

Vascular damage remote from the spinal cord itself can result in severe injury and paraplegia. An example is spontaneous or traumatic dissecting aneurysm of the thoracic aorta. The interruption of vital intercostal arteries causes ischemia in the "watershed" area of the thoracic spinal cord, approximately between T2 and T7. In traumatic rupture of the thoracic aorta, paraplegia may occur for the same reason.[42] Following surgical correction of traumatic rupture of the aorta in Herendon and King's patient,[42] the anuria and paraplegia resolved. The operation was carried out promptly following onset of neural symptoms. Tureen[84] described similar histologic as opposed to functional changes in the spinal cord during experimental temporary thoracic vascular occlusion. Damage to the spinal cord, presumably ischemic, has also been reported following injection of intercostal arteries with radiopaque dyes for visualization of spinal cord tumors and arteriovenous malformations. Spinal cord damage in these cases was thought to be due to the ischemia caused by a bolus of dye in the intercostal artery. The incidence of this complication has been reduced by injections into the aorta in the vicinity of an intercostal artery thought to be related to an intraspinal lesion instead of injection into the intercostal vessel itself.

Spontaneous dissection of the thoracic aorta is usually accompanied by severe chest or posterior thoracic pain. While the diagnosis of the attendant paraplegia is easily established, its relation to the chest lesion is sometimes difficult, but may be made by x-ray evaluation of widening of the mediastinum. Patients treated for this severe aortic problem have in some cases improved neurologically.

## ULTRASTRUCTURE

Dohrmann et al.[21,22] have shown microvasculature of the spinal cord to be very trauma sensitive. Fine structural alterations occur primarily in gray matter. Within five minutes, postcapillary venulae become distended with erythrocytes. Red cells penetrate the injured vascular endothelium within 15 to 30 minutes and, owing to endothelial gaps and ruptures in the walls, are found within perivascular spaces of postcapillary and muscular venulae. Ruptures are detected within 15 minutes after contusion but increase in number and size later. Vacuolation and swelling, hallmarks of ischemic endothelial injury, are found at four hours in the endothelium of capillary and postcapillary venulae throughout gray and white matter.

White matter also undergoes characteristic traumatic structural alterations. Five minutes after a severe injury, myelinated fibers resemble those in an uninjured animal; 15 to 20 minutes later, some fibers develop moderately enlarged periaxonal spaces. Further changes at one hour consist of altered myelin sheaths, splaying of myelin lamellae, and greatly enlarged periaxonal spaces. It is postulated that microvascular changes are characteristic of spinal cord injury, while neuronal degenerations are secondary to vascular changes and ischemia. Goodman et al.[34] showed that within five minutes of injury in monkeys, there are loss of integrity of endothelial junctions in gray matter, enlargement of the extracellular space due to vasogenic edema, and glial swelling due to cytotoxic edema. The endothelial capillary lining separates to expose the basement membrane, and formation of platelet thrombi progresses to total occlusion of the vessel. Nonperfusion in selected areas of gray matter results from occlusion of small vessels by formed blood elements.

Gledhill et al.[32] concluded that demyelination was the predominant white matter response to spinal cord compression and also reported axon cylinder reactions similar to Wallerian degeneration. Wakefield and Eidelberg[87,88] described the disappearance of microtubules, the presence of membrane-dense bodies, and Wallerian degeneration after cord compression.

Lampert and Cressman[58] studied myelin sheaths of degenerating axons from 4 to 50 days after section of ascending dorsal tracts in the thoracic spinal cord of rats following trauma. In the peritraumatic region, they noted abundant microphages rapidly engulfing degenerating axons and sheaths. Myelin lamellae were transformed into uniformly layered structures that blended with surrounding cytoplasmic membranes. The layered material then dissolved into amorphous globoid lipid bodies. In the cervical cord and lower medulla, most myelin sheaths collapsed and folded, but some were intact as late as 52 days after trauma.

Bernstein[11] studied ultrastructure of a human spinal neuroma in a paraplegic patient. The neuroma consisted of a discrete circular collection of cells and nerve fibers surrounded by a capsule of gliofibrils. Axis cylinders of nerve fibers often did not fill the myelin sheath. The myelin sheaths formed by Schwann-like cells were replete with Schmidt-Lanterman incisures and nodes of Ranvier. Bernstein[11] indicated that such a central neuroma may be of dorsal root or perivascular origin.

## CERVICAL SPINE INJURIES WITH VASCULAR COMPLICATIONS

The two carotid and two vertebral arteries upon which the brain is dependent for blood supply are vulnerable to neck injury, as are the vertebral column and spinal cord. The vertebral arteries pass through a series of lateral vertebral foramina and by virtue of their fixation within the foramina are susceptible to transient closure and damage after cervical vertebral injury. The lumen of the vertebral artery can be transiently obliterated by sudden enforced lateral rotation of the head. Vertebral artery insufficiency manifested by posterior fossa signs and symptoms has occurred in conjunction with chiropractic manipulations, injury to the vertebral body, and spinal injuries. Intimal and subintimal vertebral artery injury has been observed at postmortem examination following fatal neck trauma. Osteophytes may be a contributory factor in compression of vertebral arteries.[78] The carotid arteries, while not similarly tethered as the vertebral arteries, may nevertheless be injured by penetrating and nonpenetrating cervical trauma. Schneider and Crosby[74] describe the syndrome of vascular insufficiency of brain stem and spinal cord in conjunction with spinal trauma.

## SPINAL CORD BLOOD FLOW

There have been two theories of spinal cord blood flow. The earlier is that blood flows downward from the brain stem and cervical spinal cord to the thoracic cord and conus medullaris. The currently accepted theory[19] is that blood flows from opposite ends of the spinal cord via cervical spinal cord blood vessels, the paired posterior spinal and anterior spinal arteries. Therefore, "watershed" areas can be found at points equidistant from bifurcations of radicular arteries. It has been postulated that in the cervical area, blood flows from the posterior inferior cerebellar arteries downward. In the lower spinal cord, direction of flow in the posterior spinal arteries is upward. At the tip of the conus medullaris, the anterior spinal artery anastomoses via the "rami cruciantes" or the caudal anastomotic loop of Lazorthes with posterior spinal arteries. Thus, watershed areas occur in the upper and lower thoracic spine in which the circulation is marginal. Some authors feel that the blood supply to a given segment of the spinal cord is a dynamic and changing process varying in flow according to needs of the spinal cord. DiChiro and Fried[19] subscribe to that concept. The important artery of Adamkiewicz usually enters the spinal cord bilaterally and possibly at different levels in the area of the conus medullaris via the anterior root.

## LOCAL CIRCULATION OF THE TRAUMATIZED
## SPINAL CORD

One of the immediate events occurring with contusion of the spinal cord appears to be an alteration in intramedullary microvasculature. Histologic and electron microscopic studies reveal disruption of small blood vessels and concomitant hemorrhages within gray matter and later involvement of surrounding white matter by edema.[98] Fluorescence techniques have been used to study intramedullary blood flow patterns using Thioflavine-S and Evans blue fluorescent substances which stain walls of blood vessels through which they pass. Using one technique, after rapid intravenous injection of Thioflavine-S the contused segment of spinal cord may be examined under ultraviolet light to determine in which vessels blood is flowing at the time of the injection. Using both electron microscopy and this technique, it is observed that immediately following trauma there is extravasation of contrast material from vessels of the central gray matter. Dohrmann[23] reports tearing of muscular venulae in gray matter following spinal cord contusion. He demonstrated that no blood flow occurs in hemorrhagic areas and that by one hour after trauma the entire gray matter is in a state of hemorrhagic nonperfusion. He notes that microcirculatory alterations following a contusion sufficient to produce a permanent paraplegia differ from those of transitory lesions. Hemorrhages are more numerous and of greater magnitude. Fried and Goodkin[29] note that the most striking finding in their microangiograms of injured spinal cord segments was diminished perfusion of intrinsic arteries proportional to the severity of impact and the time interval from trauma. They also note focal dilatation and constrictions of intrinsic arteries. Wagner et al.,[85,86] using fluorescence techniques, noted a longer venous phase following trauma, which may reflect vascular stasis.

Spinal cord blood flow behaves much like cerebral blood flow. It varies with $P_{CO_2}$, although sensitivity seems to be somewhat less than that of the brain.[79] Kindt,[50] as well as Kobrine et al.,[53,55,56] suggest that there is autoregulation of spinal cord blood flow, as in the brain. They note that the changes of flow in response to $P_{CO_2}$ and blood pressure are similar. Spinal cord blood flow falls passively with decreases to 50 mm Hg and below in mean arterial pressure. At mean arterial pressures above 135 mm Hg there is a breakthrough of autoregulation and spinal cord blood flow increases with further increases in mean arterial pressure. Autoregulation of spinal cord blood flow thus resembles that of cerebral blood flow at a somewhat lower level.[55,56]

## ISCHEMIA

There has been a controversy concerning the role of ischemia following spinal cord injury. Walker and Yashon[89,90,91] found experimental hypotension caused decrease in metabolically significant blood flow in the spinal cord. Feldman et al.[27] showed that lactate accumulated in primate spinal cord much as it did in a cerebral model during circulatory arrest. Locke et al.[61] showed that ischemia was immediately evident following trauma to the spinal cord and persisted for about 18 hours. Kobrine,[53] using a hydrogen clearance method, found that in monkeys blood flow more than doubled in the lateral funiculus of white matter within four hours after injury, but returned to normal by eight hours and remained in the normal range for 24 hours. They challenged the notion that spreading ischemia of white matter is an important factor in pathophysiology of experimental spinal cord injury.[55,56] With pretreatment by antihistamine drugs, Kobrine et al.[54] found that the rise in blood flow did not occur, so they concluded that histamine was the mediator of the previously demonstrated increase in funicular blood flow. Likewise, Bingham et al.,[12] using indicator fractionation techniques, also could not support the concept of ischemia of white matter as a factor in paraplegia after trauma. Griffiths[39] found that autoregulation was lost following a spinal cord injury, but also that following a 300 g/cm force injury, a marked and progressive reduction in spinal cord blood flow occurred in both gray and white matter. His work supports the notion of ischemia as a cause for secondary damage following spinal injury.

Shay[77] studied experimental ischemia of the cat spinal cord with electron microscopy, and found that mitochondria of neuron cell bodies, axon terminals, and astrocytic processes were two to three times larger following ischemia. Only a small number of mitochondria of axons and axon terminals as well as astrocytic processes lost their matrix density compared to the larger number of mitochondria of neuron cell bodies. The ischemia caused no significant changes in mean sizes of axons or axon terminals. Lysosomes in neurons were unchanged by the electron microscopy methods. Astrocytic processes increased in size more than threefold.

Ducker and Perot[24] used analysis of xenon-133 desaturation curves as well as mass spectrometry to measure changes in tissue oxygen by polarographic techniques, and found that there was considerable ischemia following spinal trauma. Yashon et al.[99] found considerable elevation of lysosomal enzymes and in some cases nonlysosomal enzymes following spinal trauma. This could be secondary to ischemia or other primary mechanism.

## EDEMA FOLLOWING TRAUMA

Edema in the nervous system has been assessed by histologic techniques and by electron microscopy. Perhaps the best evaluation is by chemical analysis in which the amount of increase in fluid can be measured. The dry weight remaining after desiccation of a given weight of control and experimental tissue enables calculation of the amount of fluid evaporated. Edema is therefore demonstrated by increase in water content in injured tissue. Yashon et al.[98] found that edema began early and persisted up to the fifteenth day following spinal trauma. Lewin et al.[59] found that in cats, edema began a day after injury and increased significantly to a maximum in three to six days after trauma, and began to recede on the ninth day. They found that cats treated with dexamethasone within 24 hours of injury exhibited significantly better recovery and less histologic abnormality than untreated cats. This was true of post-traumatic edema also.

Hansebout et al.[41] found that dexamethasone prevents a loss of intracellular potassium from injured spinal cord in cats. They felt that the level of potassium within spinal cord correlates with the functional state of the experimental animal. Perhaps membrane stability is enhanced by steroids, thus preventing leakage of potassium out of the cell. Green et al.[35] and Green and Wagner,[36] using the fluorescent indicator Evans blue, found that edema was significant following experimental trauma. Likewise, Griffiths and Miller[37] found extreme vascular permeability leading to vasogenic edema. Griffiths,[38] using a similar Evans blue albumin fluorescent technic, felt that increased permeability following release of chronic compression may result from reactive hyperpyremia.

Kobrine[54] used an I[131] serum albumin method to mark extravasation of serum proteins into the extraneurocellular spaces. He and others stated that a possible reason for fluid extrusion into tissues is breakdown of the pentilaminar tight junctions of capillary endothelium into surrounding white matter. Parker et al.,[68] as well as Nolan,[65] advocate the use of mannitol in the treatment of the acute phase of injured spinal cord. DeCrescito et al.[18] bring up an interesting concept that ethanol potentiates traumatic cerebral edema. It is possible that this could also be true in the spinal cord, thus resulting in more severe injury in an alcohol-intoxicated individual. This is only speculative, but deserves further research.

# REFERENCES

1.  Ahmann PA, Smith SA, Schwartz JF, Clark DB: Spinal cord infarction due to minor trauma in children. Neurology 25:301–307, 1975
2.  Bailey FW: Histological changes in the spinal cord of man in cases of fatal injury. II. Alterations in the neurocytons. Bull Los Angeles Neurol Soc 24:204–213, 1959
3.  Bailey FW: Histological changes in the spinal cord of man in cases of fatal injury. III. Alterations in the nerve fibers. Bull Los Angeles Neurol Soc 25:147–160, 1960
4.  Bailey FW: Histological changes in the spinal cord of man in cases of fatal injury. IV. Alterations in the classical neuroglia. Bull Los Angeles Neurol Soc 26: 32–40, 1961
5.  Balentine JD: Central necrosis of the spinal cord induced by hyperbaric oxygen exposure. J Neurosurg 43:150–155, 1975
6.  Barnett HJM, Botterell EH, Jousse AT, Wynn-Jones M: Progressive myelopathy as a sequel to traumatic paraplegia. Brain 89:159–174, 1966
7.  Barnett HJM, Jousse AT: Nature, prognosis and management of posttraumatic syringomyelia. In Barnett JHM, Foster JB, Hudgson P (eds): Syringomyelia. Philadelphia, Saunders, 1973
8.  Barnett HJM: Syringomyelia consequent on minor to moderate trauma. In Barnett HJM, Foster JB, Hudgson P (eds): Syringomyelia. Philadelphia, Saunders, 1973
9.  Barnett HJM, Jousse AT, Ball MJ: Pathology and pathogenesis of progressive cystic myelopathy as a late sequel to spinal cord injury. In Barnett HJM, Foster JB, Hudgson P (eds): Syringomyelia. Philadelphia, Saunders, 1973
10.  Bedbrook GM: Some pertinent observations on the pathology of traumatic spinal paralysis. Paraplegia 1:215–227, 1963
11.  Bernstein JJ: Ultrastructure of a human spinal neuroma. J Neurol Sci 18:489–492, 1973
12.  Bingham WG, Goldman H, Friedman SJ, et al: Blood flow in normal and injured monkey spinal cord. J Neurosurg 43:162–171, 1975
13.  Boden G: Radiation myelitis of the brain-stem. J Fac Radiol 2:79, 1950
14.  Breithaupt DJ, Jousse AT, Wynn-Jones M: Late causes of death and life expectancy in paraplegia. Can Med Assoc J 85:73–77, 1961
15.  Burke MJ, Hicks AF, Robins M, Kessler H: Survival of patients with injuries of the spinal cord. JAMA 172:121–124, 1960
16.  Cooper IS, MacCarty CS, Rynearson EH: Gynecomastia in paraplegic males. J Neurosurg 7:364–367, 1950
17.  Cooper IS, Hoen TI: Metabolic disorders in paraplegics. Neurology 2:332–340, 1952

18. DeCrescito V, Demopoulos HB, Flamm ES, Ransohoff J: Ethanol potentiation of traumatic cerebral edema. Surg Forum 25:438–440, 1974
19. DiChiro G, Fried LC: Blood flow currents in spinal cord arteries. Neurology 21: 1088–1096, 1971
20. Dietrick RB, Russi S: Tabulation and review of autopsy findings in fifty-five paraplegics. JAMA 166:41–44, 1958
21. Dohrmann GJ, Wagner FC, Bucy PC: The microvasculature in transitory traumatic paraplegia. An electron microscope study in the monkey. J Neurosurg 35:263–271, 1971
22. Dohrmann GJ, Wagner FC, Bucy PC: Transitory traumatic paraplegia: electron microscopy of the early alterations in myelinated nerve fibers. J Neurosurg 36: 407–415, 1972
23. Dohrmann GJ, Wick KM, Bucy PC: Spinal cord blood flow patterns in experimental traumatic paraplegia. J Neurosurg 38:52–58, 1973
24. Ducker TB, Perot PL, Jr: Local tissue oxygen and blood flow in the acutely injured spinal cord. Proc 18th Vet Admin Spinal Cord Inj Conf, October 1971, pp 29–32
25. Ducker TB, Kindt GW, Kempe LG: Pathological findings in acute experimental spinal cord trauma. J Neurosurg 35:700–708, 1971
26. Emminger-Augsburg E: Zur pathologischen anatomie des schleudertraumas der halswirbelsaule. Arch Link Chir 316:445–457, 1966
27. Feldman RA, Yashon D, Locke GE, Hunt WE: Lactate accumulation in primate spinal cord during circulatory arrest. J Neurosurg 34:618–620, 1971
28. Freed MM, Bakst HJ, Barrie DL: Life expectancy, survival rates, and causes of death in civilian patients with spinal cord trauma. Arch Phys Med 47:457–463, 1966
29. Fried LC, Goodkin R: Microangiographic observations of the experimentally traumatized spinal cord. J Neurosurg 35:709–714, 1971
30. Froscher W: Die Strahlenschadigung des Ruckenmarks. Fortschr Neurol Psychiatr 3:94, 1976
31. Gilmore SA: Long-term effects of ionizing radiation on the rat spinal cord: intramedullary connective tissue formation. Am J Anat 137:1–18, 1973
32. Gledhill RF, Harrison BM, McDonald WI: Demyelination and remyelination after acute spinal cord compression. Exp Neurol 38:472–287, 1973
33. Goodkin R, Campbell JB: Sequential pathologic changes in spinal cord injury: A preliminary report. Surg Forum 20:430–432, 1969
34. Goodman JH, Bingham WG, Jr, Hunt WE: Edema formation and central hemorrhagic necrosis following impact injury to primate spinal cord. Surg Forum 25: 440–442, 1974
35. Green BA, Wagner FC, Bucy PC: Edema formation within the spinal cord. Trans Am Neurol Assoc 96:244–245, 1972
36. Green BA, Wagner FC: Evolution of edema in the acutely injured spinal cord: A fluorescence microscopic study. Surg Neurol 1:98–101, 1973
37. Griffiths IR, Miller R: Vascular permeability to protein and vasogenic edema in experimental concussive injuries to the canine spinal cord. J Neurol Sci 22:291–304, 1974
38. Griffiths IR: Vasogenic edema following acute and chronic spinal cord compression in the dog. J Neurosurg 42:155–165, 1975
39. Griffiths IR: Spinal cord blood flow after acute experimental cord injury in dogs. J Neurol Sci 27:247–259, 1976
40. Grollmus J, Hoff J: Spontaneous spinal epidural haemorrhage: Good results after early treatment. J Neurol Neurosurg Psychiatry 38:89–90, 1975
41. Hansebout RR, Lewis MG, Pappius HM: Evidence regarding the action of steroids in injured spinal cord. In Reulen HJ, Schurmann K (eds): Steroids and Brain Edema. New York, Springer-Verlag, 1972, pp 153–155

42. Herendeen TL, King H: Transient anuria and paraplegia following traumatic rupture of the thoracic aorta. J Thorac Cardiovasc Surg 56:599–602, 1968
43. Holmes G: The Goulstonian lectures on spinal injuries of warfare. Br Med J 2:769–774, 1915
44. Horenstein S: Intramedullary cyst formation with progressive gliosis (traumatic syringomyelia) following spinal cord injury. Trans Am Neurol Assoc 95:263–266, 1970
45. Jackson R: Case of spinal apoplexy. Lancet 2:5–6, 1869
46. Jellinger K: Zur morphologie and pathogenese spinaler lasionen bei verletzungen der halswirbelsaule. Acta Neuropathol 3:451–468, 1964
47. Jones A: Transient radiation myelopathy. Br J Radiol 37:727, 1964
48. Jousse AT, Wynne-Jones M, Breithaupt DJ: A follow-up study of life expectancy and mortality in traumatic transverse myelitis. Can Med Assoc J 98:770–772, 1968
49. Keith WS: Traumatic infarction of the spinal cord. Can J Neurol Sci 1:124–126, 1974
50. Kindt GW: Autoregulation of spinal cord blood flow. Eur Neurol 6:19–23, 1971/1972
51. Kirkpatrick D, Goodman SJ: Combined subarachnoid and subdural spinal hematoma following spinal puncture. Surg Neurol 3:109–111, 1975
52. Klawans HL: Delayed traumatic syringomyelia. Dis Nerv Syst 29:525–528, 1968
53. Kobrine AI, Doyle TF, Martins AN: Local spinal cord blood flow in experimental traumatic myelopathy. J Neurosurg 42:144–149, 1975
54. Kobrine AI, Doyle TF, Rizzoli HV: Further studies on histamine in spinal cord injury and post traumatic hyperemia. Surg Neurol 5:101–103, 1976
55. Kobrine AL, Doyle TF, Rizzoli HV: Spinal cord blood flow as affected by changes in systemic arterial blood pressure. J Neurosurg 44:12–15, 1976
56. Kobrine AI, Doyle TF, Rizzoli HV: A method for estimating edema in experimental traumatic spinal cord injury. Exp Neurol 50:240–245, 1976
57. Laha RK, Malik HG, Langille RA: Post traumatic syringomyelia. Surg Neurol 4:519–522, 1975
58. Lampert PW, Cressman MR: Fine structural changes of myelin sheaths after axonal degeneration in the spinal cord of rats. Am J Pathol 49:1139–1155, 1966
59. Lewin MG, Pappius HM, Hansebout RR: Effects of steroids on edema associated with injury of the spinal cord. In Reulen HJ, Schurmann K (eds): Steroids and Brain Edema. New York, Springer-Verlag, 1972
60. Liss L: Fatal cervical cord injury in swimmers. Neurology (Minneapolis) 15:675–677, 1965
61. Locke GE, Yashon D, Feldman RA, Hunt WE: Ischemia in primate spinal cord injury. J Neurosurg 34:614–617, 1971
62. Locke GE, Giorgio AJ, Biggers SL, Johnson AP, Salem F: Acute spinal epidural hematoma secondary to aspirin-induced prolonged bleeding. Surg Neurol 5:293–296, 1976
63. Markham JW, Lynge HN, Strahlman GEB: The syndrome of spontaneous spinal epidural hematoma: Report of three cases. J Neurosurg 26:334–342, 1967
64. McLean DR, Miller JDR, Allen PBR, Ali Ezzeddin S: Post traumatic syringomyelia. J Neurosurg 39:485–492, 1973
65. Nolan RT: Traumatic edema of the spinal cord. Br Med J 1:710, 1969
66. Nurick S, Russell JA, Deck MDF: Cystic degeneration of the spinal cord following spinal cord injury. Brain 93:211–222, 1970
67. Parker AJ: Clinical significance of traumatic occlusion of segmental spinal arteries. J Am Vet Med Assoc 162:1041–1042, 1973
68. Parker AJ, Park RD, Stowater JL: Reduction of trauma-induced edema of spinal cord in dogs given mannitol. Am J Vet Res 34:1355–1357, 1973
69. Price M: Causes of death in 11 of 227 patients with traumatic spinal cord injury over period of nine years. Paraplegia 11:217–220, 1973

70. Regan TJ, Thomas JE, Colby MY: Chronic progressive radiation myelopathy. JAMA 203:128, 1968
71. Rosencrantz M: A case of fibrous dysplasia (Jaffe-Lichtenstein) with vertebral fracture and compression of the spinal cord. Acta Orthop Scandinav 36:435–440, 1965
72. Rossier AB, Werner A, Wildi E, Berney J: Contribution to the study of late cervical syringomyelic syndromes after dorsal or lumbar traumatic paraplegia. J Neurol Neurosurg Psychiatry 31:99–105, 1968
73. Russman BS, Kazi KH: Spinal epidural hematoma and the Brown-Sequard syndrome. Neurology 21:1066–1068, 1971
74. Schneider RD, Crosby EC: Vascular insufficiency of brain stem and spinal cord in spinal trauma. Neurology 9:643–656, 1959
75. Scott BB, Quisling RG, Miller CA, Kindt GW: Spinal epidural hematoma. JAMA 235:513–515, 1976
76. Senelick RC, Norwood CW, Cohen GH: "Painless" spinal epidural hematoma during anticoagulant therapy. Neurology 26:213–215, 1976
77. Shay J: Morphometry of an ischemic lesion of cat spinal cord. Am J Pathol 72:397–402, 1973
78. Simeone F, Goldberg H: Thrombosis of the vertebral artery from hyperextension injury to the neck. J Neurosurg 29:540–544, 1968
79. Smith AL, Pender JW, Alexander SC: Effects of $Pco_2$ on spinal cord blood flow. Am J Physiol 216:1158–1163, 1969
80. Spatz EL: Personal communication. In Freed MM: Life expectancy survival rates, and causes of death in civilian patients with spinal cord trauma. Arch Phys Med 47:457–463, 1966
81. Solheim OP: Radiation injury of the spinal cord. Acta Radiologica 10:474–489, 1971
82. Taylor KJW: Ultrasonic damage to spinal cord and the synergistic effect of hypoxia. J Pathol 102:41–47, 1970
83. Tribe CR: Causes of death in the early and late stages of paraplegia. Paraplegia 1:19–47, 1963
84. Tureen LL: Effect of experimental temporary vascular occlusion on the spinal cord. I. Correlation between structural and functional changes. Arch Neurol Psychiatr (Chicago) 36:789–807, 1935
85. Wagner F, Taslitz N, White RJ, Yashon D: Vascular phenomena in the normal and traumatized spinal cord. Anat Rec 163:281, 1969
86. Wagner FC, Dohrmann GJ, Taslitz N, Albin MS, White RJ: Histopathology of experimental spinal cord trauma. Proc 17th VA Spinal Cord Inj Conf, City, State, 1969, pp 8–10
87. Wagner FC, Dohrmann GJ, Bucy PC: Histopathology of transitory traumatic paraplegia in the monkey. J Neurosurg 35:272–276, 1971
88. Wakefield CL, Eidelberg E: Electron microscope observations of the delayed effects of spinal cord compression. Exp Neurol 48:637–646, 1975
89. Walker JG, Yashon D: Influence of experimental hypotension on spinal cord biochemical intermediates. Fed Proc 33:484, 1974
90. Walker JG, Yashon D, O'Neill JJ: Influence of trauma and hypotension on dog spinal cord energy state. Fed Proc 34:306, 1975
91. Walker JG, Yashon D, O'Neill JJ: Effect of experimental trauma on dog spinal cord energy state. Fed Proc 35:669, 1976
92. Watkins AL: Ruptured diaphragm: Late cause of death in paraplegia. Arch Phys Med Rehabilit 35:369–371, 1954
93. White RJ, Albin MS, Harris LS, Yashon D: Spinal cord injury: sequential morphology and hypothermic stabilization. Surg Forum 20:432–433, 1969
94. White RJ: Pathology of spinal cord injury in experimental lesions. Clin Orthop 112:16–26, 1975

95.  Wolman L: The neuropathology of traumatic paraplegia. Paraplegia 1:233–251, 1964
96.  Wolman L: The disturbance of circulation in traumatic paraplegia in acute and late stages: A pathological study. Paraplegia 2:213–226, 1965
97.  Wolman L: Post-traumatic regeneration of nerve fibers in the human spinal cord and its relation to intramedullary neuroma. J Path Bact 94:123–129, 1967
98.  Yashon D, Bingham WG, Faddoul EM, Hunt WE: Edema of the spinal cord following experimental impact trauma. J Neurosurg 38:693–697, 1973
99.  Yashon D, Bingham WG, Friedman SJ, Faddoul EM: Intracellular enzyme liberation in primate spinal cord injury. Surg Neurol 4:43–51, 1975
100.  Yashon D: Missile injuries of the spinal cord. In Vinken PJ, Bruyn GW (eds): Handbook of Clinical Neurology. New York, North-Holland 1976, p 209

# 8

## Fractures of the Upper Cervical Spine

Of the three areas in the upper cervical spine in which fracture can be identified, the most common is the odontoid fracture,[2-4] then the so-called Hangman's fracture,[82] followed by Jefferson's fracture.[47] In addition, anatomic areas such as transverse process, spinous process, as well as lamina and lateral masses may be injured. Compression fractures of the upper three vertebral bodies do occur but are uncommon. We concur with Wusthoff's[106] conclusions that injury in these fractures is usually to the head or face and not to the neck itself (Fig. 1). Most patients with upper cervical vertebral fractures sustain minimal neurologic damage because a severe spinal cord injury results in death from respiratory arrest before the patient can be treated. Pathologic fractures of the upper cervical spine occur in osteomyelitis, tuberculosis, osteogenic sarcoma, and metastatic carcinoma, as well as in association with nasopharyngeal infections (Grisel's disease).[51] Untreated fractures of the upper cervical spine may produce serious neurologic sequelae.[7] There is general accord concerning initial management with skeletal traction, usually by means of tongs. For fractures of a spinous process, transverse process, lamina, etc., a four-poster or similar collar may suffice. There is, however, considerable disagreement regarding subsequent treatment.

Embryologically, the odontoid process arises as a part of the body of the atlas but later fuses with the upper portion of the body of the axis and articulates with the posterior surface of the anterior body of the atlas. According to Plaut,[72-73] union of the odontoid process with the axis in about 23 percent of people 30 to 50 years of age is incomplete. But, in our observations of many laminagrams and polytomograms of the odontoid, we have not seen anywhere near this proportion of embryologically incomplete unions. A small island of cartilage, the vestige of the original intervertebral disc, remains at the

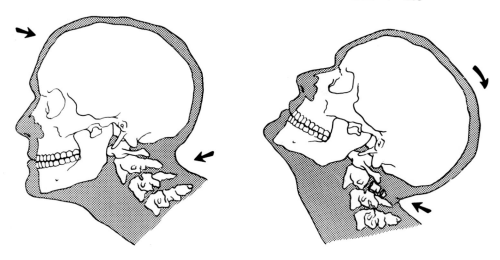

*Fig. 1.* Mechanism of injury in upper cervical spine fractures.

base of the odontoid process. This island of cartilage may contribute to some dislocations of the odontoid process.

## SIGNS AND SYMPTOMS

Most patients with upper cervical spine fractures have sustained trauma from automobile accidents or diving injuries, as well as falls from heights. A large percentage of patients exhibit neck rigidity and complain of painful torticollis, out of proportion sometimes to the injury, which may appear trivial. Such complaints, either immediately following an injury or as long as several weeks thereafter, should alert the physician to the possibility of an upper cervical spine fracture. Examination reveals neck rigidity, often tenderness over the upper cervical spine, and occasionally paraparesis or quadriparesis,[93] but hemiplegia as well as occipital neuralgia have been reported.[7] The symptoms and signs may be puzzling and atypical. As an example, Askenasy's[6] case presentation was delayed and presented as a chronic myelopathy. Sleep attacks have been described.[39]

## PATHOPHYSIOLOGY AND ANATOMY

The lateral masses of the atlas and axis, which are superimposed vertically, contain the articular facets and also foramina for the vertebral arteries.[44] The articular facets are large in proportion to the size of the vertebrae and lie nearly in a horizontal plane, sloping only very slightly in a lateral direction. The inferior facet of the atlas is flat and the superior facet of the axis is very slightly convex to permit the necessary mobility. The articular ligaments binding these facets together are vulnerable to disruption. The foramina for the vertebral arteries are located lateral to the articular facets. Emerging from the foramina of C3 and the axis, these arteries turn laterally and superiorly to reach the foramina of the atlas. Passing through the foramina of the atlas, they turn medially and superiorly in a groove on the superior surface of the atlas to enter the suboccipital triangle (Fig. 2). They then traverse the posterior occipital-atlantoid ligament[27] to enter the uppermost spinal canal, followed by the caudal posterior fossa, and anastomose to form the basilar artery. The course the vertebral arteries follow from the level of the atlantoaxial articulation to the spinal canal has two sharp turns, each almost a right angle. In severe upper cervical cord trauma, almost certainly, fatal injuries result because of vascular occlusion to the brain stem.

Schneider et al.[94] described vascular insufficiency and differential distortion of brain and spinal cord caused by cervical medullary football injuries (Fig. 2). The second cervical segment of the spinal cord was the commonest site of pathologic change on postmortem examination. A poor collateral vascular supply to the vertebral-basilar region, compression of the venous sinus-

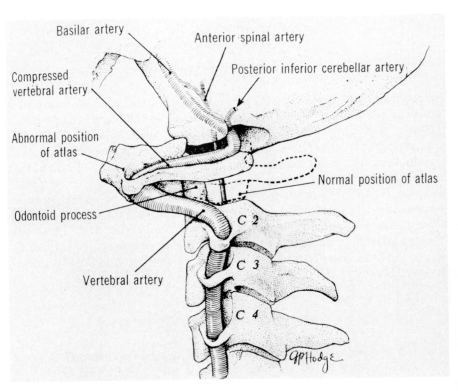

*Fig. 2.* Normal and abnormal anatomy of upper cervical spine. Note stretching of vertebral artery in odontoid fracture. (Courtesy of R. Schneider and E. Crosby. Neurology 9:643, 1959)

es, and the great disparity between the freely mobile brain and the relatively fixed cervical spinal cord form an area vulnerable to damage at the cervical medullary junction, which may lead to acute cerebral edema and tentorial or tonsillar herniation. They described vertebral basilar vascular insufficiency resulting from cervical hyperextension injuries without cervical fracture dislocation. This vertebral basilar vascular insufficiency can be caused by hyperextension injuries such as those occurring in so-called spearing tackles in which the head is used to impale the runner. In an acute hyperextension injury, it is postulated that the vertebral arteries at the C1 occipital condyle level are contused by the occipital condyles of the skull during hyperextension. This may lead to arterial vasospasm or an ascending thrombosis extending as high as the basilar artery. Such an injury with transient vasospasm might cause only a few minutes of neurologic deficit. The onset of neurologic deficit may be delayed, as it was in Schneider's[84] Case 3, in which 12 to 18 hours elapsed between injury and onset of severe neurologic deficit. Hyperextension with atlantoaxial dislocation also causes a similar syndrome (Fig. 2) because of slippage and stretching, as well as temporary or permanent occlusion, of the vertebral arteries.

Impairment of vertebral basilar artery blood flow to the brain is not uncommon after cervical cord injury. Manifestations include nausea, dizziness, unsteadiness, nystagmus, dysarthria, blurring of vision, and unconsciousness; and even death has occurred.[8,30,31] Some insufficiency may be related to chiropractic manipulations or forced torsion of the neck.[10] On occasion, it has been possible to show this angiographically. Symptoms of posterior inferior cerebellar artery insufficiency have been described by several authors. In karate, a direct blow with the radial border of the extended hand to the later C1–C2 level of the spine is effective in causing unconsciousness, probably due to transient vertebral artery insufficiency.

## FRACTURES OF THE ODONTOID PROCESS

Abnormal movement of the atlantoaxial joint or vertebrae as the result of odontoid instability has a variety of causes.[16] The most common, of course, is an actual fracture due to trauma (Figs. 3–9).[21,22,28,35,40,46,70,71,74] The odontoid may be absent or rudimentary[100,101] as a congenital anomaly.[9,18,26,33] In rheumatoid disease,[87] a fracture may result from minor trauma, or a fracture with subsequent instability of C1 upon C2 may result from odontoid reabsorption, as well as abnormal laxity of ligamentous support between the atlas and the axis due to connective tissue changes. (Figs. 10–15).[57] Infections[94] of the soft tissues of the neck, nasopharynx, and the odontoid itself, with and without actual separation of the odontoid from the body of the axis, do occur causing atlantoaxial instability. The most common site of fracture is across the neck of the odontoid at the upper C2 level (Figs. 16, 17).

Congenital anomalies of the odontoid may be of two types.[34,45,62] The entire odontoid may be absent, or the normal odontoid or an atretic odontoid

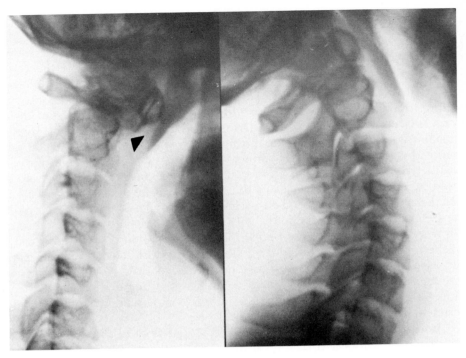

Fig. 3. Flexion-extension (stress) x-rays showing dislocation of C1 and C2 (arrow) during flexion only (left) resulting from odontoid fracture.

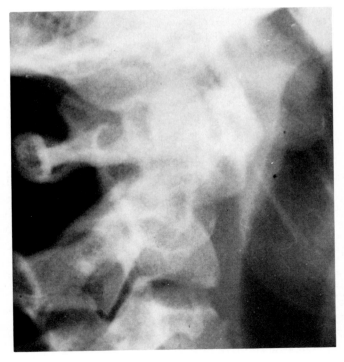

Fig. 4. Lateral x-ray showing dislocation of C1 on C2 due to odontoid fracture.

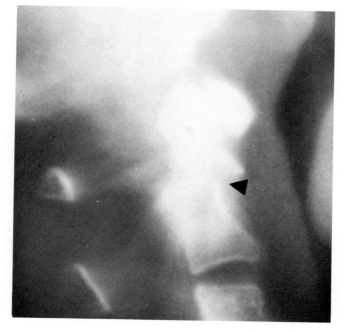

*Fig. 5.* Lateral polytome x-ray showing odontoid fracture (arrow).

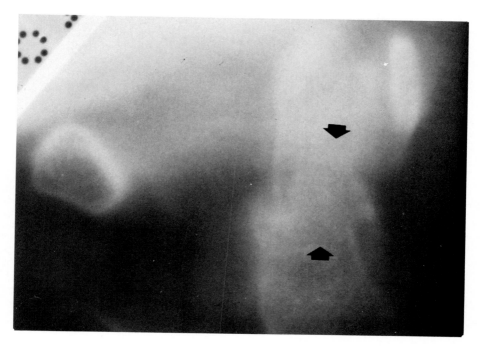

*Fig. 6.* Lateral polytome x-ray showing odontoid fracture (arrows).

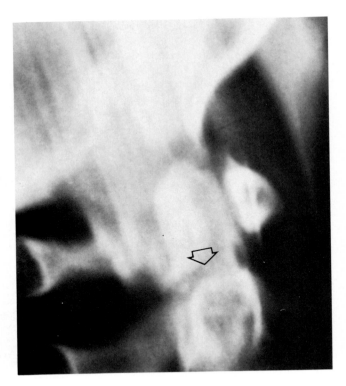

*Fig. 7.* Lateral polytome x-ray showing odontoid fracture (arrow).

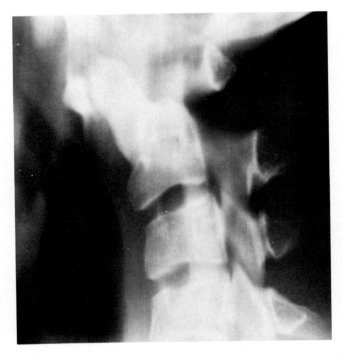

*Fig. 8.* Lateral polytome x-ray showing old healed odontoid fracture in poor alignment due to anterior angulation.

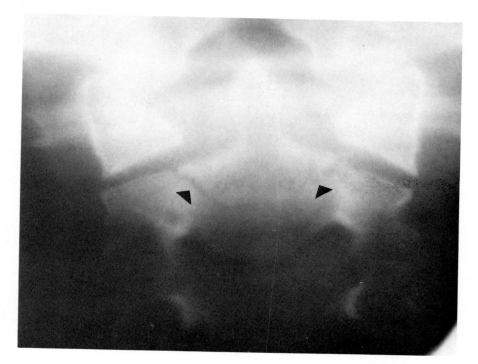

*Fig. 9.* Bilateral fractures across base of odontoid on anterior-posterior polytome x-ray (arrows).

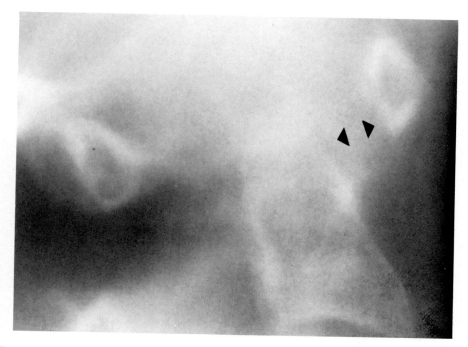

*Fig. 10.* Rheumatoid arthritis: lateral polytome x-ray demonstrating increased distance between anterior border of odontoid and anterior arch of C1 (arrows). There is erosion of bone of the odontoid process.

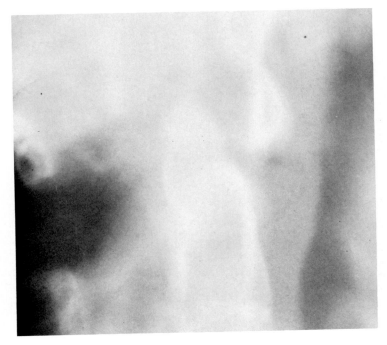

*Fig. 11.* Rheumatoid arthritis: same as Figure 10.

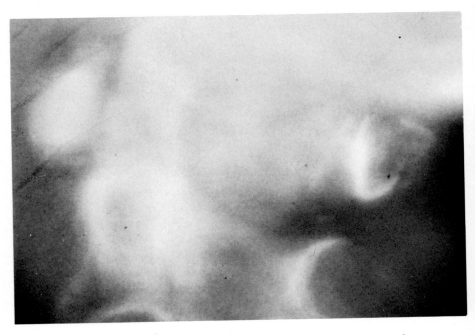

*Fig. 12.* Rheumatoid arthritis: erosion of odontoid process. Lateral polytome x-ray.

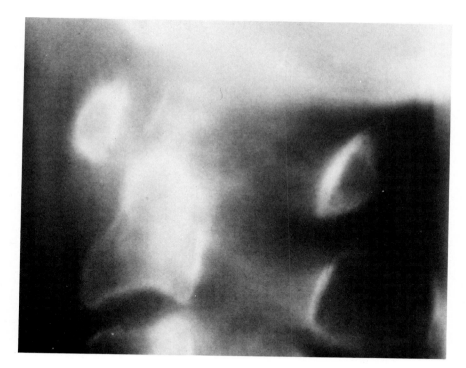

*Fig. 13.* Rheumatoid arthritis: same as Figure 12.

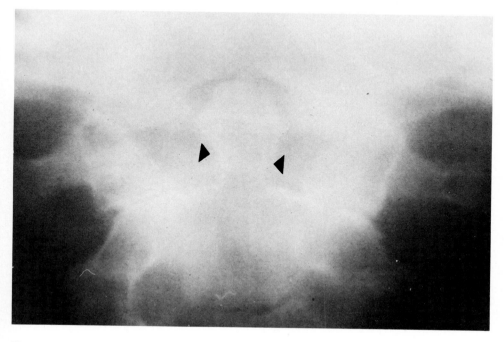

*Fig. 14.* Rheumatoid arthritis: anterior-posterior polytome showing erosion of base of odontoid (arrows).

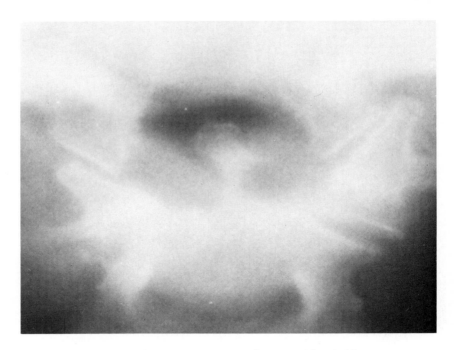

*Fig. 15.* Same as Figure 14, rheumatoid arthritis.

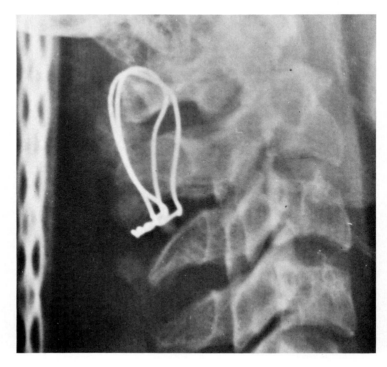

*Fig. 16.* Lateral x-ray of C1–C2 fusion with wiring. For odontoid fracture see Figure 17.

114

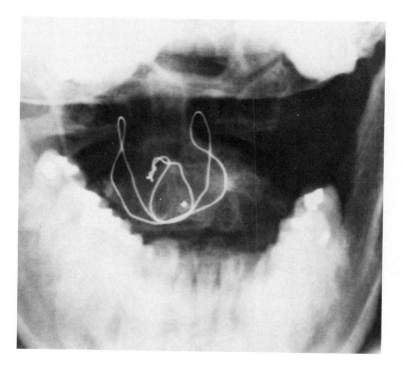

*Fig. 17.* Anterior-posterior (open mouth) x-ray of C1–C2 fusion for odontoid fracture. One wire is looped around the posterior arch of C1 in two places and fastened around spinous process of C2.

process may remain entirely separate from the body of the axis, a condition termed os odontoideum (Figs. 18, 19).[50,59,60] These anomalies are quite uncommon.[68] The articulation between the first and second cervical vertebrae is likely the most mobile joint of the vertebral column, and normally has the least stability of any other paired vertebrae. This mobile joint is located between the stable atlanto-occipital articulation above and a quite stable C2–C3 vertebral articulation below.

Fractures of the odontoid often may go unrecognized[103] because of the failure to consider the possibility, and because of inadequate x-ray examination. If an odontoid fracture goes unrecognized and there is atlantoaxial instability, the patient may complain only of a stiff neck, or he may be asymptomatic. A fibrous nonunion may result, and the patient may be extremely vulnerable to relatively minor trauma in that area. The determination of the presence or absence of union and stability after a fracture of the odontoid requires detailed x-ray examination.

In a recent study, 19 percent of 1000 patients with rheumatoid disease were found to have abnormal C1–C2 mobility.[41,52] However, only 6 of that group had neurologic signs. Rarely, abnormal atlantoaxial movement has been reported following extreme positioning of the head for anesthesia with

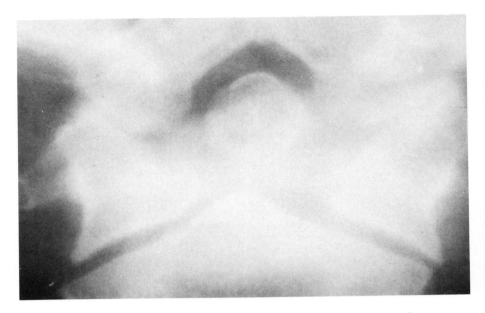

*Fig. 18.* Anterior-posterior polytome of congenital os odontoideum.

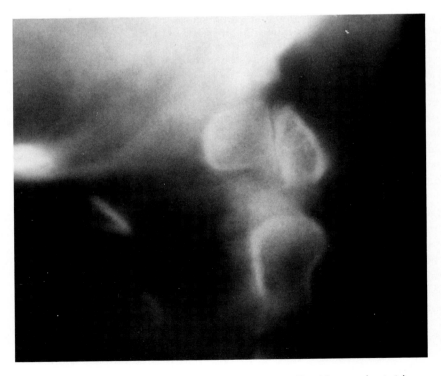

*Fig. 19.* Lateral polytome. Same patient as Figure 18 with os odontoideum.

the patient in the prone position on the operating table. Both hyperflexion and hyperextension have been implicated.

Despite a relatively capacious canal for the spinal cord in the upper cervical level, sufficient displacement of the atlas on the axis will severely damage the spinal cord.[61] It seems reasonable to hypothesize that transient ischemia of the spinal medulla or even permanent vascular damage may result from chronic or acute pathologic instability of C1 on C2, even short of that necessary to compress the spinal cord. There have been case reports of basilar artery insufficiency with brain stem ischemia resulting from C1–C2 instability.[8,13,30,31] Thus, the recurring trauma of minor compression, stretching, or angulation of the vertebral arteries may lead to thrombosis and/or ischemia.

## HANGMAN'S FRACTURE

Hangman's fracture results from hyperextension of the upper cervical spine.[95] It is an uncommon but distinctive traumatic lesion characterized by a bilateral fracture through the neural arch of the second cervical vertebra, with or without dislocation of the body of the axis upon that of the third cervical vertebra (Figs. 20–22).[102,104] The upper cervical canal is usually somewhat widened by

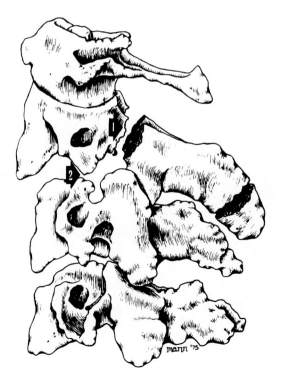

*Fig. 20.* Drawing of "hangman's fracture" showing fracture through neural arch (arrow 1) and dislocation of body of axis upon body of third cervical vertebra (arrow 2).

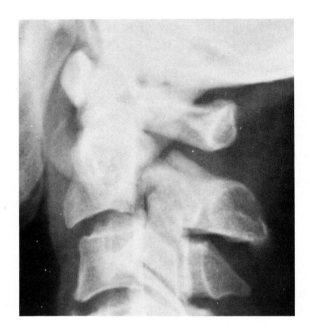

*Fig. 21.* Hangman's fracture, lateral x-ray.

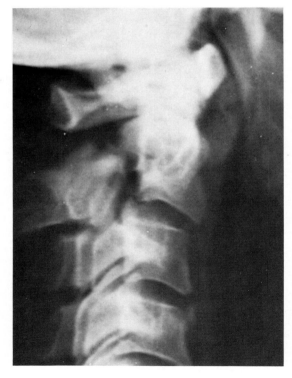

*Fig. 22.* Hangman's fracture, lateral x-ray.

nonlethal fractures. The odontoid process remains unbroken and in place, and the transverse ligament of the atlas is unruptured. The fracture is so-named because it resembles that occurring in judicial hanging,[56,98] in which the long drop and use of a submental, or less commonly, subaural knot causes such a lesion. Because of the roominess of the upper cervical spinal canal and because of a spontaneous decompression of the upper cervical cord by avulsion of the neural arch of C2, most patients have very little neurologic deficit. On the other hand, if severe spinal cord injury occurs, instantaneous death results and this is the reason for the effectiveness of judicial hanging.

Most patients with hangman's fracture respond readily to realignment of the cervical spine by skeletal traction and immobilization in a cast or brace without open reduction of the fracture or spinal fusion. Occasionally it may be advisable to perform an anterior cervical spinal fusion for the purpose of stabilization, as indicated by Schneider et al.[82] and others.[14,63]

## JEFFERSON'S FRACTURE

Force applied to the vertex of the skull is distributed centrifugally upon the ring of the atlas and, if great enough, results in fracture of this ring at its weak points, vertebral grooves, and anterior arch, with separation of the two lateral articular masses[43] (Figs. 23–26). The essential feature of the bursting fracture of the atlas lies in the transmission of force from the vertex through the occipital condyles to the vertebral column. This uncommon burst fracture is known as Jefferson's fracture because of his early description.[47] Suboccipi-

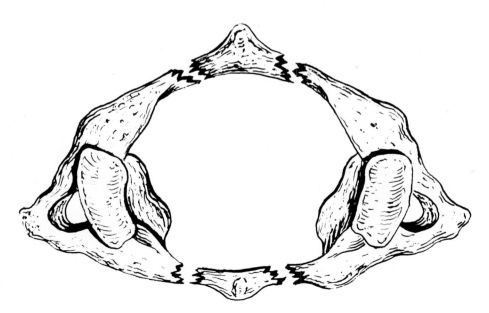

*Fig. 23.* Superior view of atlas (C1) in Jefferson's fracture.

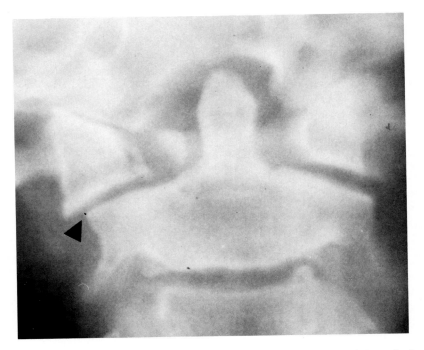

*Fig. 24.* Jefferson's fracture. Fracture of posterior arch of C1 and lateral displacement of lateral mass of C1 (arrow). Anterior-posterior x-ray.

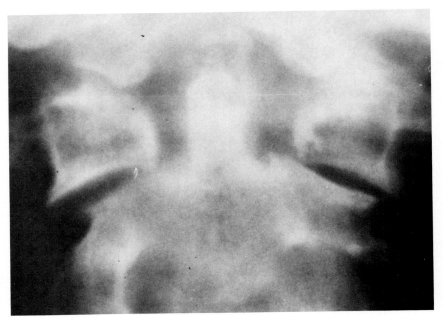

*Fig. 25.* Jefferson's fracture. Same as Figure 24.

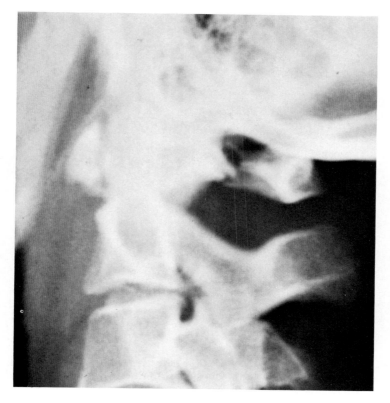

*Fig. 26.* Jefferson's fracture. Lateral x-ray. Fracture of neural arch of C1.

tal pain and nuchal stiffness are widely reported as characteristic of this fracture, as is true of other high cervical spine fractures. In addition, suboccipital pain, paresthesiae, and numbness occur. Tomograms of the atlas in the anterioposterior projection are helpful in identifying the outward separation of the lateral masses from the joints above and below. Standard open mouth views, although visualizing the odontoid well, are sometimes unsatisfactory for adequate visualization of the lateral masses. In most Jefferson fractures, there is a posterior arch fracture of the atlas, and this can sometimes be visualized on plain x-rays in the lateral projection. If such a laminar fracture is seen, tomograms should be carried out to ascertain the presence or absence of Jefferson's fracture. The posterior arch fracture in itself is generally benign, but danger lies in overlooking an associated and potentially unstable burst fracture.

Jefferson's[47] Case 2 is similar to a case we encountered, in which a gunshot wound affected the lateral portion of the occipital atlanto joint. Jefferson's patient was included because of the fracture of the atlas. Our patient had stiffness of the neck and neck pain, and follow-up polytomograms showed that the occipital atlanto joint had spontaneously fused. Our patient

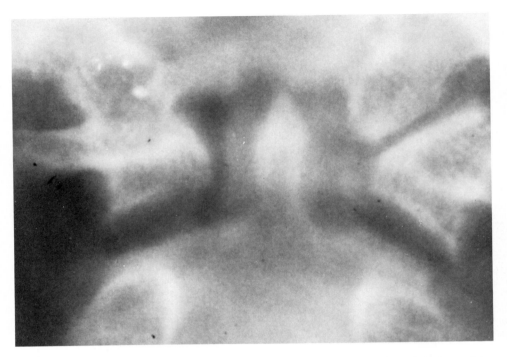

*Fig. 27.* Gunshot wound with fragments at lateral mass C1 and occipital condyle, secondary fusion resulted (see text). Anterior posterior polytome.

also complained of some hypersensitivity in the suboccipital area but was in excellent condition and had normal stability (Fig. 27).

Potentially unstable cervical fractures, such as the Jefferson's fracture and hangman's fracture, have been traditionally managed by external splinting with tongs[17] and complete bed rest while bony fusion occurs primarily. In some cases, surgical fixation with bony fusion has been advocated. In Jefferson's fracture, as with hangman's fracture, surgical fusion is rarely necessary because results obtained with immobilization at bed rest are generally excellent, although lately we have used the halo traction apparatus[66,67,108] as a preferable alternative. Cervical stability can be demonstrated approximately three months after fixation, and the patient in halo traction[96,107] may be ambulatory during this period. Early halo stabilization has been helpful economically and psychologically to our patients, and we have not yet observed any instability, although our series is small.

## RADIOGRAPHIC DIAGNOSIS

The diagnosis of atlantoid-axoid instability, odontoid fracture, hangman's fracture, or Jefferson's fracture is conclusively made by extremely detailed x-ray examination.[91] Conventional anterioposterior (AP) x-rays through the open mouth and a cone down lateral view of the upper cervical spine may reveal a bony abnormality. Unfortunately, these conventional techniques do not reveal many abnormalities, and detailed polytomography is required, both lateral and AP views of the upper cervical spine and occipital condyle foramen magnum (Fig. 27). Even excellent quality plain roentgenograms of the upper cervical spine may not reveal a fracture, so that when a stiff neck persisted after even minor injury, we have ordered polytomes and frequently found abnormalities in the upper cervical spine. Sometimes a "tear-drop" fracture (Figs. 28, 29) may signal instability.

In addition, stress films should be obtained when instability of the upper cervical spine is suspected. These are lateral films of the patient maximally flexing and extending the neck. And because of the inherent danger to the patient, the physician should not only give approval but be present for the stress x-ray examination. When a fracture is known to exist, stress films need not be made early, unless instability is deemed an indication for surgical therapy. This will be discussed in greater detail later. The lateral examination by stress films can be polytomographic or by cinefluoroscopy. Cinefluoroscopy employing either video tape or cine film is valuable in that it dynamically demonstrates instability of the upper cervical spine. In films of the odontoid process, even when a fracture is not present, there should not be more than 4 mm separating the anterior (ventral) bony portion of the odontoid process

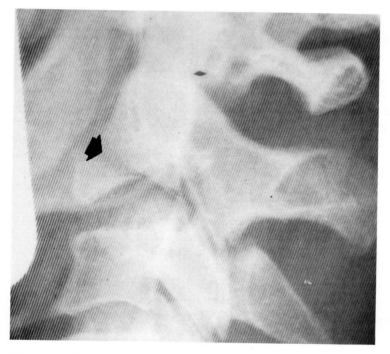

*Fig. 28.* "Tear-drop" fracture (arrow) anterior inferior lip of C2 vertebral body. Lateral x-ray.

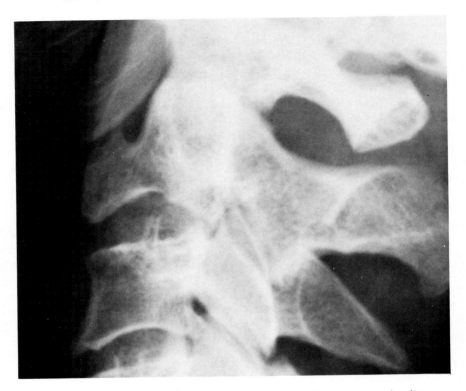

*Fig. 29.* Same patient as Figure 28 2 years later. Spontaneous healing.

and posterior bony edge of the anterior mass of C1 on lateral view. If there is more than 4 mm, C1–C2 instability may exist, although this should not be a hard and fast rule. Plain x-rays may be adequate, but in subtle cases may be inadequate. McKeever[58] states that 2 mm is the maximum separation responsible for instability, but we feel that this is perhaps too strict a criterion.

Neurologic damage from upper cervical vertebral column instability may be reflected in two ways. The first is an acute loss of neurologic function and may consist of acute quadriparesis with a multitude of neurologic signs and symptoms below the lesion, some quite unexpected and vagarious. Even sudden unexpected death may occur due to respiratory embarrassment secondary to extreme spinal cord compression. Second, it is recognized that foramen magnum tumors may cause a multitude of signs and symptoms seemingly unrelated to the lesion. This is true of chronic low-grade compression of the upper cervical spinal cord. Progressive hemiparesis, quadriparesis, and paraparesis may occur.[20,29] We have seen adult patients in whom these signs continued progressively over many years due to either congenital os odontoideum[78,80,81,92] or relatively minor trauma many years previously when the diagnosis of atlantoaxial instability was not made. When atlantoaxial instability exists chronically, it may be difficult to decide whether an odontoid nonunion is congenital or due to forgotten trauma. When the diagnosis is not made symptoms such as a stiff neck may subside for a time after treatment with cervical traction or other physical therapy measures and this can result in a false sense of security.

## TECHNIQUES OF SURGERY

In most patients skeletal tongs and traction are already in place and should remain so during the operation with continuous effective traction maintained. It is desirable to employ awake nasotracheal intubation and then place the patient carefully in the prone position following induction of anesthesia. We have used Foster and Stryker frames for this procedure. The patient can be operated upon in the bed without the use of an operating table. We advocate this since it prevents excess movement. The circular electric bed is less desirable. Changing an anesthetized patient in the upright position in a circular bed from supine to prone position necessitates caution because there may be a significant drop in blood pressure causing severe ischemia in heart, brain, or other organs. For posterior fusion,[54] both the area of the upper cervical spine and occiput are prepared as well as the posterior iliac crest, if a bone graft is to be utilized.

An incision is made from the suboccipital area to approximately the third or fourth cervical vertebra. Soft tissue and fascia are incised and the muscles reflected subperiosteally from the occiput, spinous process, and laminae of the upper cervical vertebrae. We cautiously use cutting current of the Bovie unit for incising soft tissue so as to avoid excessive movement of unstable elements. All ligamentous tissue is removed from between the occiput and ring of the atlas, as well as between C1 and C2 and C3. Using a periosteal elevator, the laminae of C1 and C2 are cleaned both above and somewhat beneath the laminae of all soft tissue, so that appropriate wires may be passed under the arch of C1. We use a high-speed drill burr to denude C1, C2, and C3 of periosteum and cortical bone. An appropriate iliac bone graft approximately two to three inches long is removed and then split in half longitudinally, using an osteotome. All soft tissue is removed from the bone graft. A thin wire is doubled and passed under the arch of C1 and hooked across and over the spinous process of C2. The two free ends (Figs. 16, 17) of the wire are fastened so that the bone graft is snugly fit into place, and the two ends of the wire are also fastened around the spinous process of C2. This is the procedure in odontoid fractures where only C1 and C2 are joined by wires. Prior to final tightening of the bone graft in place with the wire, membranous bone chips are placed in empty spaces between the lamina and bone grafts and all through the area of the graft. We have not felt it necessary to include C3 in the wire fixation graft, but we do denude the surface of C3 and allow the bone graft and chips to extend down to and include C3. We have not felt it necessary to place wires over C3, since C2–C3 are stable in odontoid fractures. Also, it is our feeling that the bony fusion will give permanent fixation, whereas the wire is only temporary until bony union takes place.[32] Others[1–3,97] have felt that C3 should be included in the wiring. Roberts and Wickstrom[77] feel that fusion of C1 and C2 is sufficient and that inclusion of C3 is not necessary. McKeever[58] has used fascia lata strips instead of wires, but we have not used this technique, and have had no problems caused by wires. Using this technique, we have had a negligible incidence of nonunion. Other reported variations include the use of heavy silk instead of wire, and only wiring of C1–C2 without bone. Postoperatively the patient is kept recumbent for a total of four to six weeks and in tong traction for the initial two to three weeks, with reduced weight of 5 to 10 pounds. Tong traction is employed primarily to keep the patient from moving rather than for reduction. An alternative is use of halo traction in the first few days postoperatively, and the patient may be ambulated thereafter. We have, on occasion, used halo traction on admission and then operated with the patient in the halo traction device, loosening some of its parts so as to make the operation possible. Following three to four months of immobilization, the last six weeks of which is in a four-poster brace, stress films are obtained to assess stability. A Minerva jacket may be utilized but is less comfortable than a four-poster.

Some authors advocate anterior fusion transorally for certain odontoid fractures.[12,25,36,37] Decompressive laminectomy has been advocated, but when neurologic signs are not present we do not feel that it is necessary or even desirable. If the odontoid process is retrodisplaced posteriorly into the spinal cord it may be necessary to remove the odontoid process transorally and then carry out a posterior fusion.[36,37] Grote et al.[38] also advocated a ventral surgical approach to the dens epistropheus (odontoid), using a transoral-transpharyngeal approach. They use this procedure for both platybasia and posterior displaced fractures of the odontoid.

Estridge and Smith[23] advocated transoral fusion of odontoid fractures. Alexander et al.[1–3] felt that operative fusion should be used in all cases. Only one fracture united of their four cases not treated surgically. Conversely, Amyes and Anderson[4] reported nonunion in only 3 of their 63 cases. They felt that the period of fixation by traction or external devices should continue until there is x-ray evidence of healing, usually four to eight months. In many of these early studies, polytomography and laminography was not carried out because such techniques were unavailable at the time. Estridge and Smith advocated fusion of the fracture line itself transorally, whereas Fang and Ong fused the lateral joints transorally.[23]

Occipital cervical fusion with bone graft had been widely used since Cone and Turner first described it in 1937.[15] This procedure is not felt to be necessary since the occipital atlanto area is not unstable. Occipital cervical fusion was also advocated by Nagashima.[65] Ashkenazy et al.[6] also advocated inclusion of the posterior rim of the foramen magnum in the fusion. Some authors have employed acrylic fixation for atlantoaxial dislocations, using wire to hold the acrylic splints in place. We feel that use of this foreign body is unnecessary, as autogenous bone is probably more effective for healing and stability.

Irreducibility of an atlantoaxial dislocation occurs on occasion and is difficult to treat. In many cases there are associated bone abnormalities from congenital and/or degenerative diseases such as Marie-Strumpell arthritis, rheumatoid arthritis, dyschondroplasia, and osteoarthritis. List[55] described atlas articular facet arthritis as a cause in a 21-year-old man with irreducible dislocation. Sherk and Nicholson[88,89] describe progressive changes in stability secondary to ossiculum terminale initially noted when the patient was six years old and who was quadriplegic at the age of 15. Three years later she died of respiratory failure. Autopsy revealed that the failure of fusion at the odontoid permitted the transverse ligament of the atlas to ride up over the body of the axis locking the atlas in an anterior dislocated position. The posterior arch of the atlas was practically in contact with the odontoid causing fatal compression of the cord to a thickness of only 1 mm. Nagashima's[64,65] case of irreducibility was probably due to osteoarthritis. In his patient, congenital fusion of C2 and C3 enhanced excessive mobility of C1 on C2. He used acrylic plastic and wire to stabilize the fracture and performed a suboccipital decompression. Progressive quadriparesis can result from atlantoaxial dislocation in patients with achondroplasia.[19] The problem may be successfully treated by skeletal traction and fusion.

There is considerable difference of opinion as to when a patient should be mobilized following upper cervical spine stabilization and fusion procedures. We have described our methods, but do not necessarily find serious fault with less or even longer immobilization. Good results with immediate postoperative mobilization have been reported. Without a halo traction device, we believe that early mobilization subjects the patient to the unnecessary risk of nonunion.

## CONSERVATIVE TREATMENT

There are several methods of conservative treatment of odontoid and other cervical spine fractures. In hangman's fracture nonoperative treatment is recommended. In Jefferson's fracture it is not definitely ascertained which is the best treatment but we have used, for the most part, nonoperative treatment. In odontoid fracture, we believe that operative treatment should be carried out, although many advocate conservative treatment. Alexander et al.[1-3] feel strongly that fusion is the treatment of choice in odontoid fractures. All agree that tong traction should be instituted, and we generally use 10 to 15 pounds of weight initially. We have used up to 60 pounds to obtain reduction, but in upper cervical spine fractures a smaller weight usually suffices (see Chap. 9). Conservative treatment of odontoid fractures consists of from 6 to 12 weeks in tongs recumbent on a frame or in a halo bracing device, after which a Minerva jacket or four-poster brace is employed. An initial trial of conservative treatment followed by an operative approach if instability or symptoms continue has been advocated. In our view, a considerable amount of time is wasted. We have encountered no morbidity or mortality from posterior fusion of odontoid fractures, and in routine cases, total immobilization rarely exceeds three to four months.

## FRACTURES OF THE ODONTOID PROCESS
## IN INFANTS AND CHILDREN

The odontoid process normally fuses with the body of the axis at age three to four years.[105] Odontoid nonunion under three years of age has been reported in only a few patients; none had neurologic deficit, and nonunion was due to trauma in only the minority. All were treated by reduction by means of dependent head traction or tong traction. None were treated surgically; they were treated with a Minerva cast or other plaster-type collar. In one case, halo traction was used. Results regarding union were equivocal in these pediatric patients. Not enough patients in this age group have been studied to justify definite conclusions. One of the problems presented by instability of the odontoid is to determine whether there is a true fracture caused by significant trauma or a congenital nonunion after minor injury.[42] Ewald[24] feels that congenital nonunion should be treated by fusion. The criteria of os odontoideum, established by Wollin,[105] may be of value in determining whether the problem is traumatic or congenital. These criteria include overdevelopment of the anterior arch of the atlas with attenuation of the posterior arch (which may be bifid). In our view, it is the degree of instability which determines whether surgery is recommended rather than the etiology, congenital versus traumatic. Operative treatment is not recommended in instability due to infection.

Keuter[51] emphasizes that children having severe persistent torticollis following a nasopharyngeal infection should be suspected of having nontraumatic atlantoaxial dislocation (Grisel's disease). This condition can also occur less commonly in adults. Occasionally, because of fever and stiff neck, the mistaken diagnosis is meningitis until the spinal fluid is found to be negative and x-rays of the odontoid show a lesion.

## PROGNOSIS

Osgood and Lund[69] reviewed the literature and reported that x-rays of the end result of odontoid healing after fracture were unsatisfactory in approximately 55 reported patients. Blockey and Purser[11] found that 22 of 25 conservatively treated fractures of the odontoid failed to achieve bony union. On the other hand, Amyes and Anderson[4] stated that only 3 of 58 odontoid fractures failed to heal. Rogers[79] reported that four of his nine odontoid fractures had nonunion. The incidence of nonunions in these series is approximately 29 percent, which is a high figure. Roberts and Wickstrom[77] found the nonunion rate of odontoid fractures with displacement was 30 percent, and those with no displacement was 17 percent. Their total series had a nonunion incidence of 20 percent. Roberts and Wickstrom[77] felt that immobilization with traction and/or Minerva jacket for 20 weeks is adequate to obtain bony union, if union is going to occur. If not, operative cervical fusion is indicated.[48]

The mortality rate of odontoid fractures has not been established. Osgood and Lund[69] reported 56 patients, of whom 29 died, a mortality rate of 52 percent. Amyes and Anderson[4] had a mortality rate of 8 percent. Jefferson,[47] in 1920, reported 13 upper cervical spine fracture patients, only 1 of whom survived. Blockey and Purser[11] reported that 1 patient of their 11 died. None of Rogers' patients died.[79] In our experience, the mortality rate after the patient reaches the hospital is extremely low; no death has occurred in which there was no associated severe injury in a large series. In general, for both hangman's and Jefferson's fractures, the prognosis for union without surgical treatment is excellent, although most published series are too small to base conclusions upon.

## REFERENCES

1. Alexander E, Jr, Masland R, Harris C: Anterior dislocation of first cervical vertebra simulating cerebral birth injury in infancy. Am J Dis Child 85:173–181, 1953
2. Alexander E, Jr, Forsyth HF, Davis CH, Jr, Nashold S, Jr: Dislocation of the atlas on the axis. The value of early fusion of C-1, C-2, C-3. J Neurosurg 15:353–311, 1958
3. Alexander E, Jr, Davis CH: Reduction and fusion of fracture of the odontoid process. J Neurosurg 31:580–582, 1969
4. Amyes EW, Anderson FM: Fracture of the odontoid process. Report of sixty-three cases. Arch Surg 72:377–393, 1956
5. Anderson LD, D'Alonzo RT: Fractures of the odontoid process of the axis. J Bone and Joint Surg 56A:1663–1674, 1974
6. Askenasy HM, Braham MJ, Kosary IZ: Delayed spinal myelopathy after atlanto-axial fracture dislocation. J Neurosurg 17:1100–1104, 1960
7. Bachs A, Barraquer-Bordas L, Barraquer-Ferre L, Canadell JM, Modolell Z: Delayed myelopathy following atlanto-axial dislocation by separated odontoid process. Brain 78:533–537, 1955
8. Bell HS: Basilar artery insufficiency due to atlanto-occipital instability. Am Surg 35:695–700, 1969
9. Berkheiser EJ, Seidler F: Non-traumatic dislocations of the atlanto-axial joint. JAMA 96:517–523, 1931
10. Blane ES: Manipulative (chiropractic) dislocations of the atlas. JAMA 85:1356–1359, 1935
11. Blockey NJ, Purser DW: Fractures of the odontoid process of the axis. J Bone Joint Surg 38B:794–817, 1956
12. Bonney G: Stabilization of the upper cervical spine by the transpharyngeal route. Proc Roy Soc Med 63:40–41, 1970
13. Carpenter S: Injury of neck as cause of vertebral artery thrombosis. J Neurosurg 18:849–853, 1961
14. Cloward RB: Anterior cervical fusion for odontoid fracture. In Hall RM (ed): Air Instrument Surgery, vol. 1. New York, Springer, 1970, p 152
15. Cone W, Turner WG: The treatment of fracture dislocation of the cervical vertebrae by skeletal traction and fusion. J Bone Joint Surg 19:584–602, 1937
16. Corner EM: Rotary dislocations of the atlas. Ann Surg 45:9–26, 1907

17. Crutchfield WG: Skeletal traction in treatment of injuries to the cervical spine. JAMA 155:29–32, 1954
18. Dastur PK, Wadia NH, Desari AD, Sinh C: Medullospinal compression due to atlanto-axial dislocation and sudden haematomyelia during decompression: Pathology, pathogenesis and clinical correlation. Brain 88:897–924, 1965
19. Des Raj G, Damodar R: Atlantoaxial dislocation with quadriparesis in achondroplasia. J Neurosurg 40:394–396, 1974
20. Dunbar HS, Ray BS: Chronic atlanto-axial dislocation with late neurological manifestations. Surg Gynecol Obstet 113:757–762, 1961
21. Elliott GR, Sachs E: Observations on fracture of the odontoid process of the axis with intermittent pressure paralysis. Ann Surg 56:876–882, 1912
22. Ely LW: Subluxation of the atlas. Report of two cases. Ann Surg 54:20–29, 1911
23. Estridge MD, Smith RA: Transoral fusion of odontoid fracture. J Neurosurg 27:462–465, 1967
24. Ewald FC: Fracture of the odontoid process in a seventeen month old infant treated with a halo. J Bone Joint Surg 53A:1636–1640, 1971
25. Fang HSY, Ong GB: Direct anterior approach to the upper cervical spine. J Bone Joint Surg 44A:1588–1604, 1962
26. Fielding JW: Disappearance of the central portion of the odontoid process. A case report. J Bone Joint Surg 47A:1228–1230, 1965
27. Fielding JW, Cochran G, Lawsing JF, Hohl M: Tears of the transverse ligament of the atlas. A clinical and biomechanical study. J Bone Joint Surg 56A:1683–1691, 1974
28. Flint A, Sr: Case of fracture of the odontoid process and body of the second cervical vertebra, with dislocation of the atlas. NY Med J 9:29–32, 1869
29. Fromm GH, Pitner SE: Late progressive quadriparesis due to odontoid agenesis. Arch Neurol (Chicago) 9:291–296, 1963
30. Ford FR: Syncope, vertigo, and disturbance of vision resulting from intermittent obstruction of the vertebral arteries due to defect of the odontoid process and excessive mobility of the second cervical vertebra. Johns Hopkins Hosp Bull 91:185, 1952
31. Ford FR, Clark D: Thrombosis of basilar artery with softenings in the cerebellum and brain stem due to manipulations of the neck. Johns Hopkins Hosp Bull 98:37–42, 1956
32. Forsyth HF, Alexander E, Jr, Davis C, Jr, Underdal R: The advantages of early spine fusion in the treatment of fracture-dislocation of the cervical spine. J Bone Joint Surg 41A:17–36, 1959
33. Freiberger RH, Wilson PD, Jr, Nicholas JA: Acquired absence of the odontoid process. A case report. J Bone Joint Surg 47A:1231–1236, 1965
34. Fullenlove TM: Congenital absence of the odontoid process. Report of a case. Radiology 63:72–73, 1954
35. Garber G: Abnormalities of atlas and axis vertebrae congenital and traumatic. J Bone Joint Surg 46A:1782–1904, 1964
36. Greenberg AD: Atlanto-axial dislocation. Brain 91:655–684, 1968
37. Greenberg AD, Scoville WB, Davey LM: Transoral decompression of atlanto-axial dislocation due to odontoid hypoplasia: report of two cases. J Neurosurg 28:266–269, 1968
38. Grote W, Romer F, Bettag W: The ventral approach to the dens epistropheus. Langenbecks Arch Chir 331:15–22, 1972
39. Hall CW, Danoff D: Sleep attacks—apparent relationship to atlantoaxial dislocation. Arch Neurol 32:57–58, 1975
40. Hamilton AR: Injuries of the atlanto-axial joint. J Bone Joint Surg 33B:434–435, 1951
41. Henderson DR: Vertical atlanto-axial subluxation in rheumatoid arthritis. Rheumatol Rehabil 14:31–38, 1975
42. Hess JH, Abelson SM, Bronstein IP: Spontaneous atlanto-axial dislocation: possible relation to deformity of the spine. Am J Dis Child 64:51–54, 1942

43. Hinchey JJ, Bickel WH: Fracture of the atlas. Review and presentation of data on eight cases. Ann Surg 121:826–832, 1945

44. Hohl M, Baker HR: The atlanto-axial joint. J Bone Joint Surg 46A(no 2):1739–1753, 1964

45. Ivie J McK: Congenital absence of the odontoid process. Report of a case. Radiology 46:268–269, 1946

46. Jackson H: The diagnosis of minimal atlanto axial subluxation. Br J Radiol 23:672–674, 1950

47. Jefferson G: Fracture of the atlas vertebra. Report of four cases, and a review of those previously recorded. Br J Surg 7:407–422, 1920

48. Kahn EA, Yglesias L: Progressive atlanto-axial dislocation. JAMA 105:348–352, 1935

49. Kamman GR: Recurring atlanto-axial dislocation with repeated involvement of the cord and recovery. JAMA 112:2019–2020, 1939

50. Karlen A: Congenital hypoplasia of the odontoid process. J Bone Joint Surg 44-A:567–570, 1962

51. Keuter EJW: Non-traumatic atlanto-axial dislocation associated with nasopharyngeal infections (Grisel's Disease). Acta Neurochirurg 21:11–22, 1969

52. Kline DG: Atlanto-axial dislocation simulating a head injury: hypoplasia of the odontoid. J Neurosurg 24:1013–1016, 1966

53. Kornbloom D, Clayton M, Nash H: Nontraumatic cervical dislocations in rheumatoid arthritis. JAMA 149:431, 1952

54. Lipscomb PB: Cervico-occipital fusion for congenital and post-traumatic anomalies of the atlas and axis. J Bone Joint Surg 38A:1289–1301, 1957

55. List CF: Neurologic syndromes accompanying developmental anomalies of the occipital bone, atlas and axis. Arch Neurol Psychiatr 45:577–616, 1941

56. Marshall JJ, De Z: Judicial hanging. Lancet 1:193–194, 1913

57. Martel W: Pathologic fracture of odontoid process in rheumatoid arthritis. Radiology 90:948–952, 1968

58. McKeever FM: Atlanto-axoid instability. Surg Clin North Am 48:1375–1390, 1968

59. Michaels L, Prevost MJ, Crang DF: Pathological changes in a case of os odontoideum (separate odontoid process). J Bone Joint Surg 51A:965–972, 1969

60. Minderhoud JM, Braakman R, Penning L: Os odontoideum: clinical, radiological and therapeutic aspects. J Neurol Sci 8:521–544, 1969

61. Mixter SJ, Osgood RB: Traumatic lesions of the atlas and axis. Ann Surg 51:193, 1910

62. Miyakawa G: Congenital absence of the odontoid process. Case report. J Bone Joint Surg 34A:676–677, 1952

63. Murray JW, Seymour RJ: An anterior, extrapharyngeal, suprahyoid approach to the first, second, and third cervical vertebrae. ACTA Orthop Scand 45:45–49, 1974

64. Nagashima C: Atlanto-axial dislocation due to agenesis of the os odontoideum or odontoid. J Neurosurg 33:270–280, 1970

65. Nagashima C: Surgical treatment of irreducible atlanto-axial dislocation with spinal cord compression. Case report. J Neurosurg 38:374–378, 1973

66. Nickel VL, Perry J, Garrett A: Application of the halo. Orthop Pros App J 14:31–35, 1960

67. Nickel VL, Perry J, Garrett A: The halo. J Bone Joint Surg 60A:1400–1409, 1968

68. Nievergelt K: Luxatio atlanto-epistrophica bei aplasie des dens epistrophei. Schweiz Med Wochenschr 78:653–657, 1948

69. Osgood RB, Lund CC: Fractures of the odontoid process. N Engl J Med 198:61–72, 1928

70. Owen-Smith MS: Fractures of the odontoid process of the axis. Proc Roy Soc Med 61:41–43, 1968

71. Pilcher LS: Atlanto-axoid fracture-dislocation. Ann Surg 51:209–211, 1910

72. Plaut HF: Fracture of the atlas in automobile accidents. The value of x-ray views for its diagnosis. JAMA 110:1892–1894, 1938

73. Plaut HF: Fractures of the atlas resulting from automobile accidents. A survey of the literature and report of six cases. Am J Roentgenol Radium Ther Nucl Med 40:867–890, 1938

74. Pouyanne L, Bombart M, Senegas J, Barouk L: Les fractures de l'axis. J Chir 98: 7–17, 1969

75. Prolo DJ, Runnels JB, Jameson RM: The injured cervical spine. JAMA 224:591–594, 1973

76. Ramadier JO: Fractures and dislocations of the cervical spine. Evol Med 13:199–209, 1969

77. Roberts A, Wickstrom J: Prognosis of odontoid fractures. Acta Orthop Scand 44: 21–30, 1973

78. Roberts SM: Congenital absence of the odontoid process resulting in dislocation of the atlas on the axis. J Bone Joint Surg 15:988–989, 1933

79. Rodgers WA: Fractures and dislocations of the cervical spine. J Bone Joint Surg 39A:341–376, 1957

80. Rowland LP, Shapiro JH, Jacobson HG: Neurological syndromes associated with congenital absence of the odontoid process. Arch Neurol Psychiatr (Chicago) 80:286–291, 1958

81. Scannell RC: Congenital absence of the odontoid process. A case report. J Bone Joint Surg 27:714–715, 1945

82. Schneider RC, Livingston KE, Cave AJE: "Hangman's fracture" of the cervical spine. J Neurosurg 22:141–145, 1965

83. Schneider RC: Trauma to the spine and spinal cord. In Kahn EA, Crosby EC, Schneider RC (eds): Correlative Neurosurgery, 2nd ed. Springfield, Charles C. Thomas, 1969, pp 597–649

84. Schneider RC, Gosch HH, Norrell H, et al: Vascular insufficiency and differential distortion of brain and cord caused by cervico medullary football injuries. J Neurosurg 33:363–375, 1970

85. Schwarz GA, Wigton RS: Fracture-dislocations in the region of the atlas and axis, with consideration of delayed neurological manifestations and some roentgenographic features. Radiology 28:601–607, 1937

86. Scoville WB, Palmer AH, Samra K, Chong G: The use of acrylic plastic for vertebral replacement of fixation in metastic disease of the spine. J Neurosurg 27: 274–279, 1967

87. Sharp J, Purser GW: Atlanto-axial dislocation in ankylosing spondylitis and rheumatoid arthritis. Ann Rheum Dis 20:47, 1961

88. Sherk HH, Nicholson JT: Rotary atlanto-axial dislocation associated with ossiculum terminale and mongolism: A case report. J Bone Joint Surg 51A:957–964, 1969

89. Sherk HH, Nicholson JT: Fractures of the atlas. J Bone Joint Surg 52A:1017–1024, 1970

90. Sherk HH, Nicholson JT: Gunshot wound with fracture of the atlas and arteriovenous fistula of the vertebral artery. Case report. J Bone Joint Surg 56A: 1738–1740, 1974

91. Shotemor SH, Kashigina EA: X-ray diagnosis of dislocation of the atlas. Vestrik Rentg Radiol 45:9–16, 1970

92. Stiefel DM: Congenital absence of the odontoid process. Report of a case. J Bone Joint Surg 32A:946–947, 1950

93. Stratford J: Myelopathy caused by atlanto-axial dislocation. J Neurosurg 14:97–104, 1957

94. Sullivan AW: Subluxation of the atlanto-axial joint; sequel to inflammatory processes of the neck. J Pediatr 35:451–464, 1949

95. Termansen NB: "Hangman's fracture." ACTA Orthop Scand 45:529–539, 1974

96. Thompson H: The "halo" traction apparatus. A method of external splinting of the cervical spine after injury. J Bone Joint Surg 44B:655–661, 1962

97. Torres H, Ferguson L, Norton T: Fractures of the odontoid process. Neuro-chirurg 14:81–82, 1971
98. Vermooten W: A study of the fracture of the epistropheus due to hanging with a note on the possible cause of death. Anat Rec 20:305–311, 1921
99. Watson-Jones R: Fractures and Joint Injuries, 4th ed, vol 2. Baltimore, Williams and Wilkins, p 981
100. Watson-Jones R: Spontaneous hyperemia dislocation of the atlas. Proc Roy Soc Med 25:586, 1934
101. Weiler HG: Congenital absence of odontoid process of the axis with atlantoaxial dislocation. J Bone Joint Surg 24:161–165, 1942
102. Williams TG: "Hangman's fracture." J Bone Joint Surg 57B:82–88, 1975
103. Wilson HA: Fracture dislocation of the atlas without symptoms of spinal cord injury. Ann Surg 45:632–635, 1907
104. Wolfe R: Injury to the cervical vertebrae as a result of judicial hanging. J Med Ass S Afr 2:460–462, 1928
105. Wollin DG: The os odontoideum. Separate odontoid process. J Bone Joint Surg 45A:1459–1471, 1963
106. Wustohoff R: Uber die luxationsfraktur im unteren kipfgelenk (atlas-epistro-pheus-gelenk). Dtsch Z Chir 183:73–98, 1923
107. Zuerling MT, Riggins RS: Use of the halo apparatus in acute injuries of the cer-vical spine. Surg Gynecol Obstet 138:189–193, 1974
108. Zimmerman JE, Grant J, Vise WM, Yashon D, Hunt WE: Treatment of Jefferson fracture with a halo apparatus. J Neurosurg 44:372–375, 1976

# 9

## Skeletal Traction in the Treatment of Cervical Spine Injuries

The use of skull tongs to reduce fracture dislocation and to maintain alignment of cervical spine fractures is now universal (Figs. 1–7).[19,28] It is also now generally agreed that skeletal traction and reduction offer an important means of protecting and internally decompressing the cervical spinal cord and nerve roots following fracture dislocation (Figs. 1A–C, 2).[17] Halter traction is also a widely accepted tool in the treatment of minor neck injures and is valued as a temporizing maneuver until skeletal traction can be established. Traction for thoracic and lumbar spine injuries is not feasible because the enormous forces required for distraction and realignment render it impractical.

Halter traction was first employed in 1929 by Taylor,[31] and its use has since become so widespread that most authors do not explore its origin. The use of halter traction is discussed in the sections on emergency treatment and chronic care. Many implanted skeletal devices were described in the early twentieth century. The tongs primarily used by physicians today were described by Crutchfield (Fig. 3).[9–13] Many modifications of these tongs have been designed and presently available types are illustrated. In 1938, Crutchfield[12] reported 43 patients treated with tongs, with the single complication being osteomyelitis at the tong site in a patient with preexisting infection. Jamieson et al.[22] reported a cerebral abscess secondary to skull traction.

All types involve fixation in some manner of the skull (Figs. 3–7).[26] Neubeiser[25] described his use of debarbed fish hooks placed under each zygomatic arch and attached to a spreader bar connected to 6 to 15 pounds of traction. Selmo[30] and Peyton et al.[27] stated their preference for the zygoma-hook

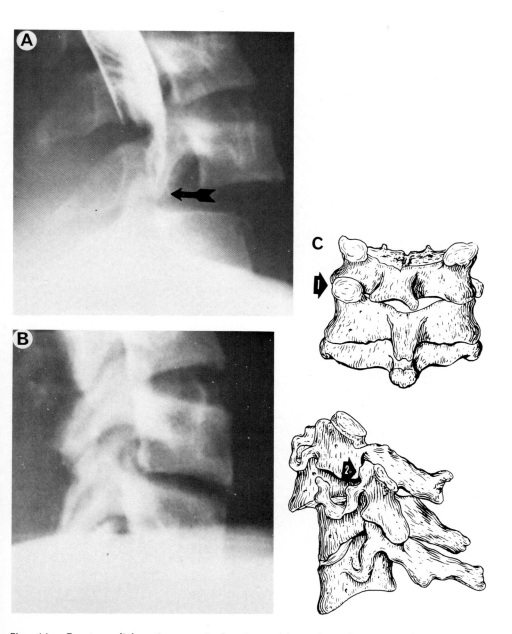

*Fig. 1A.* Fracture-dislocation cervical spine with unilateral jumped facet (arrow). Complete block to pantopaque introduced at C1–C2. *1B.* Laminectomy with intraoperative reduction and restoration of normal position of facets. Same patient as 1A. *1C.* Sketch of jumped facet in 1A (arrow 1) dorsal view top, lateral view with jumped facet (arrow 2), and dislocation (bottom).

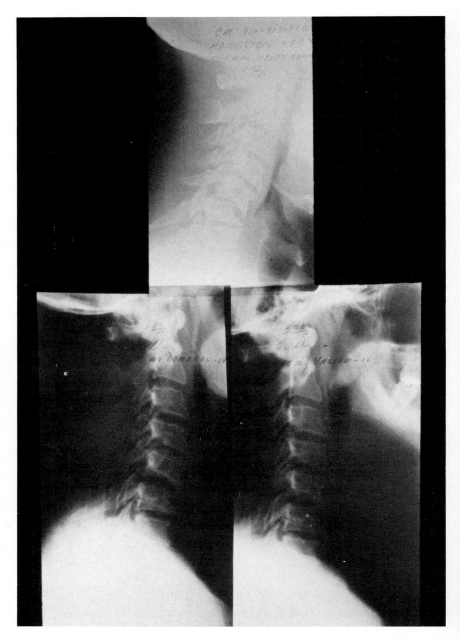

*Fig. 2.* Reduction series with good realignment in 1 hour utilizing 60 pounds.

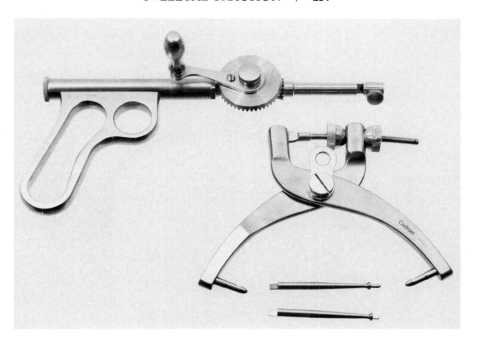

*Fig. 3.* Crutchfield tongs with drill. (Courtesy Codman & Shurtleff Inc.)

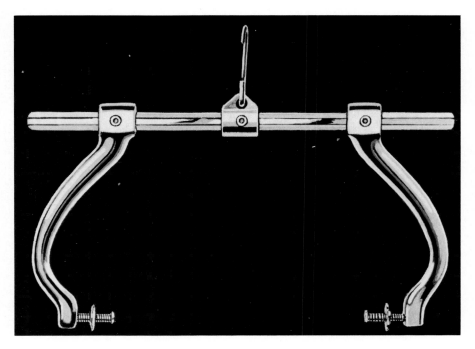

*Fig. 4.* Blackburn tongs. (Courtesy Orthopedic Equipment Company Inc.)

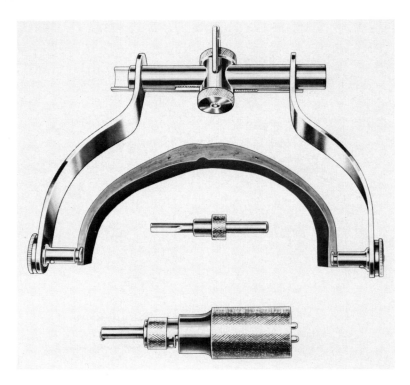

*Fig. 5.* Vinke tongs with applier. (Courtesy Zimmer USA)

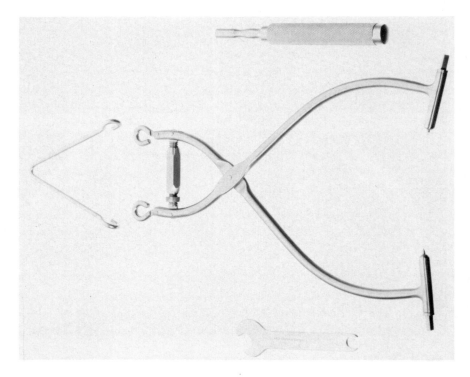

*Fig. 6.* Cone skull tongs. (Courtesy Codman and Shurtleff Inc.)

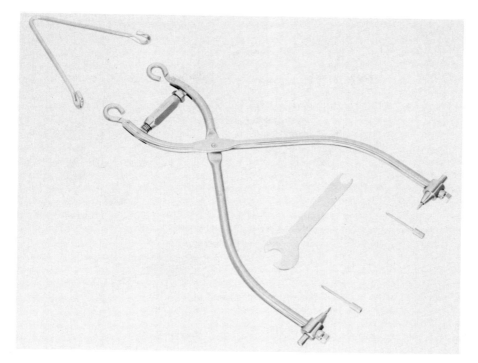

*Fig. 7.* Barton skull tongs. (Courtesy Codman and Shurtleff Inc.)

method. Hoen,[20] in 1936, placed wires underneath the skull bone and above the dura through burr holes that were connected to a spreader bar using up to 22 pounds of traction. Cone and Turner[7] reported favorably on a series of patients treated in this fashion. In 1938, Barton[4] reported a modification of the previously described tongs for skull traction. In 1948, Vinke[33] described a new set of tongs based on Barton's tongs but which had interlocking devices between the inner and outer tables of bone. We prefer Crutchfield tongs but we have also used Vinke and Barton tongs.[34,35]

Tongs should be placed as soon as possible after the injury since in essence realignment effects an internal decompression of the spinal contents.[1,32] Delay in treatment following an injury poses a philosophical question much akin to that concerning laminectomy, as to whether tongs should be placed and reduction carried out. We generally place tongs even after one week has elapsed, since adequate bone healing diminishes the chance of further neurologic damage even if that damage is confined to a single nerve root in a tetraplegic patient. Also, adequate bone healing lessens the possibility of pain later. The second indication for placement of tongs is immobilization. We utilize turning frames exclusively (Fig. 8A–C) in treatment and advise against circoelectric beds (Fig. 9) because of excessive loading of the fracture.

The length of time that tongs should be left in place is variable. We have left tongs in place for 12 weeks without ill effect. The tong sites are treated daily with antibiotic ointment and kept clean with soap and water. Tongs

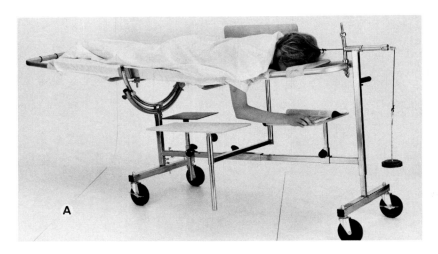

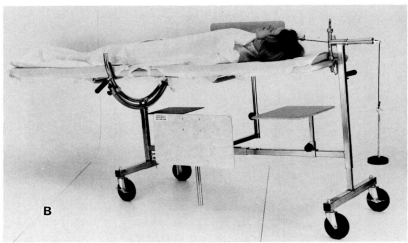

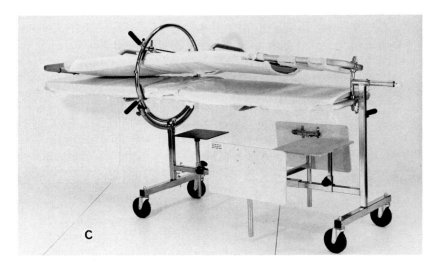

*Fig. 8A, B, C.* Stryker frame. (Courtesy Stryker Corp.)

must be gently tightened daily or every other day. Skull x-rays can be valuable in detecting complications. The position may be changed if skull penetration or osteomyelitis becomes a problem. In Crutchfield's patient, described in 1933, tongs were left in place for 36 days. At present, in our hospital tongs are left in place up to eight weeks, depending on the fracture. They are used during cervical surgery (both fusion and laminectomy) for maintenance of alignment and are left in place until fusion occurs spontaneously or is surgically induced. In upper cervical spine fractures we have used tongs initially until halo traction devices could be applied. On occasion, when doubt exists about the presence of a fracture dislocation or stability, tongs have been installed only to be removed shortly thereafter when the physician felt that they were unnecessary. When stability is questionable it is perhaps prudent to place tongs.

In deciding the amount of weight to be utilized it should be remembered that skeletal traction is employed for alignment and reduction. For alignment maintenance, 10 to 25 pounds of weight is recommended. An even lesser amount can be utilized if it is demonstrated that reduction and maintainence of alignment can be effected.

Reduction involves consideration of one, the rapidity with which reduction should be carried out, and two, the amount of weight to be utilized.

In the four decades since Crutchfield[9] reported tong traction to reduce a fracture dislocation of the upper cervical spine, most proponents of various tongs, wires, and hooks have used traction weights of no more than 35 pounds to reduce cervical fracture dislocations over several hours or even days.[6−9,12,13,18,20,23−25,27] Although greater weights have been used to reduce cervical fracture dislocations complicated by locked facets,[5,14,29] Bailey,[2,3] Bovill et al.,[5] and Hollin and Gross[21] have suggested that weights greater than 45 to 50 pounds are excessive, and that operative reduction is indicated when such weights fail to produce satisfactory vertebral alignment in 24 to 48 hours.

Indeed, Crutchfield[12,13] cautioned against using heavy weights to achieve more rapid reduction, believing that force sufficient to speed reduction would add further injury to supporting tissues and endanger the spinal cord. Instead he advocated a minimal corrective pull of up to 18 pounds,[13] followed by gradual completion of reduction with no more than double this weight. Others[3,8,12,29,31] have concurred with the principal of gradual reduction.

There is at least a theoretical argument in favor of more rapid reduction and this is our preference.[34,35] Cervical fracture dislocations often represent emergencies[15] in which the extent and duration of neurologic dysfunction may depend upon the time interval between injury and spinal cord decompression.[15,16] A minimum of 60 to 90 minutes commonly elapses before a patient with a cervical fracture dislocation is brought to the Emergency Service and placed in skull traction. Although shorter intervals unusually occur, most often there are delays upwards of six hours. In many cases, there is little useful information concerning improvement or deterioration in the patient's neurologic status during this period. Also, at least theoretically, prompt closed

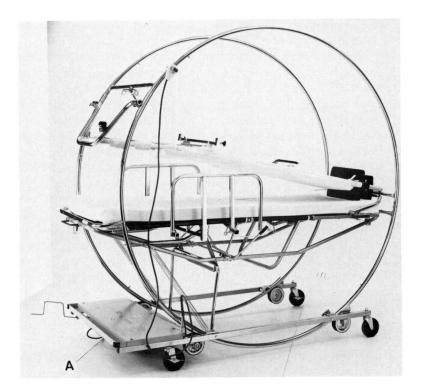

internal reduction provides relief of direct bony pressure on the spinal cord, thus diminishing damage.

In the presence of severe cord injury and radiographic evidence of a cervical fracture dislocation with or without locked facets, application of a minimal corrective pull to protect neural structures from further injury may represent less than optimal acute treatment. When no neurologic functional loss is apparent, such rapidity is not necessarily indicated. In our clinic we attempt to reduce the dislocation as completely as possible, no longer than two hours after traction is applied.[34,35] Our goal is to quickly decompress the spinal cord by restoring the anteroposterior diameter of the cervical spinal canal and by achieving satisfactory positioning of bone fragments.

The technique consists of intravenous administration of muscle relaxants to reduce paraspinous muscle spasm, elevation of the head of the bed to exert countertraction, and initial application of 20 to 30 pounds to appropriate tongs inserted in a coronal plane determined by the cervical transverse processes and the external auditory meati. Traction force is thus exerted along the longitudinal axis of the vertebral bodies with the neck in a neutral position. It should be noted that Crutchfield exerted traction in the plane of the articulating facets, using the mastoid processes as landmarks.[11] He criticized a more anterior placement of the traction apparatus on the skull,[13] although others have preferred it;[3,4,17,20,23,25,27] 5 to 10 pounds are added every 10 minutes,

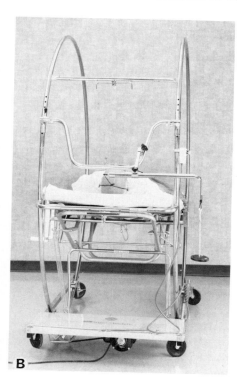

*Fig. 9A, B, C.* Circoelectric bed, see text. (Courtesy Stryker Corp.)

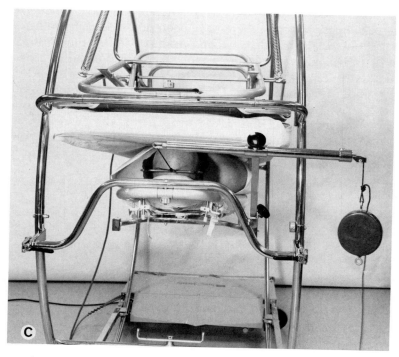

and brief appropriate neurologic examination and lateral cervical spine films are repeated after each increment. Occasionally manual traction on the occiput and jaws is required. Once reduction is achieved, traction is maintained with minimum weight (10 to 30 pounds). It should be emphasized that during reduction attention must be paid to the patient's description of additional neurologic symptoms, such as parasthesia, pain, and neurologic loss. In patients without neurologic deficit the same technique and precautions may be employed, but haste is not so important.

Among patients in our hospital successfully treated in this manner over past years, the greatest amount of weight used in the first hour was 75 pounds. Operative reduction and decompression is considered in patients with severe neurologic signs in whom we cannot restore the anteroposterior diameter of the cervical spinal canal to within approximately 3 mm of normal[8] with 60 to 70 pounds of traction over one to two hours. The inability to establish appropriate alignment by traction usually signifies locked or jumped facets,[14] which probably should be unlocked by an open surgical maneuver with reduction accomplished on the operating table. However, this remains a controversial issue. The acceptance of imperfect alignment is necessitated occasionally for practical reasons.

Because of variables such as subsequent operative intervention (decompressive laminectomy, fusion, stabilization), it cannot be proved that rapid reduction of cervical fracture dislocations by means of skull traction ultimately yields a better neurologic result than gradual reduction. However, in over 50 patients with significant neurologic deficit whom we have treated with this technique in the past 12 years, there have been no cases of neurologic deterioration that could be attributed to traction itself. It is our opinion that the low incidence of neurologic complications reported for reduction of cervical fracture dislocations with skeletal traction[13,29] is not the result of speed of reduction or the amount of weight used, but rather that neurologic examination is performed carefully and sequentially during the procedure. Our concern for possible harm to supporting soft tissue structures is diminished both by our greater concern for preservation and restoration of neurologic function and by our tendency to insure stability by subsequent operative fixation and fusion.[33]

## REFERENCES

1. Abbott KH, Hale N: Cervical Trapeze. J Neurosurg 10:436–437, 1953
2. Bailey RW: Fractures and dislocations of the cervical spine. Surg Clin NA 41: 1357–1366, 1961
3. Bailey RW: Fractures and dislocations of the cervical spine. Orthopedic and Neurosurgical Aspects. Postgrad Med 35:588–599, 1964
4. Barton LG: The reduction of fracture dislocations of the cervical vertebrae by skeletal traction. Surg Gynecol Obstet 67:94–96, 1938
5. Bovill EG, Eberle CF, Day L, Aufranc OE: Dislocation of the cervical spine without spinal cord injury. JAMA 218:1288–1290, 1971
6. Cave E: Immediate fracture management. Surg Clin NA 46:771–788, 1966

7. Cone W, Turner WG: The treatment of fracture dislocations of the cervical vertebrae by skeletal traction and fusion. J Bone Joint Surg 19:584–602, 1937
8. Crenshaw AH (ed): Campbell's Operative Orthopedics, vol I. St. Louis, Mosby, 1971, pp 616–630
9. Crutchfield WG: Skeletal traction for dislocation of cervical spine: Report of case. Southern Surg 2:156–159, 1933
10. Crutchfield WG: Further observations on the treatment of fracture dislocations of the cervical spine with skeletal traction. Surg Gynecol Obstet 63:513–517, 1936
11. Crutchfield WG: Fracture-dislocations of the cervical spine. Am J Surg 38:592–598, 1937
12. Crutchfield WG: Treatment of injuries of the cervical spine. J Bone Joint Surg 20:696–704, 1938
13. Crutchfield WG: Skeletal traction in treatment of injuries to the cervical spine. JAMA 155:29–32, 1954
14. Dowman C: Reduction of cervical fracture dislocation with locked facets. JAMA 219:1212, 1972
15. Ellis VH: Injuries of the cervical vertebrae. Proc R Soc Med (Section of Orthopaedics) 40:19, 1946
16. Evans DK: Reduction of cervical dislocations. J Bone Joint Surg 43B:552–555, 1961
17. Gallie WE: Skeletal traction in the treatment of fractures and dislocations of the cervical spine. Ann Surg 106:770–776, 1937
18. Gallie WE: Fractures and dislocations of the cervical spine. Am J Surg 46:495–499, 1939
19. Harris P, Wu PH: The management of patients with injury of the cervical spine using Blackburn skull calipers and the Stryker turning frame. Paraplegia 2:278–287, 1965
20. Hoen TI: A method of skeletal traction for treatment of fracture dislocation of cervical vertebrae. Arch Neurol Psychiatr 36:158–161, 1936
21. Hollin SA, Gross SW: Management of cervical spine dislocations with locked facets. Surg Gynecol Obstet 124:521–524, 1967
22. Jamieson KG, Yelland JG: Cerebral abscess due to skull traction. Aust NZ J Surg 34:301–302, 1965
23. Loeser JD: History of skeletal traction. J Neurosurg 33:54–59, 1970
24. McKenzie KG: Fracture, dislocation, and fracture-dislocation of the spine. Can Med Assoc J 32:263–269, 1935
25. Neubeiser BL: A method of skeletal traction for neck extension. J Miss State Med Assoc 30:495, 1933
26. Nicholson MW: Treatment of cervical spine dislocation. JAMA 219:1764, 1972
27. Peyton WT, Hall HB, French LA: Hook traction under zygomatic arch in cervical spine injuries. Surg Gynecol Obstet 791:311–313, 1944
28. Prather GC, Mayfield FH: Injuries of the Spinal Cord. Springfield, Ill, Charles C Thomas, 1953
29. Rogers WA: Fractures and dislocations of the cervical spine. J Bone Joint Surg 39A:341–376, 1957
30. Selmo JD: Traction on the zygomatic process for cervicovertebral injuries. Am J Surg 46:405, 1939
31. Taylor AS: Fracture dislocation of the cervical spine. Ann Surg 90:321–340, 1929
32. Veibiest H: Anterolateral operations for fractures and dislocations in the middle and lower parts of the cervical spine. J Bone Joint Surg 51A:1489–1530, 1969
33. Vinke TH: A skull-traction apparatus. J Bone Joint Surg 30A:522–524, 1948
34. Yashon D, White RJ: Injuries of the vertebral column and spinal cord. In Feiring EH (ed): Brock's Injuries of the Brain and Spinal Cord and Their Coverings. New York, Springer, 1974, pp 688–743
35. Yashon D, Tyson G, Vise WM: Rapid closed reduction of cervical fracture dislocations. Surg Neurol 4:513–514, 1975

# 10

## Lower Cervical, Thoracic, and Lumbar Spinal Cord Injuries

Many concepts concerning general management of lower cervical, thoracic, and lumbar spinal cord injuries have been considered elsewhere, especially in the chapter on high cervical spinal cord injuries, but some will be repeated in this chapter.

Nonsurgical versus surgical treatment of spinal injuries without neurologic deficit has been the subject of debate for many years.[22] Controversy exists even among those advocating surgical treatment as to whether anterior or posterior fusion and/or decompression should be carried out. All agree on a few points. The spinal cord that has been injured must be protected from further damage. Correction and prevention of bony deformities is desirable, and many agree that stabilization is required to accomplish this.

The definition of stability is also under much debate. Among orthopedists, physiatrists, and neurosurgeons, there is considerable variance, even within the groups, as to what constitutes a stable or an unstable spine, even in a specific patient. Cheshire[14] defined stability as the absence of abnormal mobility between any pair of vertebrae, with or without pain or other clinical manifestations when lateral x-rays of the cervical spine (or other regions of the spine) are taken in flexion and extension at the conclusion of conservative treatment for vertebral fracture. Penning[55] defined instability as abnormal mobility that can be expressed in degrees at one or more levels and in one or more positions of the vertebral column. There is no question that if on flexion-extension radiographs, vertebral bodies move on one another, instability exists.

146

Another concept of instability is the gradual increase in angulation that occurs over months to years, most commonly seen in thoracic fractures but which may occur in cervical fractures hitherto thought stable. San Giorgi[62] stressed that the continued existence of a dislocation may not per se mean instability. In our view, gradual or acute movement between vertebral bodies constitutes instability. Gradual onset of such instability is sometimes impossible to recognize except in retrospect with serial radiographic observations. Stern[70] describes neurosurgical aspects of injuries of the thoracic and lumbar spine, emphasizing the aforementioned controversies concerning treatment.

## CERVICAL SPINE (FIGS. 1–14)

The cervical spine is inherently the most mobile and least stable of all spinal vertebral elements.[62] Anteriorly, there is an amphiarthrodial joint secured by the anterior and posterior longitudinal ligaments. Posteriorly, there are two disarthrodial joints, joint capsules, ligamentum flavum, interspinous ligaments, and supraspinous ligaments. Instability may be anterior or posterior,

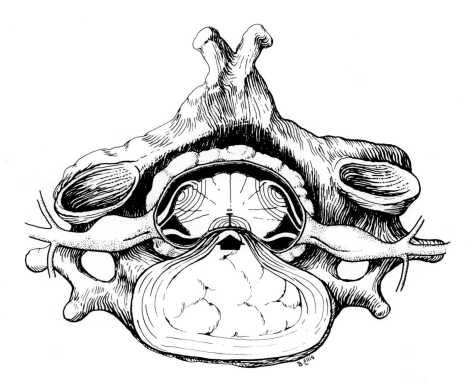

*Fig. 1.* Traumatic herniated disc (arrow) causing anterior spinal cord injury syndrome (see text). Note circumferential lines of stress laterally by restraining dentate ligaments, anteriorly by herniated disc.

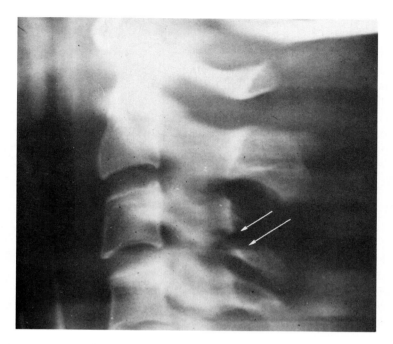

*Fig. 2.* Fracture across base of spinous process of C3 (arrows). Lateral midline polytome. No neurologic deficit.

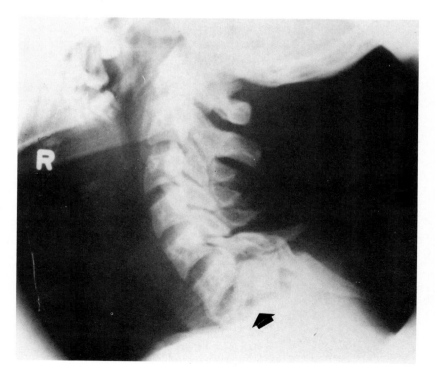

*Fig. 3.* Fracture dislocation C7 (arrow) with quadriplegia. The lateral x-ray just preceding showed vertebral bodies down to C6 emphasizing the necessity to visualize all 7 cervical vertebrae.

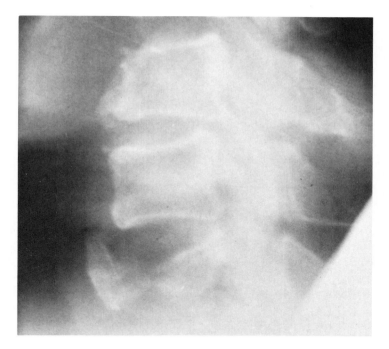

*Fig. 4.* Bursting fracture C6 without posterior displacement. Midline lateral polytome.

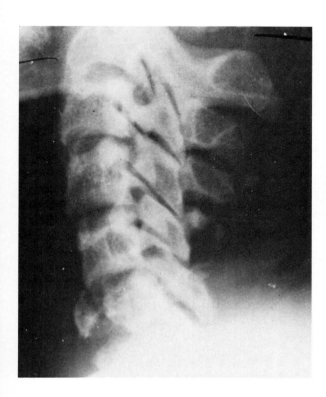

*Fig. 5.* Bursting fracture C5 with posterior dislocation.

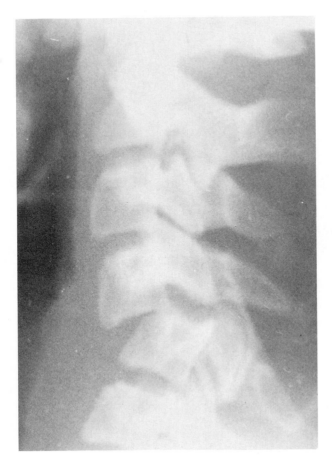

*Fig. 6.* Dislocation C5 with quadriplegia.

depending on mechanism of injury. In flexion injuries, force is expended on the vertebral body, the longitudinal ligaments with posterior ligaments usually remaining intact. Bick[7] reviewed the history of spinal fusion. In 1891, Hadra[20] reported the first successful stabilization of a cervical fracture by utilizing wire to secure spinous processes. Other earlier attempts made use of celluloid,[39] steel bars,[40] silk,[49] and bone.[7,34] Both Hibbs[33] and Albee[1] introduced the modern spinal fusion in 1911.

Burke and Tiong[11] reported that of 175 patients with cervical spine and spinal cord injuries, only 4.2 percent required delayed spinal fusion for instability after initial conservative treatment. The criteria for instability is the issue, and according to our experience, this represents an extremely low incidence of instability.

Del Sel et al.[18] discussed stability following fracture dislocation of the cervical spine based on observation of over 150 cases, and concluded that conservative orthopedic treatment yields the best results. They emphasized importance of skull traction and of a well-molded Minerva plastic jacket. On

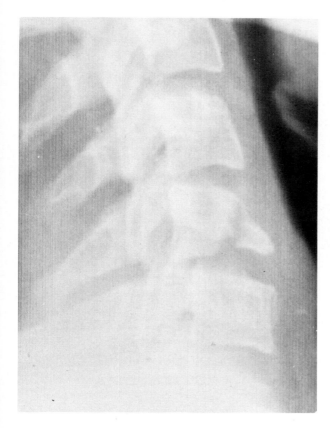

*Fig. 7.* Tear-drop fracture C5 with posterior displacement.

the other hand, Stauffer and Rhoades[69] stated that the decision whether to stabilize the cervical spine surgically after trauma and the choice of method to be used must be made separately for each case. They suggested that unstable injuries be treated surgically. Bedbrook[4] studied 420 patients with vertebral injuries who did not have surgical fusion and found that only 20 were unstable after three months. Bedbrook does admit that criteria for stability varied. He believes that a fracture dislocation should not be judged unstable earlier than eight weeks or even 12 weeks after injury. He suggested that late instability is the only indication for anterior spinal fusion. Many physicians caring for spinal injured patients disagree with this concept and recommend early fusion so that subsequent mobilization can be earlier. Bedbrook[5] states that 90 percent of fractures of the dorsal and lumbar spine with paraparesis or paraplegia can be treated and reduced by closed methods. Strict posturing techniques are the most important part of the reduction he states. The remaining 10 percent of cases should be treated by gently active surgical techniques, such as manipulation under general anesthesia or open reduction. He believes the use of spinal rods and clamps is rarely indicated, thus emphasizing the controversies in this field. He also stated that surgical techniques may be

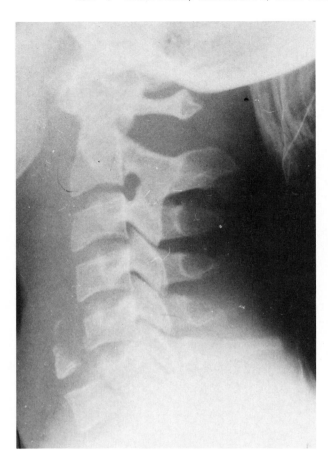

*Fig. 8.* Tear-drop fracture C5, bursting fracture C6 with quadriplegia.

advisable later for treatment of nonunion or spinal stenosis, as well as failure to improve.

White et al.[76] defined clinical instability as a loss of ability of the spine under physiologic loads to maintain relationships between vertebrae in such a way that there is neither damage nor irritation to the spinal cord or nerve roots, and, in addition, no development of deformity with excessive pain. In a good discussion of instability and fusion, they stated, and we agree, that despite disagreement in the literature, the spine is probably unstable when all anterior or posterior elements in a motion segment are destroyed or incapable of function. They also stated that many simple unilateral facet dislocations and most bilateral facet dislocations are unstable. The presence of distinct spinal cord or root damage following spinal trauma should alert the clinician to the probability of spinal instability. They believe that manipulation may be a useful technique for closed reduction of unilateral facet dislocations without neurologic involvement, but that neurologic deficit and bone or foreign material in the spinal canal are indications for laminectomy. Other indications included radiologic evidence of an extradural block and good clinical evidence

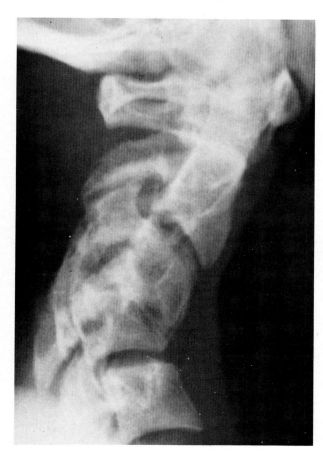

*Fig. 9.* Ancient cervical fracture dislocation with laminectomy demonstrating marked angulation.

of an incomplete progressive neurologic lesion. They felt that a decision should be made and decompression carried out without delay.

Instability can be evaluated by the measurement with calipers of angles between the anterior bodies of the involved vertebrae on stress radiographs. Any increase or decrease in angulation with flexion or extension means abnormal movement, or instability.

Every conflict, particularly the world wars, has precipitated a spate of papers concerning spinal cord injuries, and following World War II, many excellent reports were published. The review by Martin[44] is extensive and the entire problem of spinal injury is discussed. During that period the treatment of spinal cord injury was generally conservative, except that open or compound injuries caused by missiles were treated by debridement. However, Raff[57] stated that laminectomy should be done only if neurologic signs indicate that the cord lesion is progressing, if an incomplete cord lesion with evidence of pressure on the cord is indicated by x-ray, if spinal fluid block is present, or if it can be demonstrated that the spinal fluid pathways, open following injury, become blocked. We do not necessarily agree. Evans and

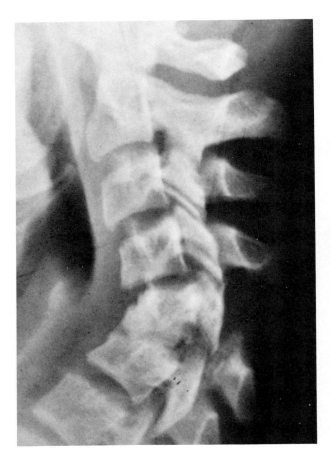

*Fig. 10.* Ancient cervical bursting fracture C5 without laminectomy or fusion demonstrating marked angulation.

Rosenauer[21] stated that spinal manometric studies are of virtually no practical value in making a judgement concerning operative management. They further stated that they were unable to adduce positive evidence that decompressive laminectomy was of value in their patients undergoing operation. Similarly, Mayfield and Cazan[45] stated that results of Queckenstedt's test should not be a major factor in the selection of cases for laminectomy. They consider laminectomy in compression injury of the cord only if there is an incomplete lesion and the patient shows progressive loss of function. Wannamaker[73] reported spinal cord injuries during the Korean conflict and emphasized the low mortality rate in patients received at Army hospitals.

Davidoff[17] was also conservative in recommending laminectomy, stating that it is seldom indicated, but that when indication does exist, the procedure should seldom be done as an emergency. His thesis was that only in patients with complete manometric block not relieved by hyperextension should a laminectomy be considered within the first two days after injury. Even in these patients, when the examiner is convinced that a complete transverse lesion exists, no good purpose is served by operation. In the presence of a complete block and an incomplete spinal lesion, operation should be carried out within 24 to 48 hours of the injury. In an incomplete lesion, when symptoms grow worse rather than better and a spinal block develops in the course of weeks or months, laminectomy is also indicated because of possible development of adhesions. On the other hand, Bedbrook[3] was against virtually all operations, particularly laminectomies in any spinally injured patient. But many physicians do advise laminectomy immediately when severe neural damage is present.

Holdsworth,[35] in a study of 1000 spinal injury patients, said that if the paraplegia below the cord lesion remains complete for 24 hours, recovery never occurs. There is much truth to this, but isolated cases of moderate to marked improvement have been observed. Livingston and Newman,[42] reporting on spinal cord concussion in war wounds, observed that in 33 of 821 (4 percent) wounded, quadriplegia was transient. This transient nature justified the term "concussion" as it is applied to the cerebral cortex. In all 33 patients the wounding agent was a missile. It has been pointed out in the chapter on missile wounds that such transient lesions are uncommon in civilian injuries.[79,80] Holdsworth[35] also stated that with the possible exception of a partial paraplegia that shows signs of becoming complete, laminectomy is never indicated.

Although vertebral injuries can occur in adjacent bodies, it is uncommon for spinal or vertebral injuries to occur at two or more levels distant from one

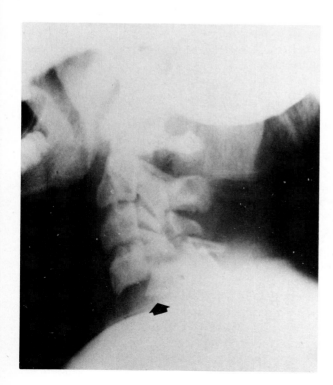

*Fig. 11.* Complete dislocation C5 (arrow).

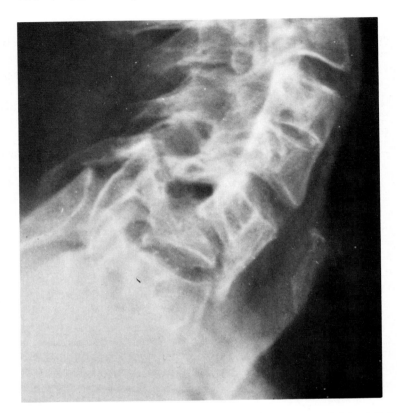

*Fig. 12.* Ancient fracture-dislocation C5–C6 in ankylosing spondylitis. Minimal neurologic deficit (same patient as Figure 13).

another. Bentley and McSweeney[6] describe several such cases and review the literature. This is distinctly uncommon, but should be considered.

Comarr and Kaufman[16] surveyed neurologic results in 858 patients with spinal cord injuries. Of 579 patients undergoing laminectomy, 16 percent were significantly improved; of 279 patients not operated upon, 29 percent improved. The authors felt that patients treated by laminectomy had suffered more extensive injuries. Patients with a complete block on spinal puncture who were not operated upon did not improve. Recovery in cauda equina lesions was more frequent than in spinal cord lesions. It is well known that lesions of the cauda equina show a greater propensity to improve. They also noted that gross observation of the cord at surgery did not constitute a reliable indicator of prognosis unless the cord was transected. Many patients described as having a normal-appearing cord did not improve, and many patients with subtotal or minimal anatomic lesions at surgery did improve. Suwanwela et al.[71] discussed prognosis in spinal cord injury with special reference to patients with motor paralysis and sensory preservation. These patients could possibly have had acute central cord or anterior cord syndromes.

They reported that of 28 patients with complete motor and sensory paralysis, none recovered, although 13 were seen within the first 24 hours after injury. Laminectomy was performed on 16 patients.

In another group,[16] 16 patients had complete motor paralysis but some sensory preservation below the injury level and were examined within 24 hours. Of the 8 who had preservation of touch below the injury level, 3 had laminectomy (2 had a normal cord and 1 had a swollen cord at operation); 4 of the 8 patients recovered partially, 2 did not recover, the fate of the other 2 was unknown, and the other 4 had only sacral or perineal sensation, of which 2 had good recovery, one partial recovery, and one no recovery. Laminectomy was performed in 3 of these patients, and 2 had a normal cord, while in 1 the cord appeared swollen.

Of six patients with complete motor paralysis and sensory preservation first examined seven days to two years after injury, three had good recovery and three had none.[16] This emphasizes the fact that when some function is preserved, improvement is likely to occur.[16] In patients with severe paralysis and even some functional preservation, it has been our experience that significant improvement does not occur.

Burke[10] described hyperextension injuries of the spine. This is a relatively

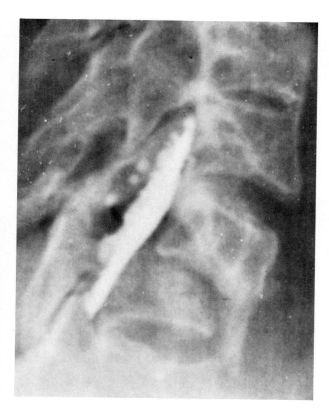

*Fig. 13.* No myelographic block (same patient as Figure 12).

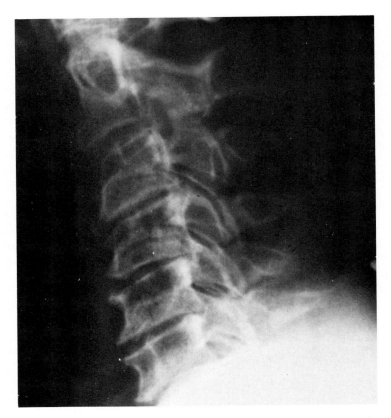

*Fig. 14.* Severe generalized cervical spondylosis contributing to the central cord syndrome (see text).

common mechanism of injury in the cervical spine but is uncommon in the thoracolumbar spine. Of 154 patients with thoracolumbar lesions, only 4 were of the hyperextension type and all had complete and permanent paraplegia.

Munro[51] compared fusion and nonfusion therapy in cervical cord and root injuries. He concluded that treatment by internal fixation and operative fusion has greater mortality, causes more undesirable symptoms, and is less effective than treatment by skeletal traction without either internal fixation or fusion. He did feel that delayed operative bony fusion is permissible and probably mandatory when observation has demonstrated that irrecoverable extensive paralysis of the paraspinal muscles prevents support of the head on the neck or the torso when the patient is erect. This condition is quite uncommon in our experience. Delayed operative bony fusion is also a means of treating postinjury pain. He stated that internal fixation by wiring is not helpful, is not as effective as traction, is not reliable, and alters mechanics of the cervical spine. We feel that wiring is a temporary measure to allow the bony structures to heal. It is not a permanent fixation device. We also disagree with

Munro[51] in that we believe fusion is an important means of avoiding further damage and preventing pain with little, if any additional morbidity or mortality. We emphasize that bony union is important and that wiring only provides temporary stability for it to take place. This emphasizes the controversy regarding treatment and the fact that many other types of treatment are advocated by other physicians. Many have validity.

McWhorter et al.[46] described use of rib grafts in six children who required posterior cervical fusion. Four of these suffered cervical spine injuries in accidents. Tucker[72] used a metal clamp between laminae of dislocated spine to fixate subluxation. In our view, this is only temporary; although a piece of metal gradually tightened in place will allow bone healing, unless bone healing does eventually occur, we believe the clamp will be ineffective. Bone itself may be required for fusion. Weiss[74] advocated a dynamic spring-loading internal fixation device for thoracic and lumbar fracture dislocation. This so-called dynamic alloplasty causes steady gradual correction of the spinal deformity. Gait training may begin within two weeks after insertion.

Munro[50] emphasized the relation between spondylosis of the cervical spine and injury. He stated that in a patient over 60 years of age with previously quiescent spondylosis of the cervical spine who suffers an acute injury of the cord, prognosis is more serious than in a younger person without spondylosis. The central cord syndrome is more common in patients having preexisting cervical spondylosis. In this regard a congenitally narrowed cervical canal, as measured on lateral view and allowing 10 to 20 percent for magnification, predisposes the cervical spinal cord injury. Braakman and Vinken[9] described unilateral facet interlocking in the lower cervical spine, stating that the clinical symptoms of cervical hemiluxation are not specific. Pain is common but may be mild. The head may be held in a position of flexion or rotation and there may be muscle spasms. They point out that this condition is rare, occurring approximately only one per two million population per year. Their method of treating facet interlocking was skull traction with tongs and operative reducton when closed methods failed.

In a discussion of serious and fatal neurosurgical football injuries, Schneider[67] stated that although it had been thought that football fatalities occurred in sandlot players not protected by equipment, he found in his series only 26 sandlot players, or 11.8 percent of the group, who had not worn equipment. This was an unexpectedly small number. Statistics included both spinal and cerebral injuries with injuries occurring in the spinal cord and vertebral column, including ruptured discs and brachial plexus injuries.

Schneider et al.[66] described the effects of chronic recurrent spinal trauma in high diving. They studied cervical x-rays of Acapulco's high divers. It was deduced from studies of momentum at impact that these athletes suffered chronic recurrent cervical trauma. Of six divers studied, although histories and neurologic signs were normal, x-rays of the cervical spine showed chronic bone changes in four. The three cervical spines that showed the greatest spondylitic changes were those of divers who had slightly longer, less heavily muscled necks, and who struck the water with hands outstretched thereby absorbing the shock of impact directly upon their heads. Trauma to the cervical spine and head was lessened if the hands were clasped above the head so that the hands took the brunt of the impact. Chrisman et al.[15] described lateral flexion neck injuries incurred in athletic competition. This injury, the so-called nerve pinch, was considered a sprain with associated stretching of lower cervical nerve roots and limitation of lateral motion on the side of the sprain. Long-term spondylitic symptoms can result, and protective prevention consists of use of appropriate neck and shoulder padding.

The syndrome of acute anterior cervical spinal cord injury was emphasized by Schneider (Fig. 1).[64] The syndrome is characterized by immediate complete paralysis with hypesthesia and hypalgesia to the level of the lesion. There is preservation of touch, motion, positon, and vibration sense. This syndrome can be caused by anterior spinal cord compression or destruction of the anterior portion of the cord. Compression of the anterior spinal artery may contribute to the observed signs. Since a surgically significant lesion causing spinal cord compression is not distinguishable from a lesion considered nonsurgical, these patients should have exploratory laminectomy or at least myelography. A herniated disc is the most common offender (Fig. 1).

The latter is not to be confused with the syndrome of acute central cervical spinal cord injury.[63] The patient exhibiting this syndrome may have pre-existing cervical spondylosis, and the injury is characterized by disproportionate weakness in the upper as compared to the lower extremities, with some impairment of bladder function. Associated pain and temperature loss is present in the early phase, and in more severe cases there may be impairment of touch, motion, position, and vibration sensation. The important point is that the hands are weaker than the legs. The shoulders and arms are usually stronger than the hands. The prognosis for significant functional recovery is generally good, with motor power returning to lower extremities first and motion of the fingers the last to return. Sensory recovery does not pursue an orderly course as does motor function. Extension is usually the mechanism of injury. Compression of the spinal cord occurs simultaneously from both anterior and posterior surfaces on hyperextension. There is bilateral damage to the anterior horn cells in the gray matter supplying hand and arm function as well as damage to hand and arm portions of the corticospinal tract, which is most medial in the cervical spine; hence, the designation "central cord syndrome."

Harris et al.[32] describe traumatic disruption of cervical discs from hyperextension injury (Fig. 1). These patients present with symptoms compatible with herniated disc and nerve root compression. The electromyogram and the myelogram usually show a herniated disc, and surgery may relieve symptoms. Marar[43] studied the pathogenesis of cord damage in hyperextension injuries of the cervical spine by clinical x-ray and observation of autopsy material. The studies show that the cord is damaged in an anterior-posterior direction by a squeezing effect produced between a backward subluxating vertebral body at the disc space, or through a complete fracture of the vertebral body just below the vertebral pedicle and the enfolded ligamentum flavum posteriorly. The mechanism of injury was thought to be a combination of hyperextension and backward shearing forces. Forsyth[23] also described extension injuries of the cervical spine, while Petrie[56] described consequences of flexion injuries of the cervical spine.

In rheumatoid arthritis, chronic proliferative inflammatory changes may involve all synovial tissue in the cervical spine. Although chronic dislocation at the C1–C2 area is most common, it also occurs at other levels.[47] These processes cause laxity of ligaments with consequent hypermobility and instability. Fracture dislocations of the ankylosed thoracic spine in rheumatoid spondylitis (ankylosing spondylitis, Marie-Strumpell disease) are uncommon, but do occur. There have been very few case reports in the literature. Hansen et al.,[29] in a review of the literature and report of three patients of their own, advocated internal and external fixation to avoid spinal injury. Isolated fractures of the articular processes of the lower cervical spine can occur. Nieminen[53] described 28 patients treated conservatively in a total of 285 injuries of the lower cervical spine. Usually these patients present with pain and a stiff neck but no neurologic signs. Treatment consists of nonsurgical measures, primarily those for relief of pain, including a soft or hard collar, analgesics, and various physical therapy modalities.

Saldeen[61] described severe neck injuries caused by use of diagonal safety belts. Although this type of seat belt reduces the total number of injuries by at least 50 percent and is particularly effective in preventing head injuries and injuries to the upper torso and limbs, the neck is still free to flex violently.[2] In addition, the victim may slip out of the diagonal safety belt and be ejected from the car with the belt catching the neck causing severe injury. Saldeen stressed risks in the event of a collision involving the combination of inadequate car door locks and a diagonal belt.

A "tear-drop" anterior vertebral body fracture caused by acute flexion is characterized by crushing of one vertebral body by the vertebral body superior to it in such a manner that the anterior part of the involved centrum is not only compressed, but often completely broken away. In many cases this fragment resembles a drop of water dripping from the vertebral body; hence it is frequently termed "tear drop." In severe cases, the inferior margin of the fractured vertebral body may be displaced backward into the spinal canal and may cause compression of the anterior portion of the spinal cord. The most common location for this fracture is the cervical spine. Recognition of such lesions, particularly minor ones, is important in that it may signal instability even though vertebral alignment appears normal.[65] Instability may be due to torn anterior and posterior ligaments. Even some time later, instability may occur because the ligaments heal by scarring and tend to stretch and become relaxed so that abnormal motion may be apparent on late stress films.

## THORACIC, THORACOLUMBAR, AND LUMBAR SPINE INJURIES

There is a significantly increased incidence of fractures of the spine due to osteoporosis in the later years of life (Fig. 15). On relatively minor trauma,

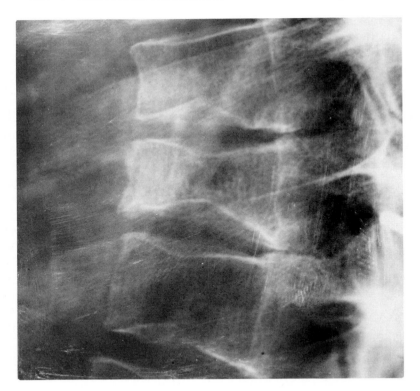

*Fig. 15.* Collapsed midthoracic vertebrae. Osteoporosis with minor trauma. No neurologic deficit.

compression fractures with vertebral collapse are common in older people. After age 70 in the asymptomatic population, the incidence of such fractures is 20 percent. In the aging spine, the etiology of such fractures may be spontaneous and obscure without a major traumatic event. They may occur with sneezing, raising windows, or lifting weights. The patient can then experience severe pain in the spine, although absence of discomfort is common. Minor falls may produce such fractures. In addition to having back pain, these patients may have local tenderness and may be reluctant to move in bed in order to avoid further pain. Some patients may have root pain, and a very small minority may have injury to the spinal cord. About 15 percent of such patients may develop paralytic ileus particularly in association with fractures of T12 and L1. It is generally considered that retroperitoneal hemorrhage is the underlying factor in the production of the ileus either by the size of the hemorrhage or irritation of the celiac plexus. In our view, these patients should be treated with simple analgesics and early ambulation.

Management of patients with acute traumatic paraplegia after thoracic and lumbar fracture and fracture-dislocation continues to be controversial. Many pertinent concepts have been discussed earlier in this chapter. Fracture or fracture-dislocation of the spine of sufficient severity to cause traumatic paraplegia implies the possibility of a degree of bone and ligamentous injury which can result in an unstable spine (Figs. 15–24). Progressive deformity in an unstable spine may result in gibbus formation which causes skin break-down, infection, pain, and impaired sitting and standing balance. With deformity may come progressive loss of neurologic function. Guttmann[27] opposed any surgical treatment whatsoever, including laminectomy and stabilization, and advocated conservative therapy including postural reduction. In his opinion, open reduction and internal fixation are indicated at the thoracolumbar junction in rare instances, such as those with marked lateral dislocation or repeated redislocation following conservative treatment. Patients who had open reduction and internal fixation showed results no better than those treated by nonoperative means. Holdsworth[35] distinguished between stable and unstable injuries, and there is considerable controversy regarding his concepts. Holdsworth recognized that rehabilitation may be impaired if the spine is grossly angulated. Continued angulation can cause further injury to roots that may have escaped initial damage, but may be prevented by internal fixation with plates bolted to the spinous processes. Bolting of the vertebra with metal is for temporary stability only, in most qual-

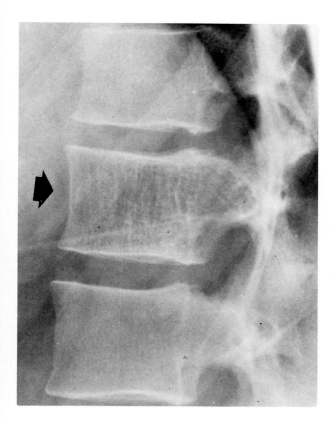

*Fig. 16.* Hemangioma (arrow) of thoracic vertebral body unrelated to trauma.

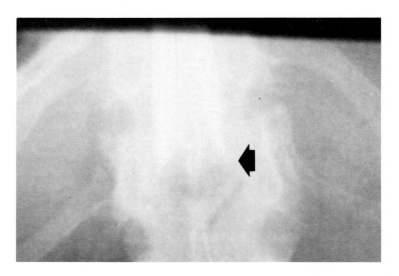

*Fig. 17.* Complete block of myelographic contrast (arrow) T12. Contrasted instilled C1–C2. Patient paraplegic.

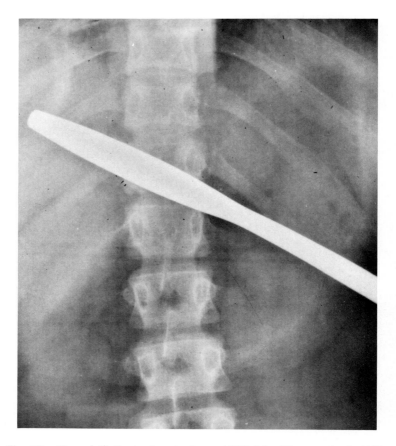

*Fig. 18.* Gearshift through spinal canal T12–L1 with paraplegia (AP).

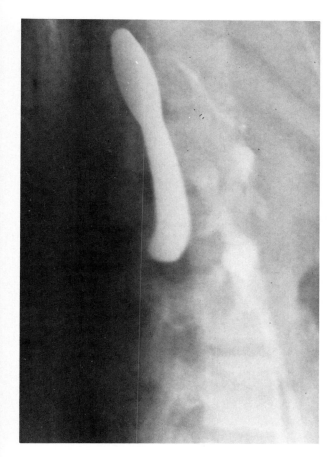

*Fig. 19.* Same patient as Figure 18 (lateral view).

ified opinions, since final stability is achieved only by spontaneous interbody bony union. Kelly and Whitesides[37] recommended posterior fusion and anterior vertebral body removal for decompressive purposes with insertion of a bone graft in place of the damaged vertebral body. Removal of the anterior vertebral body via a thoracic or abdominal approach is uncommonly done at the present time, but the rationale seems sound. Likewise, Paul et al.[54] recommended anterior transthoracic surgical decompression of acute thoracic spinal cord injuries (see Chap. 12). Kaufer and Hayes[36] reported that back pain and increasing deformity were late problems in patients who had fracture-dislocation at the thoracolumbar junction with paraplegia. They reported that of 10 patients with unstable fracture-dislocations, spontaneous vertebral body fusion occurred in only 2.

Principles of management of fractures of the thoracic and lumbar spine are similar to those in the cervical spine. In the first place, there may be fractures of almost any element of the bony vertebral column without involvement of nervous tissues. For example, Melamed[48] reported fractures of the pars interarticularis in lumbar vertebra. He stated that some cases of spon-

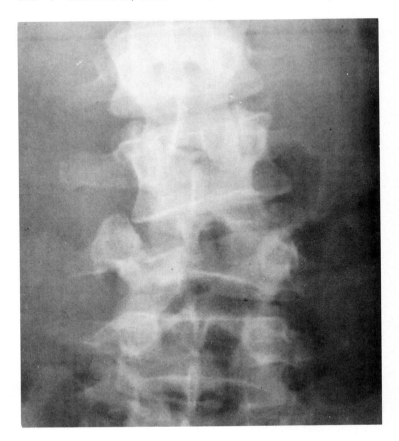

*Fig. 20.* AP showing traumatic collapse of L3.

dylolysis and spondylolisthesis may, in fact, be due to unrecognized or ancient trauma. Usually fractures of bony structures, such as spinous processes,
transverse processes, and pedicles are accompanied by pain. In the later
stages, the patient may have traumatic arthritis and be subject to pain as a
result of the ancient injury.

The most common place for thoracolumbar fractures is at the T12–L1 interspace level, with L1–L2 second. Kaufer and Hayes[36] considered that most
fracture-dislocations of the lumbar spine are unstable and have the potential
to produce a neural deficit where initially none existed, or to cause an increase in a previously incomplete neurologic deficit. In the lumbar area, neural injury is to the cauda equina and not to the spinal cord itself because of
the anatomy of the spinal cord. At T12–L1 the conus medularis is involved;
below that, the cauda equina. Kaufer divided lumbar fracture-dislocations
into five groups. In the first type, there was dislocation of both articular processes and of the vertebral bodies without associated fracture, a pure dislocation. This is a rare injury. In the second type, there was dislocation of both

articular processes and of the vertebral bodies combined with compression fracture of one or more vertebral bodies. This type accounted for about 50 percent of cases. The third type consisted of dislocation of both articular processes without dislocation of the vertebral body. There was in some instances compression of a small portion of the vertebral body. This accounted for about 25 percent of cases. Type 4 dislocations involved only one pair of articular processes. These accounted for about 20 percent of patients. Type 5 dislocation occurred in 5 percent of cases; this was a bilateral fracture through the pedicles or pars intra-articularis with slight dislocation.

Kaufer and Hayes[36] reported that 53 percent of patients had neural deficit. This is compared to a 60 to 70 percent incidence of neural deficit reported in most series. In two of Kaufer and Hayes'[36] patients there was progression between the time of trauma and definitive treatment. In a third patient who had no deficit initially, a mild deficit did develop. Decrease in neural deficit in the interval between injury and definitive treatment did not occur.

Kaufer and Hayes' patients had three types of treatment:[36] (1) laminec-

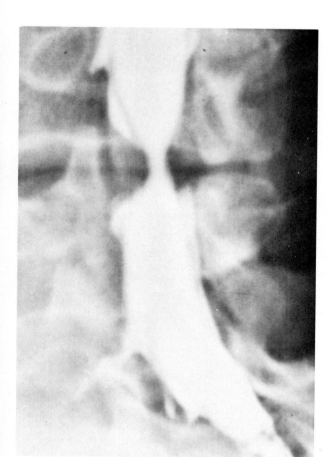

*Fig. 21.* Acute lumbar herniated disc L4–L5. Oblique myelogram.

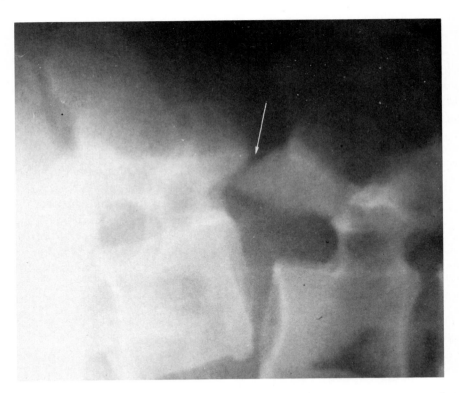

*Fig. 22.* Superior articulating facet of L4 jumped (arrow) over inferior articulating facet L3 with dislocation. See Figures 23 and 24.

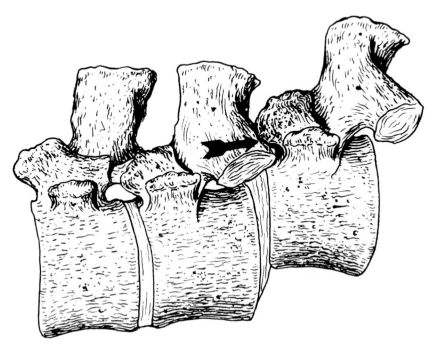

*Fig. 23.* Artist's depiction of jumped facets (arrow) with dislocation.

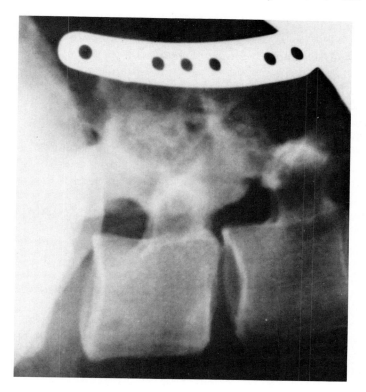

*Fig. 24.* Same patient as Figure 22. Operative reduction, stabilization, and fusion.

tomy, (2) closed reduction, and (3) early open reduction, internal fixation, and fusion. It is not possible to compare results of these three types of treatments because of disparity in types of cases and the small number. Closed reduction was attempted by hyperextension, but only partial reduction could be obtained. Open reduction was carried out in 10 patients. Complications of open reduction and laminectomy consisted of ileus and transient worsening of neurologic status. In our experience, closed reduction is not effective and possibly may even be unsafe. Kaufer and Hayes agree with this.

It has been our practice to carry out immediate decompressive laminectomy in patients with thoracic and lumbar spinal cord injury with severe neurologic deficit. We have felt that this does not damage the patient further if done carefully, and lateral transverse process fusion can then be carried out, or at least insertion of rods can be accomplished to stabilize the patient while bony healing progresses. Although we cannot prove that this has greater benefit than no treatment at all, as advocated by Guttmann[27,28] and others, it does assure the patient that everything that could be done during the acute stage is done.

As a note of caution, Roberts and Curtiss[58] suggested that in patients with thoracic spine fractures in the erect position on a circle bed, there is considerable vertical loading, and unstable fractures can displace, especially when the patient is turned. Without strong axillary supports, use of the circle bed may be similar to allowing a patient with an unstable fracture to stand erect, and this can cause severe damage to the unsupported spinal cord.

Lewis and McKibbin[41] compared results of treatment in a retrospective study of conservatively managed patients without operative treatment but with postural reduction and patients who had routine open reduction and plating of unstable thoracolumbar spine injuries. They could detect no difference in neurologic recovery between the two groups, but while a number of conservatively treated patients had significant residual spinal deformity and subsequently developed serious pain, this did not occur in any patients treated by metallic plating. On the other hand, Burke and Murray[12] had 8 of 26 patients undergoing surgical treatment for thoracic and thoracolumbar injury who had chronic severe pain. In both groups, about 25 percent showed significant neurologic improvement. Burke and Murray generally advised against early operation.

Weitzman[65] described the treatment of stable thoracolumbar spine compression fractures without dislocation. He advocated early ambulation without body casts or braces. There was no neurologic deficit in his patients. In our opinion, wedge fractures without dislocation may be treated in that manner, as they generally do well with any type of therapy. It appears that pain is reduced with early ambulation.

Whitesides and Shah[77] described their management of unstable fractures of the thoracolumbar spine, utilizing anterior decompression and fusion with posterior stabilization with Meurig-Williams plates or Harrington rods. Hardy[30] compared results of conservatively and operatively treated patients in a large series of fracture-dislocations of the lumbodorsal spine and found no difference between the two groups. The operative group had greater severity of bony injury, and he felt that the ease of handling this group was greatly improved by operative procedures.

Boshes et al.[8] managed wartime spinal cord and cauda equina injuries with laminectomy. Most of these were caused by missiles, however. Myers[52] reported posterior dislocation of the L4 body accompanied by a massive extrusion of the intervertebral disc above and below the level. The patient was treated by laminectomy and did well.

Landau et al.[38] emphasized that the question of surgery in cases of traumatic spinal lesions involving the conus medullaris and the cauda equina is highly complex and controversial. They stated that in the opinion of many, late surgical intervention is usually unrewarding from the point of view of reversal of neurologic deficit. They presented nine patients having neurologic deficits as a result of traumatic lesions involving the conus medullaris or cauda equina who were operated upon at intervals from one month to 17 years following injury. In seven, the improvement was functionally significant; in all, compressive lesions were removed. There were bony spicules through the dura, bony compression, loose bone fragments, considerable scar, and lysis was performed in many cases. The onset of improvement varied widely between eight hours and nine months. In one case, the recovery of normal bladder function with clearing of previously chronic urinary tract infection six years after injury was dramatic. They also suggested that the fact that laminectomy had been carried out at some earlier date did not preclude the possibility of further improvement by later procedures. They also stressed the psychologic effect of the chance of recovery as a result of surgery as an important factor.

Compression fractures of the lumbar vertebrae occur in some cases with relatively minor trauma. There is often a history of lifting heavy loads, or stooping, or some unusual movement. In some cases, there is a history of a sudden, sharp pain or snapping noise with a sensation of movement in the area of injury. Physical examination reveals only spinal muscular spasm, with or without scoliosis, but the patient complains of pain. There may be localized tenderness over the spinous processes in the area of the compression fracture. X-ray verifies the fracture. The treatment is generally bedrest and early ambulation, although there is considerable difference of opinion. In the treatment of stable fractures, bedrest is not necessary for more than a few days at the most, in our view.

Yau and Chan[81] reported stress fractures in the fused lumbodorsal spine in ankylosing spondylitis. Fracture occurs through a former interspace, which has been fused by the spondylitic process. They treated three patients by anterior spinal fusion, and indicated that these fractures were stress fractures originating posteriorly. Pseudoarthrosis may occur and may simulate a tuberculous lesion. Operative fusion averts pain and further neurologic deficit.

## LUMBAR SPINE INJURIES ASSOCIATED WITH LAP-TYPE SEAT BELTS

It is said that the use of lap-type seat belts decreased the incidence of fatal vehicular accidents by 25 percent, but a new pattern of injuries did evolve, and many articles have appeared.[24–26,68] In addition to spinal and vertebral injuries, there have been reports of splenic rupture, hernias through muscle, intra-abdominal lesions, bowel perforations, uterine ruptures, mesentery lacerations, and vascular lesions including liver fractures. The spinal injuries occur generally from the second lumbar to the fifth lumbar vertebrae and can involve any or all or many parts of one or more vertebrae.

In 1948, Chance[13] described an unusual fracture of the vertebral body consisting of a horizontal splitting of the spine, neural arch, and the vertebral body just in front of the neural foramen.[59] With acceptance of the lap-type seat belt, this "Chance fracture" has been diagnosed with increasing frequency as a result of injury sustained while wearing this device. The injury is produced by the seat belt acting as a fulcrum over which the vertebral body is split transversely; the fracture is also known as a fulcrum fracture. Approximately 15 percent of these fractures are associated with intra-abdominal injuries, and another 15 percent are associated with injuries to the spinal cord or cauda equina. Implications in the literature are that seat belt injuries may be prevented by proper positioning of the lap-type belt or by substitution of the bandolier or shoulder-type belt, but there is no evidence that the lap-type seat belt injury can in fact be prevented by proper positioning.

## FRACTURES OF THE SACRUM

Isolated fractures of the sacrum are uncommon and may be overlooked because of inadequate x-ray examination. Rowell[60] reviewed the literature and reported a case. Complications of the fracture may be vascular, resulting in hematoma in the presacral retroperitoneal area, probably due to rupture of the middle sacral artery or its branches. Uncommonly, such a hematoma may compress the rectal ampulla. Another complication may be cauda equina lesion, particularly of the sacral nerves, causing urinary incontinence. The rectum may be injured by the fracture, since it is in close proximity. The fracture may be compound externally, but this is a rare occurrence. Most often, the patient complains of localized pain, which may be worse on defecation or coughing. Rectal examination may reveal a hematoma or mass, and there may be severe pain on movement of the coccyx. On neurologic examination, there may be saddle anesthesia with or without sphincter disturbances. A patient reported by Rowell[60] had cerebral spinal fluid leakage through an open wound after a severe injury. Traumatic dislocation of the fifth lumbar vertebra on the sacrum is rare. Dewey and Browne[19] reported two such cases. One patient was treated conservatively and survived, the other was treated by operative decompression and died of fat embolism.

## DISC-SPACE INFECTIONS

Intervertebral disc surgery and trauma are occasionally followed by pain and varying degrees of bone destruction and sclerosis without clinical or bacteriologic evidence of infection. If the pain persists and the postoperative x-ray changes are marked, the process is called a disc-space infection. Williams et al.[78] called such infections pseudoinfections, since the etiology is not well understood and in most cases infections are low grade and aseptic. Abnormalities of the vertebrae adjacent to an intervertebral disk may be either destructive or sclerotic. At one end of the spectrum, the x-ray changes are primarily destructive with little or no sclerosis. These are usually frank infections and may be proved bacteriologically. There may be systemic signs of infection, such as elevation of sedimentation rate, fever, and elevated white blood count. At the other end of the spectrum, there is purely sclerotic change with disc space narrowing, but no bone destruction. Biopsy can be carried out if required via a needle into the involved area. Both types of patients respond favorably to rest and antibiotics. Williams et al.[78] tried radiotherapy, but the results were equivocal, and we do not recommend such therapy. Osteomyelitis is unusual in spinal cord injury.

# REFERENCES

1. Albee FH: Transplantation of a portion of the tibia into the spine for Pott's disease: A preliminary report. JAMA 57:885, 1911
2. Backstrom CH: Traffic injuries in south Sweden with special reference to medico-legal autopsies of car occupants and value of safety belts. Acta Chir Scand Suppl 308:5–104, 1963
3. Bedbrook GM: Spinal injuries. Lancet 2:247, 1963
4. Bedbrook GM: Stability of spinal fractures and fracture dislocations. Paraplegia 9:23–32, 1971
5. Bedbrook GM: Treatment of thoracolumbar dislocation and fractures with paraplegia. Clin Orthop 112:27–43, 1975
6. Bentley G, McSweeney T: Multiple spinal injuries. Br J Surg 55:565–570, 1968
7. Bick EM: An essay on the history of spine fusion operations. Clin Orthop 35:9–15, 1964
8. Boshes B, Zivin I, Tigay EL: Recent methods of management of spinal cord and cauda equina injuries. Neurology 4:690–704, 1954
9. Braakman R, Vinken PJ: Unilateral facet interlocking in the lower cervical spine. J Bone Joint Surg 49B:249–257, 1967
10. Burke DC: Hyperextension injuries of the spine. J Bone Joint Surg 53B:3–12, 1971
11. Burke DC, Tiong TS: Stability of the cervical spine after conservative treatment. Paraplegia 13:191–202, 1975
12. Burke DC, Murray DD: The management of thoracic and thoracolumbar injuries of the spine with neurological involvement. J Bone Joint Surg 58B:72–78, 1976
13. Chance GQ: Note on type of flexion fracture of spine. Br J Radiol 21:452–453, 1948
14. Cheshire DJ: The stability of the cervical spine following the conservative treatment of fractures and fracture-dislocations. Paraplegia 7:193–203, 1969
15. Chrisman OD, Snook GA, Stanitis JM, Keedy VA: Lateral-flexion neck injuries in athletic competition. JAMA 192:613–615, 1965
16. Comarr AE, Kaufman AA: A survey of the neurological results of 858 spinal cord injuries. J Neurosurg 13:95–106, 1956
17. Davidoff LM: Spinal cord injuries. Surg Clin North Am 21:433–441, 1941
18. Del Sel JM, Cibeira JB, Espagnol RO, Del Sel GM, Del Sel HJ: Stability following fracture-dislocations of the cervical spine. Paraplegia 13:203–207, 1975
19. Dewey P, Browne PSH: Fracture-dislocation of the lumbosacral spine with cauda equina lesion. J Bone Joint Surg 50B:635–638, 1968
20. Eggers GWN: Berthold Earnest Hadra (1842–1903): A biography. Clin Orthop 21:32–39, 1961
21. Evans JP, Rosenauer A: Spinal cord injuries. Arch Surg 72:812–816, 1956
22. Feuer H: Management of acute spine and spinal cord injuries. Arch Surg 111:638–645, 1976
23. Forsyth HF: Extension injuries of the cervical spine. J Bone Joint Surg 46A:1792–1797, 1964
24. Friedman MM, Becker L, Reighmister JP, Neiviaser JS: Seat belt spinal fractures. Am Surg 35:617–618, 1969
25. Fletcher BD, Brogdon BG: Seat belt fractures of the spine and sternum. JAMA 200:177–178, 1967
26. Greenbaum E, Harris L, Halloran WX: Flexion fracture of the lumbar spine due to lap-type seat belts. Calif Med 113:74–76, 1970
27. Guttmann L: Initial treatment of traumatic paraplegia. Proc R Soc Med 47:1103–1190, 1954
28. Guttmann L: Initial treatment of traumatic paraplegia and tetraplegia. Spinal injuries. In Phillip Harris (ed): Proceedings of a Symposium, Royal College of Surgeons of Edinburgh, 7-8 June 1963. London, Morrison and Gibb Limited, 1963
29. Hansen ST, Taylor TKF, Honet JC, Lewis FR: Fracture-dislocations of the ankylosed thoracic spine in rheumatoid spondylitis. J Trauma 7:827–837, 1967

30. Hardy AG: The treatment of paraplegia due to fracture-dislocations of the dorsolumbar spine. Paraplegia 3:112–123, 1965
31. Harris JL, Cummingham EB: Stress fractures of the lumbar vertebrae. J Occup Med 7:255–256, 1965
32. Harris WH, Hamblen DL, Ojemann RG: Traumatic disruption of cervical intervertebral disk for hyperextension injury. Clin Orthop 60:163–167, 1968
33. Hibbs RA: An operation for progressive spinal deformities: A preliminary report of three cases from the service of the Orthopedic Hospital. NY Med J 93:1013, 1911
34. Henle A: Die operative Schierung der spondylitischen Wirbelsaule. Munch Med Wochenschr 71:1169, 1924
35. Holdsworth F: Fractures, dislocations, and fracture-dislocations of the spine. J Bone Joint Surg 52A:1534, 1551, 1970
36. Kaufer H, Hayes JT: Lumbar fracture-dislocation. J Bone Joint Surg 48A:712–730, 1966
37. Kelly RP, Whitesides TE, Jr: Treatment of lumbodorsal fracture-dislocations. Ann Surg 167:705–717, 1968
38. Landau B, Campbell JB, Ransohoff J: Surgical reversal of the effects of long-standing traumatic lesions of the conus medullaris and cauda equina. Proc Am Clin Spinal Cord Injury Conf 17:27–33, 1967
39. Lange F: Operative behandlung der spondylitis. Munch Med Wochenschr 35:1817–1818, 1909
40. Lange F: Support for the spondylitic spine by means of buried steel bars attached to the vertebrae. Am J Orthop Surg 8:344–361, 1910
41. Lewis J, McKibbin B: The treatment of unstable fracture-dislocations of the thoracolumbar spine accompanied by paraplegia. J Bone Joint Surg 56B:603–612, 1974
42. Livingston WK, Newman HW: Spinal cord concussion in war wounds. West J Surg Obstet Gynecol 54:131–139, 1946
43. Marar BC: Hyperextension injuries of the cervical spine: The pathogenesis of damage to the spinal cord. J Bone Joint Surg 56A:1655–1662, 1974
44. Martin J: The treatment of injuries of the spinal cord. Int Abst Surg, Surg Gynecol Obstet 84:403–416, 1947
45. Mayfield FH, Cazan GM: Spinal cord injuries. Analysis of six cases showing subarachnoid block. Am J Surg 55:317–325, 1942
46. McWhorter JM, Alexander E, Jr, Davis CH, Jr, Kelly DL, Jr: Posterior cervical fusion in children. J Neurosurg 45:211–215, 1976
47. Meijers KA: Dislocation of the cervical spine with cord compression in rheumatoid arthritis. J Bone Joint Surg 56B:668–680, 1974
48. Melamed A: Fracture of pars interarticularis of lumbar vertebra. Am J Roentgen 94:584–586, 1965
49. Mixter SJ, Osgood RB: Traumatic lesions of the atlas and axis. Am J Orthop Surg 7:348, 1910
50. Munro D: Relation between spondylosis cervicalis and injury of the cervical spine and its contents. N Engl J Med 262:839–846, 1960
51. Munro D: Treatment of fractures and dislocations of the cervical spine complicated by cervical-cord and root injuries. N Engl J Med 264:573–582, 1961
52. Myers P: Posterior dislocation of the L4 body accompanied by massive extrusion of the disc above and below. Proc Ann Clin Spinal Cord Injury Conf 15:89–90, 1966
53. Nieminen R: Fractures of the articular processes of the lower cervical spine. Ann Chir Gynaecol Fenn 63(3):204–211, 1974
54. Paul RL, Michael RH, Dunn JE, Williams JP: Anterior transthoracic surgical decompression of acute spinal cord injuries. J Neurosurg 43:299–305, 1975
55. Penning L: Cited in San Giorgi SM: Orthopaedic aspects of the treatment of injuries of the lower cervical spine. Acta Neurochir 22:227–233, 1970
56. Petrie JG: Flexion injuries of the cervical spine. J Bone Joint Surg 46A:1800–1806, 1964

57. Raaf J: Treatment of the patient with spinal cord injury. Am J Surg 67:119–279, 1945
58. Roberts JB, Curtiss PH, Jr: Stability of the thoracic and lumbar spine in traumatic paraplegia following fracture or fracture-dislocation. J Bone Joint Surg 52A:1115–1130, 1970
59. Rogers LF: The roentgenographic appearance of transverse or chance fractures of the spine: The seat belt fracture. Am J Roentgenol Radium Ther Nucl Med 111:844–849, 1971
60. Rowell CE: Fracture of sacrum with hemisaddle anaesthesia and cerebro-spinal fluid leak. Med J Aust 1:16–19, 1965
61. Saldeen T: Fatal neck injuries caused by use of diagonal safety belts. J Trauma 7:856–862, 1967
62. San Giorgi SM: Orthopaedic aspects of the treatment of injuries of the lower cervical spine. Acta Neurochir 22:227–233, 1970
63. Schneider RC, Cherry G, Pantek H: The syndrome of acute central cervical spinal cord injury. J Neurosurg 11:546–577, 1954
64. Schneider RC: The syndrome of acute anterior spinal cord injury. J Neurosurg 12:95–122, 1955
65. Schneider RC, Kahn EA: The significance of the acute-flexion or "tear-drop" fracture-dislocation of the cervical spine. J Bone Joint Surg 38A:985–997, 1956
66. Schneider RC, Papo M, Alvarez CS: The effects of chronic recurrent spinal trauma in high-diving. A study of Acapulco's divers. J Bone Joint Surg 44A:648–656, 1962
67. Schneider RC: Serious and fatal neurosurgical football injuries. Clin Neurosurg 12:226–236, 1964
68. Smith WS, Kaufer H: A new pattern of spine injury associated with lap-type seat belts: A preliminary report. Univ Mich Med Cent J 33:99–104, 1957
69. Stauffer ES, Rhoades ME: Surgical stabilization of the cervical spine after trauma. Arch Surg 111:652–657, 1976
70. Stern WE: Neurosurgical aspects of injuries of the thoracic and lumbar spine. Surg Clin North Am 52:769–782, 1972
71. Suwanwela C, Alexander E, Jr, Davis CH, Jr: Prognosis in spinal cord injury with special reference to patients with motor paralysis and sensory preservation. J Neurosurg 19:220–227, 1962
72. Tucker HH: Technical report: Method of fixation of subluxed or dislocated cervical spine below C1-C2. Can J Neurol Scie 2:381–382, 1975
73. Wannamaker GT: A review of the early treatment in 300 consecutive cases during the Korean conflict. J Neurosurg 11:517–524, 1954
74. Weiss M: Dynamic spine alloplasty (spring-loading corrective devices) after fracture and spinal cord injury. Clin Orthop 112:150–158, 1975
75. Weitzman G: Treatment of stable thoracolumbar spine compression fractures by early ambulation. Clin Orthop 76:116–122, 1971
76. White AA, Southwick WO, Panjabi MM: Clinical instability in the lower cervical spine. A review of past and current concepts. Spine 1:15–29, 1976
77. Whitesides TE, Jr, Shah SGA: On the management of unstable fractures of the thoracolumbar spine. Spine 1:99–107, 1976
78. Williams JL, Moller GA, O'Rourke TL: Pseudoinfections of the intervertebral disk and adjacent vertebrae. Am J Roentgen 103:611–615, 1968
79. Yashon D: Missile injuries of the spinal cord. In: Proceedings of the Nineteenth Veterans Administration Spinal Cord Injury Conference, Scottsdale, Arizona, October 31, 1973. Washington DC, US Government Printing Office, February 1977
80. Yashon D: Missile injuries of the spinal cord. In Vinken PJ, Bruyn GW (eds): Injuries of the Spine and Spinal Cord Handbook of Clinical Neurology. New York, Elsevier, 1976, pp 209–220
81. Yau ACMC, Chan RNW: Stress fracture of the fused lumbo-dorsal spine in ankylosing spondylitis. A report of three cases. J Bone Joint Surg 56B:681–687, 1974

# 11

## Anesthesia

### INDUCTION

The risk of damaging the spinal cord by the slightest movement of the neck or head after cervical injury is a prime concern of the surgeon and anesthesiologist.[8] Movement after thoracic and lumbar injuries is similarly of considerable concern. Because damage may occur during transport, induction of anesthesia, intubation, or positioning, the anesthesiologist is extremely careful to avoid excessive moving of the patient. In cervical cord injuries, skeletal traction along the spinal axis to stabilize the head and to protect against inadvertent movement is maintained during induction and intubation as well as throughout the operative procedure, and is continued postoperatively.

In patients undergoing emergency operation, a full stomach is an added hazard during induction of anesthesia.[8] Regurgitation is more probable than vomiting, because of paralysis of abdominal muscles. Factors that predispose to regurgitation include head-down tilt, airway obstruction, intermittent positive pressure breathing before intubation, and the use of depolarizing muscle relaxants. Emptying of the stomach by nasogastric tube before induction of anesthesia not only does not guarantee an empty stomach, but, in fact, may facilitate regurgitation if the tube is left in place during induction. Head-up tilt decreases the likelihood of regurgitation, but may initiate or aggravate hypotension and may add to the technical difficulty of intubation.[9]

Awake intubation is widely advocated because it protects against possible failure to intubate the trachea, with loss of patent airways, and somewhat decreases the risk of inhalation of vomitus.[9] But attempts to visualize the larynx and intubate the trachea by direct oropharyngeal laryngoscopy in an awake patient with severe cervical muscle spasm may be difficult and traumatic. Therefore, blind nasotracheal intubation is viewed as the procedure of choice by many. Gilbert et al.[14,15] described a technique for blind nasotracheal intubation in awake patients with cervical cord injuries which involved bilateral superior laryngeal nerve block and use of topical transtracheal and nasalanesthetic spray. The procedure is time consuming. They also advised a hypnotic dose of Thiopentone, to be given only after the blocking agent to avoid laryngeal spasm. Shapiro[26] recommended awake oral endotracheal intubation under neuroleptanalgesia obtained with fentanyl (a short-acting narcotic) and droperidol (a major tranquilizer), along with local anesthesia of the pharynx and larynx. This may lead to hypotension, however.

Blind nasal intubation does not require a deep level of anesthesia, and, in fact, can be done without anesthesia. Blind nasal intubation obviates the need for muscle relaxants and traumatic endoscopy; the tube is easier to fix in place than the oral tube and is well tolerated by the conscious patient after operation. Suctioning the trachea is more difficult through a nasotracheal tube. Risk of damage to the mucous membrane of the nose and nasal pharynx is high, but this is balanced against the greater importance of nontraumatic intubation. Lubrication of the tube with a nonanesthetic bland jelly and prespraying of the nose with a 5 percent cocaine solution to shrink nasal mucosa will lessen the likelihood of epistaxis. A tube about 1 to 2 mm smaller than an oral tube with its bevel directed toward the nasal septum is most easily introduced.

Awake intubation may be carried out by nasal passage of the endotracheal tube. Blind oral or nasal intubation while the patient is awake helps to prevent additional injury, since the awake patient can report untoward neurologic symptoms. The patient can be examined during and after intubation. Elective tracheostomy can be performed in unusual cases, but, by and large, this has been unnecessary on our service.

A patient positioned on the Stryker frame may be anesthetized, intubated, and then turned to the prone position for surgery. A folded towel or sandbag under the chest causes the head to angulate so that adequate flexion for C1–C2 fusions and laminectomy can be accomplished with the head in the neutral position. The Stryker frame is ideal for such procedures; the circoelectric bed is not recommended because blood pressure may fall while the patient is erect, and loading of the fracture with consequent further damage can occur with change in position. While the patient is prone, prolonged pressure to the eyes must be avoided. Such pressure may exceed the normal retinal artery pressure and result in thrombosis of the retinal artery, causing permanent blindness. Severe uneven and prolonged pressure on the face may result in necrosis about the face, especially in the areas of the zygomatic arch, the supraorbital ridges, and the mandible. Other areas of concern are the feet, the breasts, and the genitalia.

To prevent spinal cord injury during procedures such as the Harrington operation for idiopathic scoliosis, intraoperative evaluation of spinal cord function is advisable but not widely practiced. The risk of paraplegia in operative correction of scoliosis is slight but definite. Crawford et al.[7] utilized hypnosis to assist in the anesthetizing and the awakening of the patient during the surgical procedure to perform voluntary movements for the assessment of motor function.

## CARDIOVASCULAR CONSIDERATIONS

Cardiovascular instability, due mainly to the loss of the influence of higher centers on sympathetic innervation of the heart and blood vessels, is a serious aspect of spinal injury. Bradycardia and peripheral vasodilatation with hypotension may be encountered. The flaccid muscles are not able to facilitate venous return by their normal massaging effect and cardiac output fails. Circulatory disturbances may be intensified by anesthetics or narcotic analgesics which have myocardial depressant and vasodilator effects. Therefore, the level of anesthesia should be light, and doses of sedatives and analgesics minimal.

Hypovolemia due to blood loss is poorly tolerated by quadriplegic patients, and its cause should be identified and remedied immediately during the operation. It is essential to replace blood as it is lost as well as to maintain postoperative fluid balance. However, transfusion of blood solely because of hypotension caused by impaired sympathetic activity is not justified.

The central venous pressure level may be misleading in quadriplegic patients, because it may reflect a balance between changes in cardiac output and diminished venous return. Therefore, any tendency of central venous pressure to rise owing to cardiac depression or hypervolemia might be masked by venous pooling resulting from reduction of peripheral venous tone. Severe hypotension in the absence of hypovolemia can be corrected by temporary use of a vasopressive drug having both cardiac and peripheral action. For bradycardia, atropine may be given.

One must be alert to hypertensive crises due to autonomic hyperreflexia during anesthesia in patients with spinal injuries. Thorn-Alquist[31] reported three patients with high spinal lesions who showed signs of severe hypertension during cystoscopy under anesthesia. The hypertension was controlled with an intravenous drip of Arfonad (trimethaphan). Fatal cerebral hemorrhage can occur during the hypertensive crisis. This syndrome occurs in patients with a lesion located above thoracic level six. In addition to paroxysmal systemic hypertension, symptoms include bradycardia, sweating, severe headache, and pilomotor erection. The syndrome may be initiated by almost any stimulus including distention of the bladder and rectum, and pain. Ciliberti et al.[3] felt that removal of the trigger stimulus, if it is possible, is the best method of treatment. Bors and French[1] discussed management during anesthesia when spontaneous systemic hypertension occurs. Johnson et al.[19] reviewed the syndrome of autonomic hyperreflexia and made a strong plea for those managing spinal cord injury patients to be aware of this syndrome and its consequences.

Drinker and Helrich[11] discussed a mass autonomic reflex phenomenon during halothane anesthesia in a quadriplegic patient, and reported that an increased concentration of halothane was useful in bringing down the blood pressure. The anesthesiologist should be ready to control such events by ganglionic blockers, such as trimethaphan, or direct-acting vasodilators, e.g., nitroprusside.

Stone et al.,[29] as well as others, warned against massive hyperkalemia in patients with musculoskeletal disease such as quadriplegia following relaxation with succinylcholine. A likely explanation for increase in serum potassium is that the denervated muscle cell membrane is altered, resulting in an atypical response to the depolarization produced by succinylcholine. The increased sensitivity to succinylcholine commences on about the sixth day after injury and may continue for over 12 weeks. Snow et al.[28] reviewed the literature on cardiovascular collapse following use of succinylcholine in paraplegic patients.

Frankel et al.[12] reviewed mechanisms of reflex cardiac arrest in tetraplegic patients. They presented four patients not under anesthesia who suffered cardiac arrest within six weeks of a complete high cervical spinal cord injury. All required intermittent positive pressure ventilation in the stage of spinal shock; stimuli to the trachea induced bradycardia, and in two patients, cardiac arrest resulted. Bradycardia occurred when the patients were hypoxic, and seemed to be due to vasovagal reflex. This reflex is normally opposed by sympathetic activity, but during hypoxia by increased pulmonary vagal reflex activity due to increased breathing. In spinally injured patients, compensatory sympathetic activity is prevented, and increased pulmonary vagal reflex activity occurs because ventilation is mechanical and does not increase with hypoxia. Treatment of such emergencies includes administration of atropine and adequate oxygenation.

Desmond and Laws[10] studied blood volume and capacitance vessel compliance in 27 quadriplegic patients, using radio I-131 albumin and upper limb plethysmography, and found that blood volume may be reduced considerably. They suggested that failure of the capacitance side of the circulation to respond normally to application of respiratory stress is due to disordered control of autonomic receptors. The capacitance system is abnormally dilated. Such failure of compliance of the capacitance side of the circulation increases the serious implications of reduction of blood volume during surgery in quadriplegics. Further, they noted that in those patients having reduced blood volume, the red blood cell volume is disproportionately reduced in relation to plasma and total blood volume. On that basis, they suggested that wound healing may be deficient. Further, a large dose of induction medication such as thiopentone might cause undue dilatation of the resistance and capacitance system, with a profound drop in blood pressure.

Intraoperative shock in paraplegic patients was emphasized by Williams and Walker,[32] who found that 57 percent of patients had an incident of profound hypotension or shock during surgery. This is an extremely high percentage. Shock is uncommon in our patients. Freyschuss and Knutsson[13] studied circulatory responses of patients with long-standing tetraplegia to vasomotor stimuli prior to and after cholinergic and alpha-adrenergic block. They observed that patients with functional interruption of the cervical cord well above the sympathetic outflow from the spinal cord (upper thoracic cord) regulate heart rate by varying vagal tone, but are able to induce sympathetic vasoconstriction. The pathways of this sympathetic discharge are unknown.

Thompson and Witham[30] reported on paroxysmal hypertension occurring in spinal cord injuries and reviewed the literature to 1948.

On the other hand, LaBan et al.[22] found that in 14 patients with traumatic spinal cord dysfunction, blood volume, measured by radioiodinated serum tracer methods, was significantly elevated. Patients with cauda equina injury had the highest blood volume, although the higher the lesion in the spinal cord, the less the increase in blood volume. They stated that important factors contributing to overall blood volume increases are an increase in venous capacity, alteration in the muscle–fat ratio, and a strenuous program of physical therapy. Cole et al.[4] investigated the loss of cardiovascular control in quadriplegic patients in two situations: the first during postural change in which a large portion of the body was moved from horizontal to a dependent position, or vice versa; and the second during autonomic hyperreflexia. They found that the cardiovascular system of a chronic quadriplegic patient is well able to tolerate the usual activities of daily living.

In 15 quadriplegic patients, Silver[27] studied blood pressure, forearm and hand blood flow, and heart rate in response to deep breathing, bladder distension, and tilting with and without arterial cuffs. During spinal shock, inspiratory vasoconstriction and autonomic hyperreflexia in response to filling of the bladder was, in fact, present. Past the spinal shock stage, the response to tilting was a fall in blood pressure and forearm blood flow accompanied by tachycardia, and this response was modified by application of arterial cuffs to the lower limbs. Silver suggested that reflex autonomic control of blood vessels could be mediated by isolation of the spinal cord from the medullary centers during stages of spinal shock.

Kunin[20] studied blood pressure in 152 adult male paraplegic and quadriplegic patients known to have chronic urinary tract infection. Contrary to the widely held belief, elevated blood pressure was rare. He emphasized that hypertension is present in patients late in the disease when death is close. He considered hypertension to be a late manifestation of severe pyelonephritis and renal amyloidosis.

Greenhoot[16,17] demonstrated alterations in the electrocardiogram and fuchsinophilic degeneration of myocardial cells following experimental spinal cord injury in dogs. He suggested that sympathetic discharge was the primary event occurring within seconds of injury and caused the cardiac lesions because of associated hypertension and tachycardia. Cardiac abnormalities have not been a problem in our patients.

## PULMONARY CONSIDERATIONS

In the presence of cervical spinal cord injury, ventilatory capability may be assessed with spirometry and arterial gas studies before induction of anesthesia.

Halothane, although a suppressant of sympathetic activity, is potent in low concentration, so that it is preferred for maintenance of an easily controlled level of anesthesia. Halothane also has the advantage of being nonirritant to the respiratory tract, effecting early depression of pharyngeal and laryngeal reflexes, thus facilitating intubation under anesthesia.

Intermittent positive pressure ventilation (IPPV) interferes with venous return by increasing intrathoracic pressure. Normally the valsalva maneuver in the presence of elevated mean intrathoracic pressure compensates for the decreased venous return by increasing peripheral vascular tone, thus maintaining the pressure gradient between intrathoracic veins and peripheral circulation. This compensatory response is a reflex mechanism mediated through baroreceptors in the aorta and carotid sinuses. These receptors send afferent impulses to the vasomotor center in the medulla which, in turn, sends down activating impulses for sympathetic outflow. The latter efferent pathways are interrupted in cervical cord injury.

In the use of IPPV in paralyzed patients, the inspiratory phase should be reduced to a minimum (one second) with a longer than normal expiratory pause (three seconds). The incorporation of a subatmospheric pressure phase during expiration is claimed to help venous return and augment cardiac output. However, when the operative site lies above heart level, a subatmospheric phase increases risk of air embolism.

Haas et al.[18] studied the impairment of respiration in the chronic state following spinal injury. After cervical spinal cord injury, respiratory insufficiency develops late and is due to dysfunction of the thorax rather than to intrinsic pulmonary disease. Ventilation in these patients was worsened by the sitting position but not by the application of braces to support posture. Haas et al.[18] discussed the anesthesiologist's role in these and other emergencies in the treatment of spinal cord injury.

Pledger[24] discussed disorders of temperature regulation in acute traumatic quadriplegia, and suggested that the acute spinal cord injury deprives the patient of essentially all means of compensating for changes in environmental temperatures. He emphasized that fever in these patients may not necessarily be a sign of infection and that presence of the latter should be decided on clinical and bacteriologic grounds.

Osborne et al.[23] studied the effect of a complete lesion of the spinal cord above the fifth thoracic level upon adrenal cortical response to stress in three patients. Plasma and urinary steroid levels during and after surgical procedures were not significantly different from those in patients without spinal cord injury. They suggested that an intact suprasegmental innervation of the adrenal medulla does not seem to be essential for the normal adrenocortical response to stress. Cooper et al.[6] investigated the use of testosterone as an anticatabolic agent after injury to the spinal cord. They reported that 15 patients who received testosterone after spinal cord injury demonstrated considerably less urinary excretion of nitrogen and creatine, a more favorable status of nitrogen balance, less pronounced hypoproteinemia, and a lower incidence of decubitus ulcer than did a control group of 15 spinally injured patients who did not receive testosterone. However, testosterone has not been widely used in the care of spinal injured patients.

Brown et al.[2] studied water metabolism in 59 patients with injuries to the cervical spinal cord. Most excreted abnormal amounts of fluids; polyuria and polydipsia was reduced in three of these patients by pitressin. They concluded that interruption of cervical level neuropathways concerned in water metabolism in the intact organism is responsible for a diabetes insipidus-like syndrome. They suggested that exclusion of descending impulses from the hypothalmus to lower centers in the spinal cord is an important factor in the production of diabetes insipidus.

Rocco and Vandam[25] emphasized the importance of treating patients with amyloidosis and spinal injury for potential adrenal insufficiency in advance of anesthesia, since the adrenal may be replaced by amyloid deposits. Kurfees et al.,[21] in a review of the anesthetic management of paraplegic patients during World War II, concluded that no insurmountable problems in anesthesia are presented, provided basic principles are observed. This has been our observation also, and we do not hesitate to recommend necessary surgical procedures in patients with spinal cord injuries. Comarr and Woodard[5] reviewed 3000 operations in a 10-year survey of anesthesia in spinal cord injured patients, and concurred.

## REFERENCES

1. Bors E, French JD: Management of paroxysmal hypertension following injuries to cervical and upper thoracic segments of the spinal cord. Arch Surg 64:803–812, 1952
2. Brown M, Pyzik S, Finkle JR: Causes of polyuria and polydipsia in patients with injuries of the cervical spinal cord. Neurology 9:877–882, 1959
3. Ciliberti BJ, Goldfein J, Rovenstine EA: Hypertension during anesthesia in patients with spinal cord injuries. Anesthesiology 15:273–279, 1954
4. Cole TM, Kottke FJ, Olson M, Stradal L, Niederloh J: Alterations of cardiovascular control in high spinal myelomalacia. Arch Phys Med 48:359–368, 1967
5. Comarr AE, Woodard MM: A ten year survey of anesthesia in spinal cord injuries. J Am Assoc Nurse Anesthetists 25:31–38, 1957
6. Cooper IS, Rynearson EH, MacCarty CS, Power MH: Testosterone propionate as a nitrogen-sparing agent after spinal cord injury. JAMA 145:549–553, 1951
7. Crawford AH, Jones CW, Perisho JA, Herring JA: Hypnosis for monitoring intraoperative spinal cord function. Anesth Analg 55:4244, 1976
8. Daw EF, Svien HJ, Michenfelder JD, Terry HR: The role of the anesthesiologist in the management of acute intracranial and spinal cord emergencies. Surg Clin North Am 45:919–926, 1965
9. Demian YK, White RJ, Yashon D, Kretchmer HE: Anesthesia for laminectomy and localized cord cooling in acute cervical spine injury. Br J Anaesth 43:973–979, 1971
10. Desmond JW, Laws AK: Blood volume and capacitance vessel compliance in the quadriplegic patient. Can Anaesth Soc J 21:421–426, 1974
11. Drinker AS, Helrich M: Halothane anesthesia in the paraplegic patient. Anesthesiology 24:399–400, 1963
12. Frankel HL, Mathias CJ, Spalding JMK: Mechanisms of reflex cardiac arrest in tetraplegic patients. Lancet 2:1183–1185, 1975
13. Freyschuss U, Knutsson E: Cardiovascular control in man with transverse cervical cord lesions. Life Sci 8:421–424, 1969

14. Gilbert RGB, Brindle GF, Galindo A: Anesthesia for Neurosurgery. Boston, Little, Brown, 1966, p 162
15. Gilbert RGB, Brindle GF, Galindo A: Spinal surgery and anesthesia. Int Anesth Clin 4:863–879, 1966
16. Greenhoot JH: The effect of cervical cord injury on cardiac rhythm and conduction. Am Heart J 83:659–662, 1972
17. Greenhoot JH: Experimental spinal cord injury. Electrocardiographic abnormalities and fuchsinophilic myocardial degeneration. Arch Neurol 26:524–529, 1972
18. Haas A, Lawman EW, Bergofsky EH: Impairment of respiration after spinal cord injury. Arch Phys Med Rehabil 46:399–405, 1965
19. Johnson B, Thomason R: Autonomic hyperreflexia: A review. Milit Med 140:345–349, 1975
20. Kunin CM: Blood pressure in patients with spinal cord injury. Arch Intern Med 127:285–287, 1971
21. Kurfees JG, Whitehouse S, Cerzosimo F: Anesthesia for the paraplegic patient. JAMA 141:638–640, 1949
22. LaBan M, Johnson HE, Verdon TA, Grant AE: Blood volume following spinal cord injury. Arch Phys Med Rehabil 50:439–441, 1969
23. Osborn W, Schoenberg HM, Murphy JJ, Erdman WJ, Young D: Adrenal function in patients with lesions high in the spinal cord. J Urol 88:1–4, 1962
24. Pledger HG: Disorders of temperature regulation in acute traumatic tetraplegia. J Bone Joint Surg 44B:110–113, 1962
25. Rocco AG, Vandam LD: Problems in anesthesia for paraplegics. Anesthesiology 20:348–354, 1959
26. Shapiro HM: Neurosurgical anesthesia. Surg Clin North Am 55:913–928, 1975
27. Silver JR: Vascular reflexes in spinal shock. Paraplegia 8:231–242, 1971
28. Snow JC, Kripke BJ, Sessions GP, Fince AJ: Cardiovascular collapse following succinylcholine in a paraplegic patient. Paraplegia 11:199–204, 1973
29. Stone WA, Beach TP, Hamelberg W: Succinylcholine-induced hyperkalemia in dogs with transected sciatic nerves or spinal cords. Anesthesiology 32:515–520, 1970
30. Thompson CE, Witham AC: Paroxysmal hypertension in spinal cord injuries. N Engl J Med 239:291–294, 1948
31. Thorn-Alquist AM: Prevention of hypertensive crises in patients with high spinal lesions during cystoscopy and lithotripsy. Acta Anaesth Scand Suppl 57:79–82, 1975
32. Williams WT, Walker JW: Shock: A surgical hazard in the paraplegic. Surgery 42:664–668, 1957

# 12

## Surgical Techniques

Fracture dislocation of the vertebral column with or without involvement of the spinal cord or nerve roots or both continues to present a difficult surgical therapeutic problem. Various modes of treatment including skeletal traction with or without a plaster jacket[49,84,90] or neck brace, open fixation, posterior fusion, anterior fusion, or decompressive laminectomy followed by fusion, and immobilization in a plaster jacket or appropriate brace entail a long period of immobilization and hospitalization. The value of one treatment over another, or over no treatment at all, has been difficult to assess in terms of neurologic recovery, and, indeed, indications for operations have been controversial. All acknowledge that the salvage rate, at least as far as spinal function is concerned, has not been great. In this chapter the types of surgical treatment of the vertebral column itself are discussed.

As a result of injury to the spine, the bony structures and spinal and nerve root tissues and cells, ligaments, muscles, and other soft tissue structures may be stretched, crushed, fractured, or dislocated and the spinal cord may be crushed, contused, compressed, or severed.[3] Fracture dislocation of the cervical spine is not always accompanied by quadriparesis or tetraplegia. Often only localized paralysis and/or sensory disturbances are present, and on occasion there may be no neurologic deficit at all. Contusion and disruption of the spinal cord may be irremediable. On the other hand, secondary effects such as circulatory impairment, vasomotor disturbances, venous stasis, secondary hemorrhage, thrombosis, and edema may, for a time after the initial injury, be reversible.

Also, destruction of the intervertebral disc and herniation of the nucleus pulposus can cause injury to the spinal cord and nerve roots. Rupture of a disc may not cause a subarachnoid block to myelography or spinal puncture but may cause very severe neural damage, possibly due to compression of the anterior spinal artery.

184

The goal of surgical treatment is manifold. In the acute stage the purpose of surgical treatment is to furnish the spinal cord and nerve roots with the best possible conditions for improvement and recovery. It may include skeletal traction, described in another chapter, laminectomy, fusion, or both. One or all may be prescribed in certain circumstances, and the judgement of the physician is important. There may be legitimate differences of opinion among respected and reputable physicians concerning the optimal therapy as well as the most appropriate time to intervene. A dogmatic treatment regime is not possible in a spinal injured patient. The sparing of even a single nerve root in the cervical spine may mean an enormous amount to the quadriplegic who will spend the rest of his life partially dependent on others. The spared nerve root may give him some hand function, which can make the difference between complete dependence and the ability to care for himself. Also, it is theoretically possible that proper surgical treatment, realignment, fusion, and/or laminectomy for decompressive purposes may prevent future pain resulting from increased angulation and compression of nerve roots that are exquisitely pain sensitive. One of the late complications of spinal injury is pain from encroachment on nerve roots by excessive callus formation or osteoarthritis.

The timing of surgical procedures has been under discussion for years. It stands to reason that the earlier realignment and/or decompression can be carried out, the better.[32] Realignment might be considered a type of internal decompression. Lately many physicians have concluded that even delayed decompression of spinal injuries carries some increased benefits. Although little has been published in the English language literature, Russian authors have been advocating late laminectomy to accomplish some recovery of function even months to years following injury.[46] If the spinal cord is adequately reduced, fusion procedures can be carried out in the subacute stage. However, the earlier fusion is done following stabilization of the general condition of the patient, the less time the patient will have to remain in the recumbent position. The latter carries increased risks of pneumonia, decubiti, and other complications of the parplegic state discussed in other chapters. Lately halo traction devices have been used to make ambulation earlier.

It should be stressed that there are no absolute criteria for either operative or nonoperative treatment. Whether the patient has been operated upon or treated without surgery, spontaneous recovery and various degrees of improvement have been reported in the literature. Both points of view are strongly advocated by respected champions of various forms of treatment. It is a fact that no statistically significant study has been carrried out, and indeed it might be impossible to do so under present circumstances. That published results depend to a large degree on the training, the experience, the beliefs, the idiosyncrasies, and the prejudice of the physician can be easily verified by reviewing many of the papers contained in the reference section of this chapter.

Once surgical treatment has been carried out, there is again considerable difference of opinion concerning how long a patient should be immobilized either in the prone position with tongs (skeletal traction) or with a halo or other plaster cast or neck brace. Whether the patient should have internal fixation and how long he should be kept in bed are both extremely controversial. The decision concerning immobilization following surgical treatment for injury, for that matter, depends on the experience and beliefs of the physician caring for the patient. It stands to reason that a certain length of time is necessary for healing of soft tissue and formation of a solid bony fusion. Redislocation does occur with early mobilization and prolonged fixation or recumbency is now favored, although in the past early mobilization following fusions was advocated.[67] In our experience such patients may experience acute dislocation or slow angulation, defeating the purpose of the fusion. Andersen and Horlyck,[5] in their report of a large series of patients with dorsolumbar spine fractures, advocated early ambulation. The goal of spinal fusion is to prevent redislocation and further spinal cord damage and to correct or prevent further vertebral deformity.

In anticipation of surgery, one must consider the general condition of the patient and must be particularly aware of injury or malfunction of other organ systems. Chronic paraplegics suffer from renal disease, decubitus ulcers, metabolic disorders, decreased serum proteins, altered liver function, and autonomic hyperreflexia, and the inability of the vasomotor system to respond normally could result in shock.[88]

## ANTERIOR FUSION

Anterior fusions may be carried out in the cervical spine, incuding the C1–C2 area, the lower cervical spine, the thoracic spine, as well as in the lumbosacral spine.

## UPPER CERVICAL SPINE ANTERIOR FUSION

Several authors have described anterior approaches either through the oropharynx or via extrapharyngeal routes. Murray and Seymour[60] described an anterior extrapharyngeal suprahyoid approach to the first, second, and third cervical vertebrae. Grote et al.[38] described removal of the odontoid process (dens epistropheus) by a transpharyngeal approach. Indications for removal of the dens are very uncommon and include situations in which, when fusion is carried out posteriorly, a persistently dislocated dens impinges on the spinal cord anteriorly. With proper reduction and fusion, removal is rarely required. Stabilization of the upper cervical spine by the transoral transpharyngeal route has also been described by Bonney,[13] Fang and Ong,[28,29] Grote et al.,[38] and Estridge and Smith.[26]

There are different approaches to the transoral fusion. The patient must be intubated and have adequate airway. The palate is elevated and the mouth held open with a McIvor gag. Operative localizing x-rays can be made after a needle is inserted in the operative site if necessary. A 3 to 4 cm vertical incision is made into the pharynx. Using periosteal elevators fibrous tissue and soft tissue are scraped away from the bone. Following the technique of Estridge and Smith,[26] a dowel of bone is inserted into the actual fracture line in the odontoid, after using a high-speed burr to roughen and undercut sclerotic bone margins. The dowel graft of bone is inserted as manual traction is applied to the head. When the traction is released, the graft is locked in position. Bonney[13] recommended preoperative tracheostomy. Stabilization was secured by insertion of cortical bone grafts or insertion of cancellous bone. He stated that two struts of cortical bone can be slotted into the body of the axis and notched into the anterior arch of the atlas. The space between them can be filled with cancellous bone. Alternatively he stated that stability could be assured by packing with cancellous chips after partial decortication of the

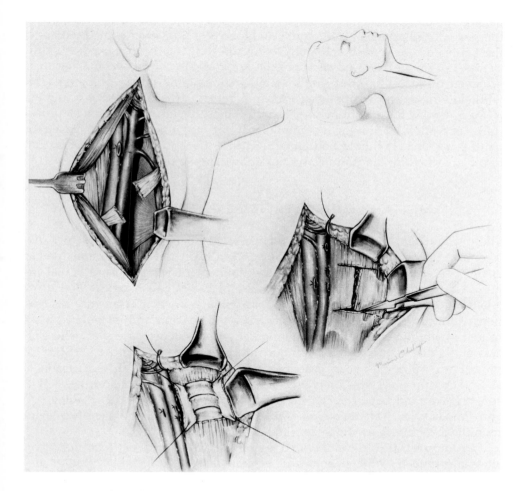

*Fig. 1.* Anterolateral approach to upper cervical spine. (After De Andrade and Mac-Nab[21])

upper vertebrae. He then used halo traction. Fang and Ong[28] and Fang et al.[29] describe several approaches to the upper cervical spine. The transpharyngeal, transoral route was advocated, and they used placement of bone from an iliac crest into the lateral masses between the atlas and axis for achievement of fusion. They removed the anterior arch of the atlas and the odontoid process in certain cases.

The anterior extrapharyngeal suprahyoid approach is used by Murray and Seymour[60] as well as Fang et al. (Fig. 1).[29] A collar incision is made along the uppermost crease of the neck at the level between the hyoid bone and the thyroid cartilage extending as far as the carotid sheaths. The sternohyoid and the sternothyoid muscles are divided and the thyrohyoid membrane exposed and detached as near to the hyoid bone as possible to avoid damage to the internal laryngeal nerve and superior laryngeal vessels. The hypopharynx is entered by cutting into the exposed mucous membrane from the side to avoid damaging the epiglottis. Traction on the hyoid bone and epiglottis exposes the posterior pharyngeal wall, and a midline vertical incision is made to bone; the bodies of the second and third or fourth vertebrae can be exposed sufficiently to remove diseased or abnormal bone or to achieve fusion. Fusion is achieved by inserting strut grafts of autogenous bone into a prepared graft with slots made in the opposing vertebral bodies. The insertion of the grafts is made easier by extending the cervical spine during the operative procedure, and then permitting resumption of the original somewhat flexed or neutral position. It should be pointed out that the upper vertebral bodies can also be reached by the routine anterior approach.

## MID- AND LOWER CERVICAL ANTERIOR FUSION

The introduction of the anterior approach to the management of fracture dislocation primarily in the cervical spine, but also in the thoracic and lumbar spine, has added a new dimension to treatment of vertebral and spinal injury. The work of Smith and Robinson[75] and Bailey and Badgley[9] first drew attention to the feasibility of the anterior approach in cervical fracture dislocations. Cloward (Figs. 2–12)[17–19] popularized the concept and introduced a set of instruments that have made this operation considerably simpler. The success and value of the anterior approach in cases of fracture and dislocation of the cervical spine has been described by Goran,[36] Riley et al.,[68] Aronson et al.,[7,8] Drompp et al.,[23] Taheri and Gueramy,[80] Cantore and Fortuna,[14] Wilson,[89] Perret and Green,[63] DePalma and Cooke,[22] Fielding et al.,[31] Riley,[67,68] and Pineda,[64] as well as others. Anderson et al.[6] describe experiences with multiple level interbody fusions in 16 patients.

Drompp et al.[23] recommended early operation, and we tend to agree, since the time that the patient will be immobilized is lessened. Taheri and Gueramy[80] describe the use of "kiel" (calf) bone in cervical interbody fusion. Cantore and Fortuna[14] agree that kiel bone can be used. In our opinion, this material is less desirable in fracture dislocations than in cervical spondylosis

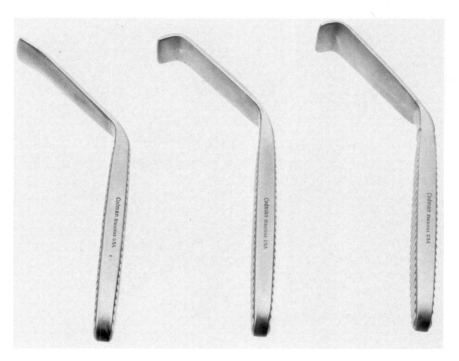

*Fig. 2.* Cloward blade retractors 18, 20, 23 mm wide. (All Cloward instrument photos courtesy of Codman and Shurtleff, Inc. Randolph, Mass 02368)

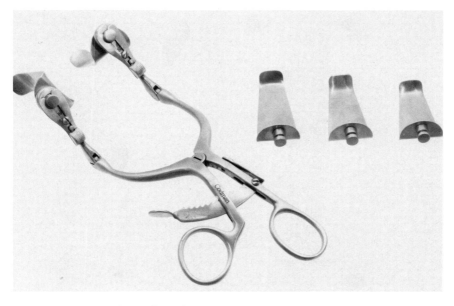

*Fig. 3.* Cloward small cervical retractor with blunt blades.

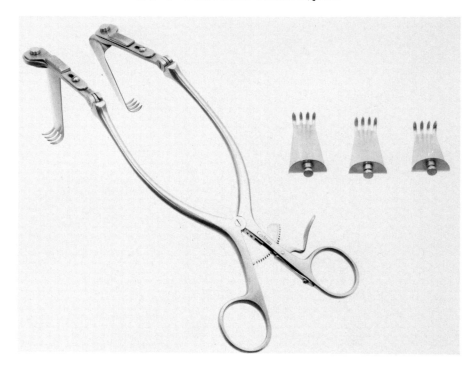

*Fig. 4.* Cloward large cervical retractor with sharp blades.

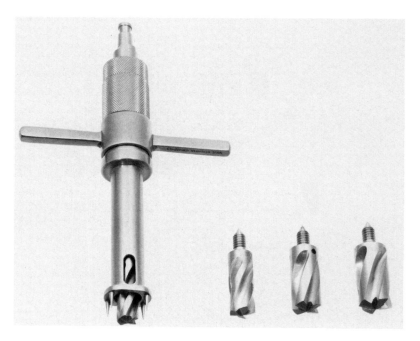

*Fig. 5.* Cloward drill shafts, drill tips, cross bar, and cervical drill guard.

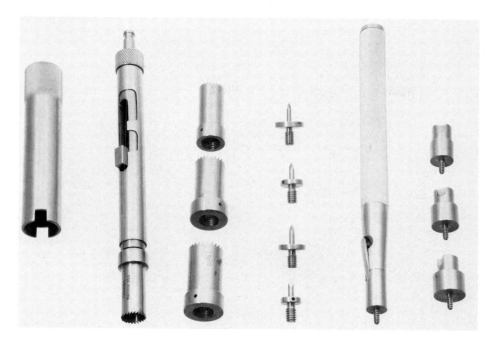

*Fig. 6.* Cloward dowel ejector, dowel cutter handle, dowel cutters and center pins, dowel handle, and impactor set.

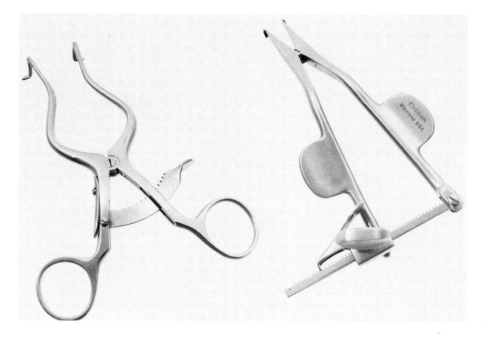

*Fig. 7.* Cloward tissue retractor and cervical interbody vertebra retractor for retracting two vertebral bodies.

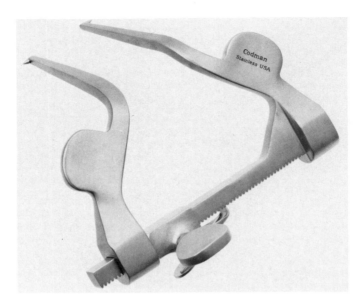

*Fig. 8.* Large Cloward intervertebral body retractor. Used when entire body is replaced. Opens wide enough to go from first to third vertebral body.

or disc disease, because we believe autologous bone heals more rapidly. The kiel bone splint makes iliac osteotomy unnecessary. But since iliac osteotomy is generally simple, we do not use the kiel bone or artificial material such as methylmethacrylate in fusions for fracture dislocation. We have not encountered complications of iliac osteotomy such as persistent pain or osteomyelitis, although these have been reported.

DePalma and Cooke[22] describe generally good results with few complications in their large series of anterior interbody fusions of the cervical spine. Their series is largely comprised of cervical spondylosis or degenerative disc disease. McFadden[50] used a stereotactic apparatus to assist in reduction of cervical fractures immediately prior to anterior fusion.

Fielding et al.[31] discussed the propriety of multiple segment anterior fusion when necessary. They feel the technique is quite satisfactory. In bursting fractures of the anterior cervical bodies, at least two levels of fusion followed by prolonged immobilization may be required for adequate healing without subsequent angulation. Posterior fusion is probably more satisfactory in bursting fractures.

Anterior cervical fusion between C3 and C7 may be performed through a transverse or a longitudinal skin incision. The transverse skin incision is sufficient for exposure of three consecutive vertebral bodies and two consecutive intervertebral discs. A longitudinal skin incision should be used in the unusual circumstance that a longer segment of the cervical spine is to be exposed. The landmark for placing either incision is the palpable anterior border of the sternomastoid muscle. A transverse skin incision should be centered over the anterior border of the sternomastoid muscle overlying the segment of the spine to be exposed. Generally the fifth, sixth, and seventh cervical segments should be approached through a transverse skin incision placed two to three finger breadths superior to the clavicle, and the third, fourth, and fifth cervical segments through a transverse incision placed three to four finger breadths superior to the clavicle.

A longitudinal incision should be made overlying the anterior border of the sternomastoid muscle and may be extended from the tip of the mastoid process to the suprasternal notch. The platysma muscle is grasped between forceps and sharply incised at the lateral limb of the transverse incision or at the caudal limb of the longitudinal incision, bluntly separated from the underlying structures by passing a blunt clamp or Metzenbaum scissors deep to the muscle, and sharply incised in line with the skin incision. If the platysma muscle is bluntly separated from the deeper structures before incising it, inadvertent incision of the underlying sternomastoid muscle will be avoided. The anterior border of the sternomastoid muscle must be clearly identified and mobilized throughout the limits of the incision. The middle layer of cer-

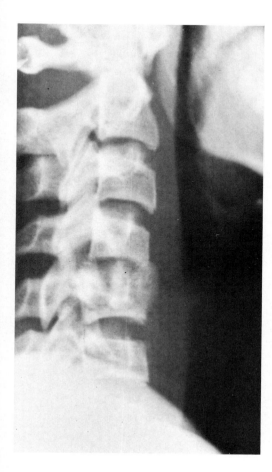

*Fig. 9.* Recent interbody fusion C4-C5. Fusion adequate but less C4 purchase than ideal.

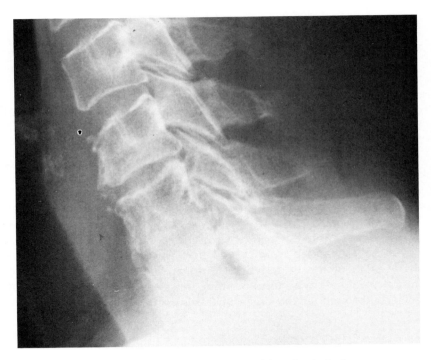

*Fig. 10.* Three-month-old cervical interbody fusion.

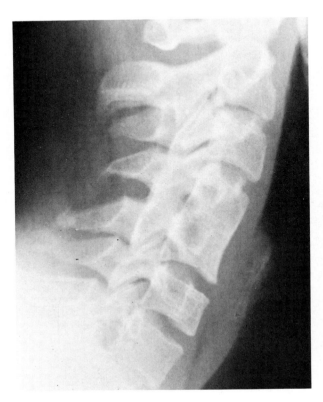

*Fig. 11.* Congenital vertebral fusion C4–C5 (block vertebrae) (no clinical significance).

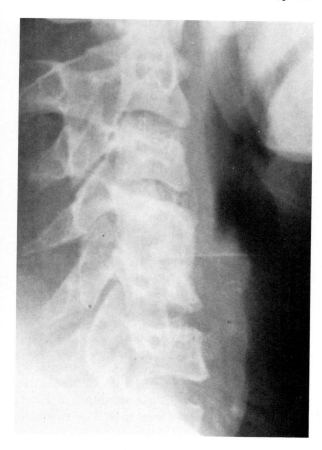

*Fig. 12.* Ancient interbody fusion C4–C5.

vical fascia is demonstrated as the sternomastoid muscle is retracted laterally. The omohyoid muscle may be seen crossing the field in the midportion of the neck at this level and may be mobilized and retracted inferiorly, superiorly, or transected to secure adequate exposure. The carotid artery is then palpated. After accurately identifying the artery, the middle layer of cervical fascia is sharply incised just medial to and parallel with the carotid sheath. As the sternomastoid muscle and the carotid sheath are retracted laterally, the anterior surface of the cervical spine may be palpated.

The esophagus lies just posterior to the trachea, or more superiorly, posterior to the larynx. After having retracted the esophagus, trachea, and thyroid gland medially, the prevertebral fasciae are incised longitudinally with cutting cautery in the midline of the neck and retracted to either side. It is important that the palpable anterior tubercles of the transverse processes not be mistaken for the vertebral bodies, or an incision, which should be made through the paravertebral fascias in the midline, may be made instead through the longus colli muscle with resulting damage to the cervical sympathetic chain or to the vertebral artery which lies deep to the longus colli muscle. The longus colli muscles may be sharply elevated from the intervertebral discs and vertebral bodies to allow more complete exposure of the entire segment of the vertebral bodies and the intervertebral discs.

The resulting exposure is sufficient for anterior cervical discectomy and fusion, and anterior decompression of the cervical portion of the spinal cord following comminuted fractures of the vertebral bodies.

Identification of the space is usually done by x-ray after inserting a needle into the disc space. At this point the graft can be prepared. The hip has been previously elevated on one sand bag. An incision is made 8 cm long parallel to and 2 to 4 cm below the crest of the ilium. Following skin retraction, the aponeurosis and muscles are cut perpendicular to the iliac crest. Dissection of the muscles from the external side of the crest is sufficient only to place the Cloward dowel cutter for removal of one or two grafts. The dowel cutter is impinged against the bone and always placed perpendicular to its surface. To ensure this, a cerebellar extension with the Hudson brace is useful. The dowel must be cylindrical in shape with the end surfaces at right angles, otherwise a poorly fitting dowel cut at an odd angle may result. This may cause poor fusion and vertebral collapse.

Returning to the neck, drilling of the selected space is then done with Cloward instruments with due consideration for the angle of the intervertebral space. The drilling should be in the plane of the space between the bodies to avoid undesirable angulation and excessive bleeding from venous channels in bone. The offset position of the dowels when two or more spaces are used is also important, as is leaving sufficient bone tissue between the drilling spaces. Initial drilling is carried to a depth of 18 mm in adults. Further drilling is done cautiously in 2 mm steps. The posterior longitudinal ligament may be removed with a Cloward angular cervical punch. Using small curettes, the remaining pieces of disc may be removed if necessary.

Using either traction or the vertebral spreader, the bone dowel is inserted. It is desirable that the anterior cortical surface of the dowel be inserted to a depth of at least 1 to 2 mm below the surface of the vertebral bodies. The strength of the fusion rests mostly on the cortical segment and not on the cancellous portion of the dowel. Closure of the incision is accomplished by approximation of the platysma muscle and skin edges.

The Smith-Robinson type of graft which is not prefitted as in the Cloward technique does not seem as efficacious in cervical spine injury.[69-71,75,77] In that technique the iliac bone is fashioned into a plate which is placed between the vertebral bodies after traction or a vertebral body spreader is used to distract the vertebral bodies (Fig. 13). Robinson emphasizes perforation of the subchondral boney end plates for vascular access to the graft.

Via the anterior approach a vertebral body which has been crushed may be excised and a replacement bone graft placed (Fig. 14). Complete excision of one or more vertebral bodies may be required when there is extensive fracture. A bony graft can then be utilized to maintain alignment and stability. With exposure of the involved vertebral body by the anterior approach, the involved vertebra is resected using rongeurs and curettes. Care must be exercised to prevent further injury to the spinal cord. Often the posterior

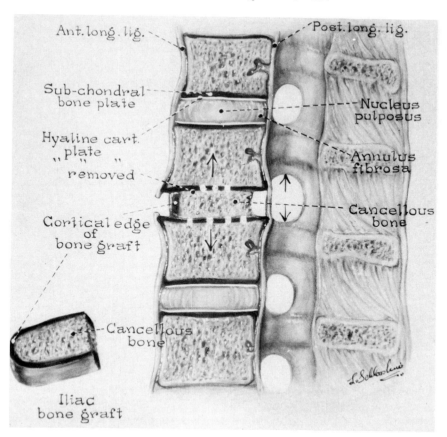

Ant. long. lig.

Post. long. lig.

Sub-chondral bone plate

Nucleus pulposus

Hyaline cart. plate " " " removed

Annulus fibrosa

Cortical edge of bone graft

Cancellous bone

Cancellous bone

Iliac bone graft

*Fig. 13.* Smith-Robinson graft. (Courtesy of J Bone Joint Surg 44A:1569–1587, 1962)

longitudinal ligament is torn or frayed. After several days, the natural line of demarcation between the posterior longitudinal ligament and the vertebral body is lost. The vertebra may be vascular and hemorrhage may be encountered. Some advocate saving of the subchondral cortical end plates of adjacent vertebrae for support for the inlayed bone graft. The graft should be fashioned so that it will fit into the defect tightly. The upper and lower intact vertebral bodies should be notched so that the graft may be fitted into a trough and lodged tightly. The cervical spine may be extended for insertion of the graft. Cancellous bone chips can then be layed over the graft prior to replacement of the longitudinal vertebral muscles. The anterior longitudinal ligaments may then be approximated.

There are certain pitfalls that must be avoided in anterior cervical spine surgery.[64] These include recurrent laryngeal nerve paralysis, collapse of vertebrae, nonfusion, and infection. Although complications are uncommon, some have occurred and paralysis has been reported.[45] Verbiest[81–83] advocated anterior fusion, and resected vertebral bodies completely or partially

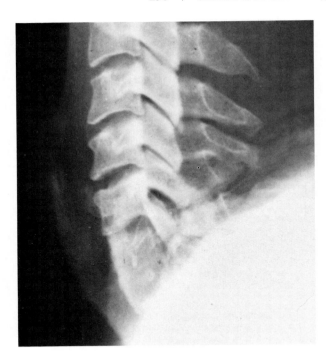

*Fig. 14.* Replacement of vertebral body after bursting fracture.

with inlay tibial grafts with good healing. Occasionally an onlay graft sutured into place was necessary to hold the inlay graft in place. Whitecloud and LaRocca[87] used a fibular graft for extensive lesions involving several segments, stating that the large amount of cortical bone yielded was advantageous. Such procedures are rarely necessary in our experience. Street[79] and Murray[59] advocated resecting the spinal cord scar resulting from the injury. The ends of the cord proved viable by biopsy of frozen section are placed in close apposition, which is made possible by resection of a portion of the vertebral column. This procedure is not recommended because spinal cord does not regenerate. Paul et al.[62] recommend transthoracic surgical decompression of acute spinal cord injuries. The thoracic cord is decompressed by removal of the pedicle. The vertebral column is stabilized by a bone graft which is fixed in place by screws. Chou and Seljeskog[16] also describe transthoracic decompression. In the lumbar region, anterior transperitoneal fusion has also been advocated.[33] This operation is uncommonly used for lumbar stabilization following fracture dislocation.

Acrylic plastics have been used for stabilization of the spine. Scoville et al.[74] employed methyl methacrylate for vertebral replacement or fixation in metastatic disease of the spine. Hamby and Glaser[41] replaced the curreted disc with methyl methacrylate with salutary results. Kelly et al.,[43] as well as Stowsand and Muhtaroglu,[78] used acrylic fixation in atlantoaxial dislocation for posterior stabilization. It is our view that in fracture dislocation use of autologous bone is preferred since it appears to be more stable in the long run and possibly has a lower incidence of infection.

## ANTEROLATERAL APPROACH TO THE UPPER CERVICAL SPINE

De Andrade and MacNab[21] described an approach to the basiocciput and anterior upper cervical spine. Figure 1 shows this lateral approach and anatomical structures involved. Access to the basiocciput anteriorly is limited by the mandible and subglottic structures superficially and by the internal carotid artery, cranial nerves, and pharynx deeper. There is limited access to this area and many potential hazards to this approach. Such an approach is generally not of use in spinal injury, but possibly could be utilized for fusion using autologous bone. A trough is fashioned and bone layed into the trough. Some advocate preliminary tracheostomy but this is not necessary in all cases. The patient should be immobilized for about a month, some of the time in skeletal traction. External stabilization is maintained by bracing until fusion is established radiographically in four to six months. Halo traction may replace a long period of recumbency. This approach can be utilized for fusion of the occiput to C1 and C2, but inclusion of the occiput is not necessary in most cases.

Southwick and Robinson[77] describe an anterior lateral approach to the upper cervical spine through a longitudinal incision parallel to the sternocleidomastoid muscle. This is a difficult approach and is similar to the one described by De Andrade and MacNab.[21]

## POSTERIOR FUSION

Posterior fusion is a widely accepted technique in the cervical, thoracic, and lumbar spines (Figs. 15–30). Indications for this procedure frequently overlap those for anterior fusion, particularly in the cervical spine. We prefer the posterior fusion only in bursting fractures of the vertebral bodies and in atlantoaxial dislocations. Thus, in the cervical spine it is not used as frequently as anterior fusion. Posterior fusion is most frequently employed in the thoracic and lumbar spine.

Several different operations have been advocated for the treatment of atlantoaxial fracture dislocations.[1,20,24,35,48,52,72] Posterior fusion of the C1 and C2 vertebrae seems to be the procedure most often chosen.[4,20,35,72] Mixter and Osgood[54] originated the concept of posterior fixation of C1 to C2. They described a technique making use of a strong silk thread wound around the posterior arch of the atlas and tied to the spinous process of the axis. Cone and Turner[20] were pioneers in the use of wires[58] and bone grafts for C1 to C2 fusions. Gallie[35] fused the adjacent articular facets while also wiring C1 to C2. Although they reported good results with early fusion for the treatment of

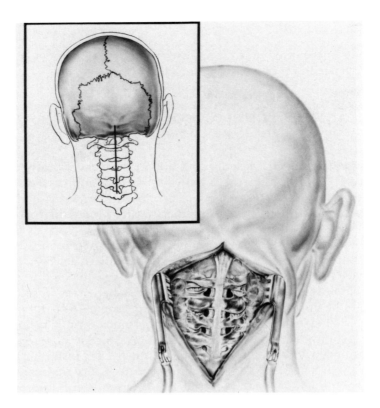

*Fig. 15.* Incision and exposure for C1–C2 fusion.

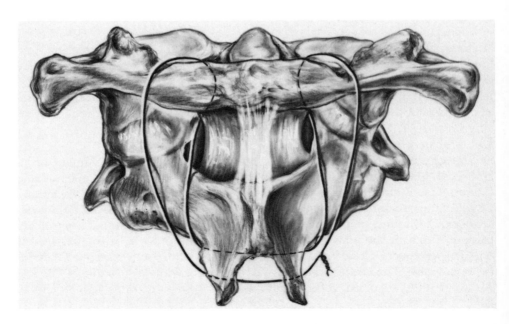

*Fig. 16.* Wiring for C1–C2 fusion.

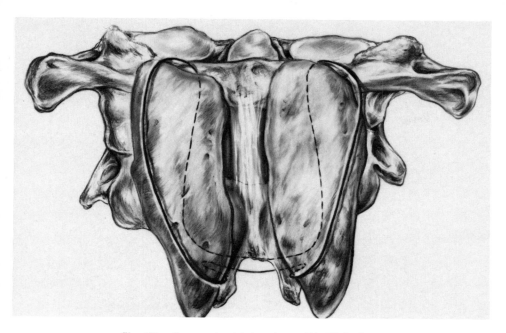

*Fig. 17.* Bone wired into place, C1–C2 fusion.

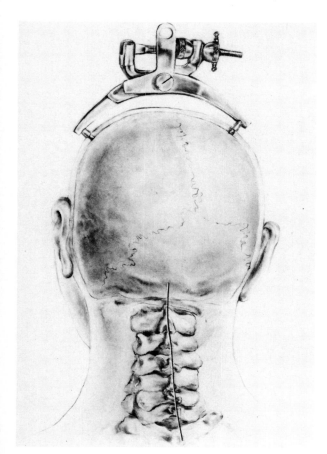

*Fig. 18.* Incision for posterior cervical fusion.

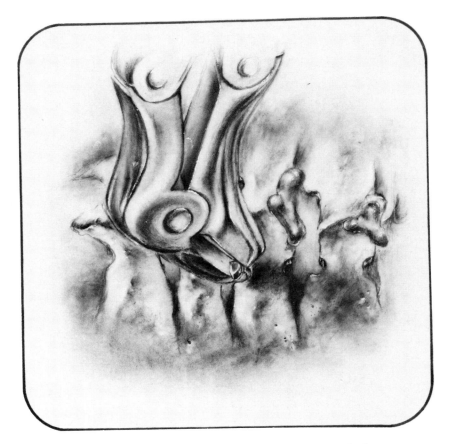

*Fig. 19.* Removing part of lamina for passage of wire.

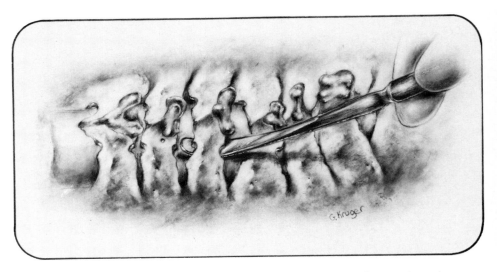

*Fig. 20.* Periosteal elevator under lamina in preparation for passing wire.

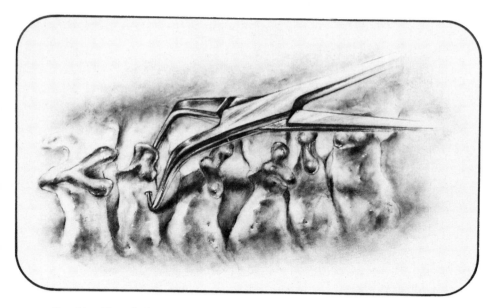

*Fig. 21.* Towel clip utilized for wire hole at base of spinous process.

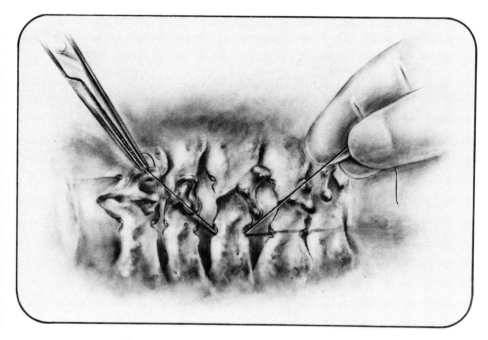

*Fig. 22.* Passing wires for posterior fusion.

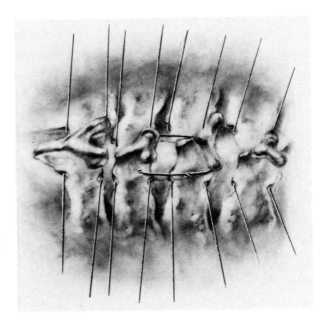

*Fig. 23.* Wires passed under laminae and at base of spinous processes. Generally wires need not be passed around each lamina as indicated in figure.

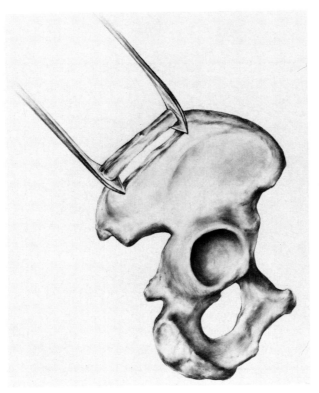

*Fig. 24.* Technique for removing bone from iliac crest.

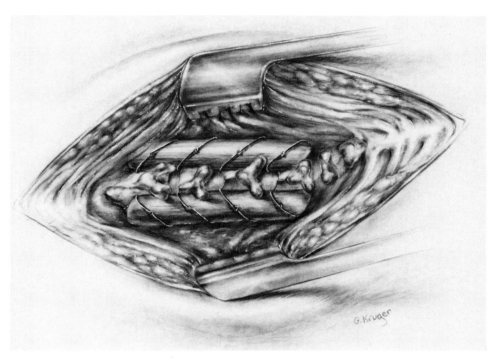

*Fig. 25.* Bone wired into place, fusion completed.

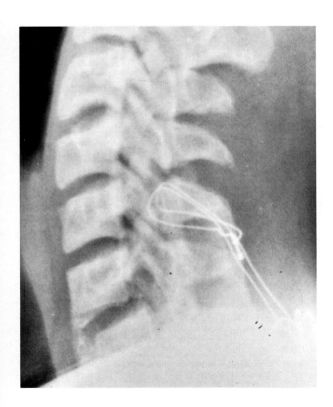

*Fig. 26.* Posterior cervical fusion, wires and bone struts visible, lateral radiograph.

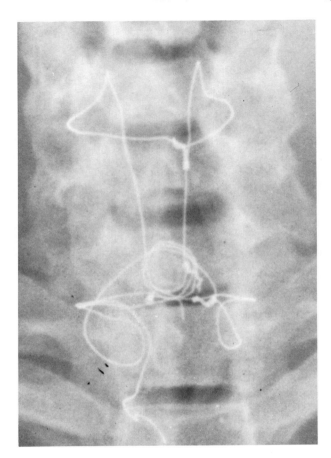

*Fig. 27.* C5–C7 fusion, anterior-posterior radiograph.

atlantoaxial fracture dislocations, neither Gallie[35] nor Cone and Turner[20] published sufficient details for comparison with other methods of treatment. Alexander et al.[1] claimed that fusion of only C1 and C2 gave unsatisfactory results. C1 to C3 fusion was advocated. In two cases recurrent dislocation occurred several months after operation. Dunbar and Ray[24] stated that C1 to C2 fusions were inadequate because they had seen "several recurrent dislocations following this procedure." Schlesinger and Taveras[73] demonstrated two cases in which wiring of C1 to C2 was ineffective; furthermore, they found that subsequent radiographs often revealed broken wires. However, Schatzker et al.[72] found generally successful results from the Gallie fusion in 14 cases. Only 2 of these cases were considered failures, from recurrent atlantoaxial dislocation, but they stressed that successful fusion did not prevent slight malalignment of the dens nor prevent nonunion of the fracture. Sound atlantoaxial fixation was the goal of their fusions. McWhorter et al.[53] described posterior fusion in children.

Once the normal relationships of the vertebrae with one another are established and following exposure of the spinous processes and lamina from

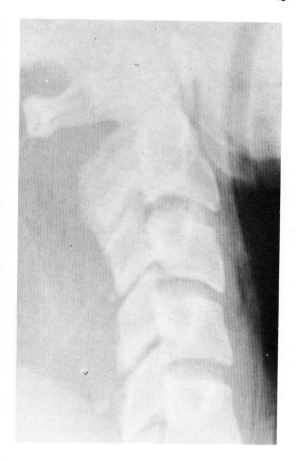

*Fig. 28.* Lateral radiograph of extensive laminectomy of cervical spine.

behind, wires are passed under the affected laminae bilaterally. An alternative approach is to pass wires around only the normal vertebrae laminae above and below the fracture site. Passage of the wire is facilitated by removal of small portions of the lamina with a Kerrison punch using no. 18 or 20 wire. The dura is separated from the lamina by a small periosteal. The cortical bone of the lamina and spinous process is denuded of periosteum and lately we have used a high-speed drill to roughen the bone edges. Autogenous bone, obtained usually from the iliac crest but sometimes from a rib or other bone, is then wired into place. The periosteum should be denuded from the graft. Small bone chips are packed in the crevices.[2,61] Fusion of the unstable cervical spine at the C1–C2 levels is frequently carried out in rheumatoid arthritis.[30] Fusion of the occiput to the atlantal arch and axis has been advocated,[40] but is not used by most surgeons at present because dislocation between the occiput and the atlas is rare. Including the occiput in the fusion for C1–C2 dislocation does not add to stability but has been carried out for nontraumatic fusions.[37]

Lewis and McKibbin[47] described treatment of unstable fracture disloca-

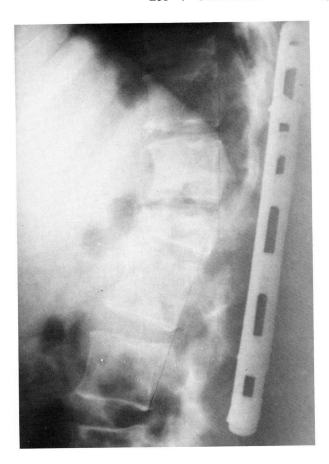

*Fig. 29.* Thoracic stabilization lateral view.

tions of the thoracolumbar spine accompanied by paraplegia. It was their conclusion that to preserve long-term spinal function, open reduction and internal fixation are indicated in displaced fractures. Although no differences in the degree of neurologic recovery could be detected between the surgically and nonsurgically treated groups, the surgically treated patients had significantly less residual spinal deformity and significantly less serious pain. In fact, they stated that no serious pain developed in any of their surgically treated patients.

## LAMINECTOMY

For many years laminectomy has been carried out to relieve compression on the injured spinal cord. Its proponents advocate its use early in spinal cord injury, but it has also been advocated in chronic phases.[46] A block to lumbar puncture or myelography has been suggested as a prerequisite. We do not subscribe to this, since an opening only the size of the spinal needle need

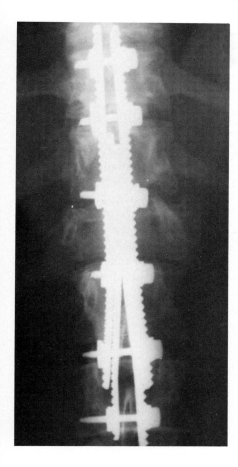

*Fig. 30.* Thoracic stabilization anterior-posterior view.

be present for normal dynamics. We have carried out laminectomy without myelography to avoid the time required for this procedure in the presence of severe neurologic deficit and severe dislocation. Another indication for laminectomy is the impossibility of performing closed reduction. A partial or complete laminectomy may then be required, to unlock facets for example, so that adequate reduction can be achieved.

In our experience, as in that of most surgeons, laminectomy has been a safe procedure. Other physiatrists and surgeons[15,39,42,55] have stated that laminectomy is dangerous or is not effective. Nevertheless, many patients do wish everything humanly possible to be done. Unsuccessful outcome after laminectomy has been reported,[44] and indeed, complete recovery from established tetraplegia is rare.

The question of whether the dura should be opened at the time of laminectomy is unanswered. If it is opened, the complication rate is increased. If it is not opened, significant hematomata may be overlooked. If the dura is opened it is frequently not possible to close, so that it must be left open or a dural substitute may be used for closure.[10] After laminectomy, posterior fusion is possible and is frequently carried out.[27] The fusion need be only lateral, involving facets and transverse processes.

## POSTERIOR LATERAL FACET FUSION

The technique employed is described by Robinson and Southwick.[70] The facet surfaces are fused from one level above the area of laminectomy to one level below using corticocancellous bone wired to the facets at each level. A small drill hole with a 7/64th-in. drill is made in the inferior articulating facet with a periosteal elevator wedged between the inferior and superior articulating facets. The wire is then brought out above the superior articulating facet and the longitudinal graft from the iliac crest is wired into place at several levels. This technique may be utilized when a laminectomy has been performed. The procedure is carried out bilaterally. The facet fusion extends over four levels. A posterior intraspinous fusion is carried out below the fused facets to the second thoracic spinous process. This prevents a subsequent development of kyphosis below the fused facets. Support in the form of tong traction or halo traction should be maintained for a considerable period of time.

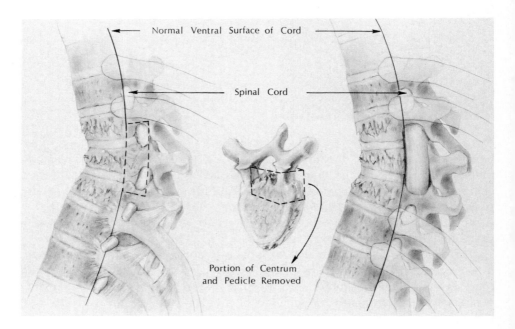

*Fig. 31.* Left: The fifth and sixth rib heads have been removed exposing the foramina between T5–T7 compression of the ventral spinal cord in the area outlined by the broken rectangle. The osteotomy begins with resection of the pedicle of T6 (center). The extent of the completed bone resection in the coronal plane is outlined by the broken line. Right: The completed resection in the longitudinal plane. Facets remain intact. (Courtesy of Paul et al: J Neurosurg 43:299, 1975)

## THORACOABDOMINAL APPROACH TO THE LOWER
## THORACIC AND UPPER LUMBAR SPINE

It is occasionally necessary to expose the lower thoracic and upper lumbar spine in continuity (Figs. 29–32). This presents a problem in exposure because of the diaphragm. A lower thoracotomy incision is made at the level of seventh to eleventh rib depending upon the desired level of the section. The incision extends from the plane of the scapula to the anterior margin of the rib cage. The latissimus dorsi muscle is transected across its fibers and the serratus anterior is divided and spread over the intended rib level. Intercostal muscles are divided and the thoracic cavity is opened utilizing a self-retaining rib retractor. The lung is deflated and retracted anteriorly and superiorly. A circumferential incision is made in the muscular portion of the diaphragm adjacent to the costal margin. This should be extended posteriorly to the area of the lateral arcuate ligament. The incision is then extended through the peritoneal reflextion of the diaphragm and the spleen and the contents of the left upper quadrant of the abdomen are exposed. The retroperitoneal space is open by blunt dissection. Abdominal organs are gently retracted medially using a Deaver retractor. The vertebral bodies and aorta are then exposed. The aorta is mobilized by a combination of sharp and blunt dissection and

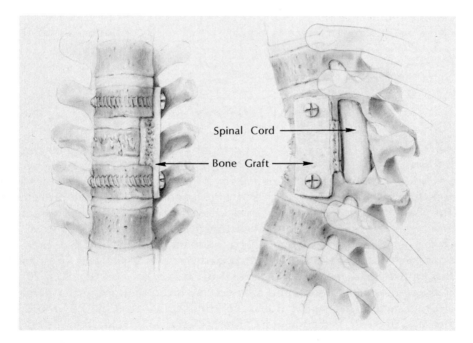

Spinal Cord

Bone Graft

*Fig. 32.* Lateral fusion after decompression illustrated in Figure 31. The template of bone is shown in both anterior-posterior and lateral views. The screws should pass from cortex to cortex of the vertebra body. Right: The relationship of the graft to the decompression. (Courtesy of Paul et al: J Neurosurg 43:299, 1975)

segmental vessels are ligated and divided to permit visualization of the involved vertebral bodies. Grafting and even resection of a vertebral body can be carried out. Fusion and inlayed bone grafting in a trough can be accomplished through this exposure. The anterior longitudinal ligament may be closed over the vertebral bodies. Various anatomic structures are reapproximated and chest tubes should be utilized and attached to water seal suction. Erickson et al.[25] advocated lateral decompression-stabilization (Figs. 33–36) for fracture dislocation.

## ANTERIOR LATERAL APPROACH TO THE LUMBAR VERTEBRAL BODIES

An anterior lateral approach to the lumbar vertebral bodies through an oblique and long flank incision can provide direct access to all lumbar vertebral bodies. In the case of spinal injury grafting can be carried out but removal of the vertebral bodies is quite difficult through this approach. A transperitoneal approach to the vertebral bodies can be carried out for anterior interbody fusion, but abdominal viscera and major vessels must be carefully retracted. In addition the hypogastric nerve plexus should be protected to avoid postoperative complications of impotence and sterility in males. The anterior lateral approach to the lumbar vertebrae is similar to that used for lumbar sympathectomy.

## MYELOTOMY

A myelotomy is an opening into the posterior substance of the spinal cord at the posterior longitudinal fissure following laminectomy and opening of the dura.[85] Allen[3] performed experimental myelotomies on a series of dogs and then on three patients in the early 1900s. Postoperatively, slight improvement in neurologic functions below the level of injury was noted in all three patients. Freeman and Wright[34] described functional recovery in dogs in whom paraplegia would otherwise have been permanent. They implied that the rapid internal decompression of traumatized necrotic tissue was responsible for the improvement in function. Benes[11] discussed his experience in 20 patients undergoing myelotomy, and seemed convinced that no further damage, beyond that incurred at injury, was done to the spinal cord by the procedure. Wagner and Rawe[56] performed an anterior cervical myelotomy, using the operating microscope and bipolar coagulation. They emphasized the ease with which hemorrhagic gray matter could be separated from normal gray and surrounding white matter. Myelotomies have been carried out for intractable pain[66,76] and for spasticity.[12,56,57]

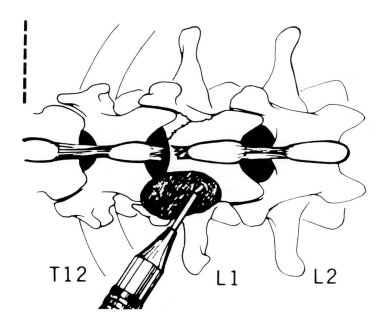

*Fig. 33.* Initiation of lateral decompression in one-stage decompression-stabilization for thoracolumbar fractures. Dorso ventral view. Note use of air drill for removal of lateral lamina, facet, and pedicle. (Courtesy of Erickson et al, Spine 2:53, 1977)

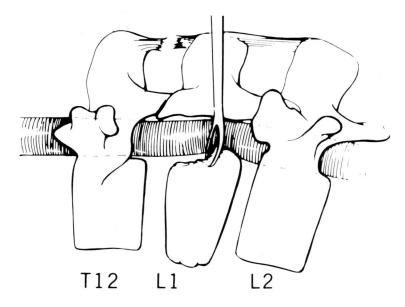

*Fig. 34.* Removal of retropulsed portion of comminuted vertebral body in one-stage decompression-stabilization for thoracolumbar fractures. Lateral view. (Courtesy of Erickson et al, Spine 2:53, 1977)

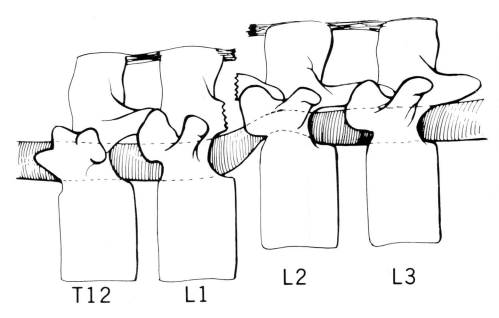

*Fig. 35.* Thoracolumbar dislocation prior to realignment, reduction, or removal of retropulsed portion of vertebral body. Lateral view. (Courtesy of Erickson et al, Spine 2:53, 1977)

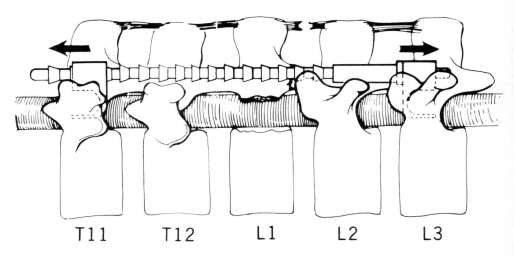

*Fig. 36.* Restoration of alignment after Harrington rod placement. Lateral view. In addition, intervening zygaphophyseal joint fusion and addition of autologous bone can enhance fusion. (Courtesy of Erickson et al, Spine 2:53, 1977)

# REFERENCES

1. Alexander E, Jr, Forsyth HF, Davis CH, Jr, Nashold BS, Jr: Dislocation of the atlas on the axis. The value of early fusion of C1, C2, and C3. J Neurosurg 15: 353–371, 1958
2. Alexander E, Jr, Davis CH, Jr, Forsyth HF: Reduction and fusion of fracture dislocation of the cervical spine. J Neurosurg 27:588–591, 1967
3. Allen A: Remarks on the histopathological changes in the spinal cord due to impact: An experimental study. J Nerv Ment Dis 41:141–147, 1914
4. Amyes EW, Anderson FM: Fracture of the odontoid process. Report of sixty-three cases. Arch Surg 72:377–393, 1956
5. Andersen PT, Horylck E: Fracture of the spine. Acta Orthop Scand 40:653–663, 1969
6. Anderson LD, Stivers BR, Park WI, III: Multiple level anterior cervical spine fusion. A report of 16 cases. J Trauma 14:653–674, 1974
7. Aronson N, Bagan M, Filtzer DL: Results of using the Smith-Robinson approach for herniated and extruded cervical discs. Technical note. J Neurosurg 32:721–722, 1970
8. Aronson N, Filtzer DL, Bagan M: Anterior cervical fusion by the Smith-Robinson approach. J Neurosurg 29:396–404, 1968
9. Bailey RW, Badgley CE: Stabilization of the cervical spine by anterior fusion. J Bone Joint Surg 42A:565–594, 1960
10. Bartal A, Schiffer J, Vodovotz D: Silicone coated dacron for enlargement of dural canal in cervical disc surgery. Neurochirurgia 13:46–49, 1970
11. Benes V: Spinal Cord Injury. Balliere, London, 1968
12. Bischof W: Zur dorsalen longitudinalen myelotomie. Zbl Neurochir 28:123–126, 1967
13. Bonney G: Stabilization of the upper cervical spine by the transpharyngeal route. Proc R Soc Med 63:40–41, 1970
14. Cantore G, Fortuna A: Intersomatic fusion with calf bone "Kiel Bone Splint" in the anterior surgical approach for the treatment of myelopathy in cervical spondylosis. Acta Neurochirurgica 20:59–62, 1969
15. Carey PD: Neurosurgery and paraplegia. Rehabilitation Jan-March: 27–29, 1965
16. Chou SN, Seljeskog EL: Alternative surgical approaches to the thoracic spine. Clin Neurosurg 20:306–321, 1973
17. Cloward RB: The anterior approach for removal of ruptured cervical discs. J Neurosurg 15:602, 1958
18. Cloward RB: Treatment of acute fractures of the cervical spine. J Neurosurg 18: 201–209, 1961
19. Cloward RB: Lesions of the intervertebral discs and their treatment by interbody fusion methods. The painful disc. Clin Orthop 27:51–77, 1963
20. Cone W, Turner WG: The treatment of fracture-dislocations of the cervical vertebrae by skeletal traction and fusion. J Bone Joint Surg 19:584–602, 1937
21. De Andrade JR, MacNab I: Anterior occipito-cervical fusion using an extra-pharyngeal exposure. J Bone Joint Surg 51:1621–1626, 1969
22. DePalma AF, Cooke AJ: Results of anterior interbody fusion of the cervical spine. Clin Orthop 60:169–185, 1968
23. Drompp BW, Siebert WE, Fulgenzi WR: Early stabilization of certain fractures and fracture-dislocations of the cervical spine. Clin Orthop 34:42–52, 1964
24. Dunbar HS, Ray BS: Chronic atlanto-axial dislocations with late neurologic manifestations. Surg Gynecol Obstet 113:757–762, 1961
25. Erickson DL, Leider LL, Brown WE: One-stage decompression-stabilization for thoracolumbar fractures. Spine 2:53–56, 1977
26. Estridge MN, Smith RA: Transoral fusion of odontoid fracture. Case Report. J Neurosurg 27:462–465, 1967

27. Fairbank TJ: Spinal fusion after laminectomy for cervical myelopathy. Proc R Soc Med 64:634–636, 1971
28. Fang HSY, Ong GB: Direct anterior approach to the upper cervical spine. J Bone Joint Surg 44A:1588–1604, 1962
29. Fang HSY, Ong GB, Hodgson AR: Anterior spinal fusion. The operative approaches. Clin Orthop 35:16–33, 1964
30. Ferlic DC, Clayton ML, Leidholt JD, Gamble WE: Surgical treatment of the symptomatic unstable cervical spine in rheumatoid arthritis. J Bone Joint Surg 57A:349–354, 1975
31. Fielding JW, Lusskin R, Batista A: Multiple segment anterior cervical spinal fusion. Clin Orthop 54:29–33, 1967
32. Forsythe HF, Alexander E, Jr, David C, Jr, Underal R: The advantages of early spine fusion in the treatment of fracture-dislocations of the cervical spine. J Bone Joint Surg 41A:17–36, 1959
33. Freebody D, Bendall R, Taylor RD: Anterior transperitoneal lumbar fusion. J Bone Joint Surg 53B:617–627, 1971
34. Freeman L, Wright T: Experimental observations of concussion and contusion of the spinal cord. Ann Surg 137:433–443, 1953
35. Gallie WE: Fractures and dislocations of the cervical spine. Am J Surg 46:495–499, 1939
36. Goran A: Fracture dislocation of cervical spine. NY State J Med 69:1050–1058, 1969
37. Grantham SA, Dick HM, Thompson RC, Jr, Stinchfield FE: Occipito-cervical arthrodesis. Clin Orthop 65:118–129, 1969
38. Grote W, Romer F, Bettag W: Der ventrale zugang zum dens epistropheus. Langebecks Arch Chir 331:15–22, 1972
39. Guttmann L: Surgical aspects of the treatment of traumatic paraplegia. J Bone Joint Surg 31B:399–403, 1949
40. Hamblen DL: Occipito-cervical fusion. Indications, technique and results. J Bone Joint Surg 49B:33–45, 1967
41. Hamby WB, Glaser HT: Replacement of spinal intervertebral discs with locally polymerizing methyl methacrylate. Experimental study of effects upon tissues and report of a small series. J Neurosurg 16:311–313, 1959
42. Harris P: The initial treatment of traumatic paraplegia. Paraplegia 3:71–73, 1965–1966
43. Kelly DT, Jr, Alexander E, Jr, Davis CH, Jr, Smith JM: Acrylic fixation of atlanto-axial dislocations. Technical note. J Neurosurg 36:366–371, 1972
44. Kewalramani LS, Orth MS, Taylor RG, Albrand OW: Cervical spine injury in patients with ankylosing spondylitis. J Trauma 15:931–934, 1975
45. Kraus DR, Stauffer ES: Spinal cord injury as a complication of elective anterior cervical fusion. Clin Orthop 112:130–141, 1975
46. Landau B, Campbell JB, Ransohoff J: Surgical reversal of the effects of long-standing traumatic lesions of the conus medullaris and cauda equina. Proc Ann Clin Spinal Cord Injury Conf 17:23–27, 1967
47. Lewis J, McKibben B: The treatment of fracture dislocation of the thoracolumbar spine. J Bone Joint Surg 56B:391, 1974
48. Lipscomb PR: Cervico-occipital fusion for congenital and post-traumatic anomalies of the atlas and axis. J Bone Joint Surg 39A:1289–1301, 1957
49. Marshall JJ: Judicial hanging. Lancet 1:193–194, 1913
50. McFadden JT: Stereotaxic realignment of the dislocated cervical spine. Surg Gynecol Obstet 133:262–264, 1971
51. McGraw RW, Rusch RM: Atlanto-axial arthrodesis. J Bone Joint Surg 55B:482–489, 1973
52. McLaurin RL, Vernal R, Salmon JH: Treatment of fractures of the atlas and axis. Wiring without fusion. J Neurosurg 36:773–780, 1972

53. McWhorter JM, Alexander E, Jr, Davis CH, Jr, Kelly DL, Jr: Posterior cervical fusion in children. J Neurosurg 45:211–215, 1976
54. Mixter WT, Osgood RB: Traumatic lesions of the atlas and axis. Am J Orthopaed Surg 7:348–370, 1910
55. Morgan TH, Wharton GW, Austin GN: The results of a laminectomy in patients with incomplete spinal cord injuries. Paraplegia 9:14–23, 1971
56. Morrison G, Yashon D, White RJ: Relief of pain and spasticity by anterior dorsolumbar rhizotomy in multiple sclerosis. Ohio State Med J 65:588–591, 1969
57. Moyes PD: Longitudinal myelotomy for spasticity. J Neurosurg 31:615–619, 1969
58. Munro D: The role of fusion or wiring in the treatment of acute traumatic instability of the spine. Paraplegia 3:97–111, 1965
59. Murray G: Surgical treatment of paraplegia. Panminerva Med 14(9):296–303, 1972
60. Murray JWG, Seymour RJ: An anterior, extrapharyngeal suprahyoid approach to the first, second and third cervical vertebrae. Acta Orthop Scand 45:43–49, 1974
61. Nieminin R, Koskinen EVS: Posterior fusion in cervical spine injuries. An analysis of fifty cases treated surgically. Ann Chir Gynaecol Fenn 62:36–48, 1973
62. Paul RL, Michael RH, Dunn JE, Williams JP: Anterior transthoracic surgical decompression of acute spinal cord injuries. J Neurosurg 43:299–307, 1975
63. Perret G, Greene J: Anterior interbody fusion. Arch Surg 96:530–539, 1968
64. Pineda A: Avoidance of certain pitfalls during cervical interbody fusion. Am Surg 34:161–164, 1968
65. Plaut HG: Fracture of the atlas in automobile accidents. The value of x-ray views for its diagnosis. JAMA 110:1892–1894, 1938
66. Putnam PJ: Severe injuries of the cervical spine treated by early anterior interbody fusion and ambulation. J Neurosurg 28:311–316, 1968
67. Riley LH: Surgical approaches to the anterior structures of the cervical spine. Clin Orthop 91:16–20, 1973
68. Riley LH, Robinson RA, Johnson KA, Walker AE: The results of anterior interbody fusion of the cervical spine. Review of ninety-three consecutive cases. J Neurosurg 30:127–133, 1969
69. Robinson RA: Anterior and posterior cervical spine fusions. Clin Orthop 35:34–62, 1964
70. Robinson RA, Southwick WO: Surgical approaches to the cervical spine. Instructional course lecture. The American Academy of Orthopaedic Surgeons. St. Louis, Mosby, XVII:299–330, 1960
71. Robinson RA, Walker AE, Ferlic DC, Wiecking DK: The results of anterior interbody fusion of the cervical spine. J Bone Joint Surg 44A:1569–1587, 1962
72. Schatzker J, Rorabeck CH, Waddell JP: Fractures of the dens (odontoid process). J Bone Joint Surg 53B:392–405, 1971
73. Schlesinger EB, Taveras JM: Lesions of the odontoid and their management. Am J Surg 95:641–650, 1958
74. Scoville WB, Palmer AH, Samra K, Chong G: The use of acrylic plastic for vertebral replacement or fixation in metastatic disease of the spine. J Neurosurg 27:274–279, 1967
75. Smith GW, Robinson RA: The treatment of certain cervical-spine disorders by anterior removal of the intervertebral disc and interbody fusion. J Bone Joint Surg 40A:607–624, 1958
76. Sourek K: Commissural myelotomy. J Neurosurg 31:524–527, 1969
77. Southwick WO, Robinson RA: Surgical approaches to the vertebral bodies in the cervical and lumbar regions. J Bone Joint Surg 39A:631–644, 1957
78. Stowsand D, Muhtaroglu U: Dorsale stabilisierug bei luxationsfrakturen des 1. und 2. halswirbels mit palacos und drahtumschlingung. Neurochirurgia (Stuttg) 18:120–126, 1975
79. Street DM: Traumatic paraplegia treated by vertebral resection, excision of spinal

cord lesion, suture of the spinal cord, and interbody fusion. Proc Ann Clin Spinal Cord Injury Conf 16:92–103, 1967

80. Taheri ZE, Gueramy M: Experience with calf bone in cervical interbody spinal fusion. J Neurosurg 36:67–71, 1972
81. Verbiest H: Anterolateral operations in cervical spinal fractures. Report of a series of 39 cases. Proc Ann Clin Spinal Cord Injury Conf 15:53–55, 1966
82. Verbiest H: Anterolateral operations for fractures and dislocations in the middle and lower parts of the cervical spine. J Bone Joint Surg 51A:1489–1531, 1969
83. Verbiest H: Anterolateral operations for fractures or dislocations of the cervical spine due to injuries or previous surgical interventions. Clin Neurosurg 20:334–366, 1973
84. Vermooten W: A study of the fracture of the epistropheus due to hanging with a note on the possible causes of death. Anat Rec 20:305–311, 1921
85. Vise WM, Yashon D, Liss L, et al: Shallow versus deep midline posterior myelotomy: A comparison of neurologic, histologic, and evoked sensory response changes. In press
86. Wagner FC, Rawe SE: Microsurgical anterior cervical myelotomy. Surg Neurol 5:229–231, 1976
87. Whitecloud TS, LaRocca H: Fibular strut graft in reconstruction surgery of the cervical spine. Spine 1:33–43, 1976
88. Williams WT, Walker JW: Shock: A surgical hazard in the paraplegic. Surgery 42:664–668, 1957
89. Wilson CB: The role of anterior interbody fusion in acute injuries of the cervical spine. Ky Med J 63:260–264, 1965
90. Wolff R: Injury to the cervical vertebrae as a result of judicial hanging. J Med Assoc S Afr 2:460–462, 1928

# 13

## Missile Injuries of the Spinal Cord and Cauda Equina

### INTRODUCTION

While there has been considerable discussion in past literature regarding war-time spinal and vertebral missile injuries,[7,29,63] similar civilian wounds have largely been neglected.[60,76,77] In general, combat injuries are more massive due to increased velocity or size of missiles and these injuries are due predominantly to shrapnel or similar projectiles as opposed to bullets. For example, Poer[62] in considering 77 military patients with spinal paralysis, found that only 17 were injured by bullets and 60 were paralyzed by shell fragments or mines. Distinction between military and civilian bullet injuries will be made in subsequent discussion. In civilian missile injuries of the spinal column, bullets projected from handguns are most common. The following paragraphs will attempt to differentiate, when practical, between various projectiles including shrapnel, military high-velocity bullets, and lower-velocity civilian bullets.

Exact statistics regarding incidence of civilian and military missile injuries are unavailable but most neurosurgeons are called to examine at least one such case per year. In this regard the author personally has recently supervised the care of 13 patients with acute spinal bullet injuries in a 12-month period while serving at a civilian trauma facility in a metropolitan area (Figs. 1–4). During periods of war, missile injuries are common, as manifest by the large quantity of related publications, as well as by an increase in the number of military men on rosters of rehabilitative facilities and listed as chronic spi-

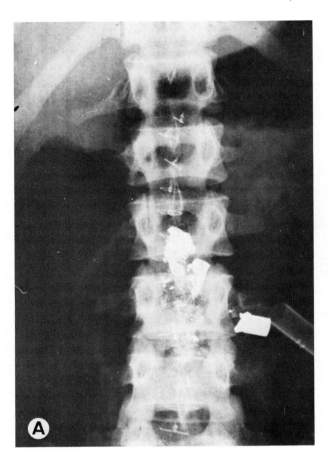

*Fig. 1A.* Anterior-posterior view of large caliber bullet in canal at lumbar 3-4. The patient had laparatomy for the concomitant abdominal injury as indicated by the wire sutures.

nal injuries. In civilian life, with the exponential increase in violent crime, there has been an increase in the incidence of spinal bullet injuries in most trauma centers. Because of their more frequent involvement in both criminal activities and military actions men, as opposed to women, overwhelmingly predominate in this group of patients.[66]

A missile may be defined as any object either purposefully or accidentally projected or thrown. Most commonly the motive is destruction of a distant target, but on occasion a missile results from accidental forces. Projectiles causing human spinal injury are frequently due to an explosive force and usually the causative instrument has been expressly designed to inflict bodily harm. The following discussion will not review the rare local vertebral blunt injury without cutaneous penetration causing temporary concussion[6] or permanent paralysis nor spinal knife wounding which will be covered elsewhere. Only penetrating missile injuries resulting from bullets, shrapnel, or other secondary projectiles will be considered.

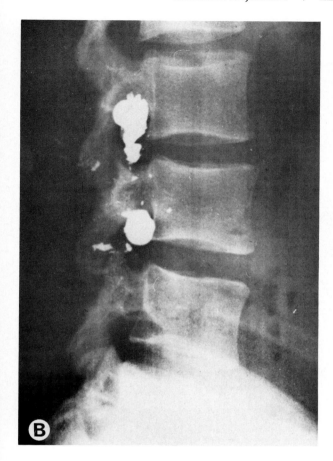

*Fig. 1B.* Same patient as in 1A. Only the most superior fragment is in the canal. Compare with 1A.

## NEUROLOGIC SYMPTOMS AND SIGNS

Neurologic symptoms and signs relate to the level and severity of injury.[44] They include motor and sensory function, as well as sphincter control. In our civilian experience,[76] four broad groups of patients can be identified: (1) immediate complete clinical loss of function of the spinal cord above the conus medullaris; (2) incomplete spinal cord signs which are nonprogressive; (3) progressive spinal cord related deficit; (4) injuries of the conus medullaris or cauda equina with an initial neurological deficit, varying in severity. Heiden et al.[36] identified groups 1, 2, and 3. Groups 1 and 4 are by far the more common. To these may be added patients described in military literature in which significant partial improvement or complete recovery occurs.[6,46] In the acute phase, flaccid paralysis is the rule. Conus medullaris and cauda equina injuries with unilateral signs are occasionally difficult to differentiate from wounds isolated to the lumbosacral plexus. Bloody cerebrospinal fluid on

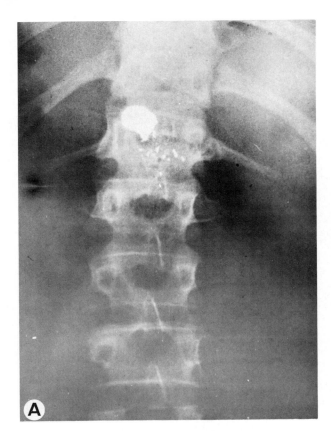

*Fig. 2A.* Large caliber bullet at T12 level.

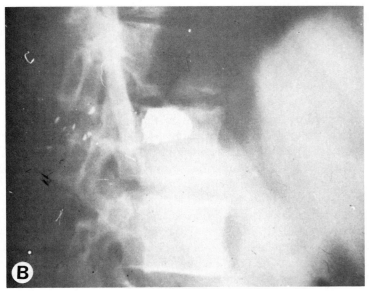

*Fig. 2B.* Same patient as 2A. Bullet lodged in vertebral body T12. Trajectory is from behind as indicated by fragments.

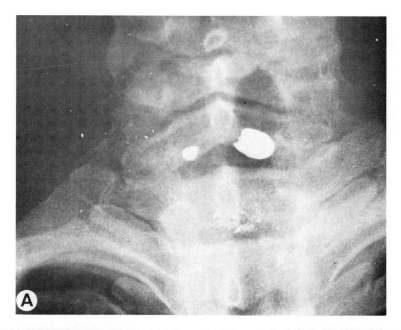

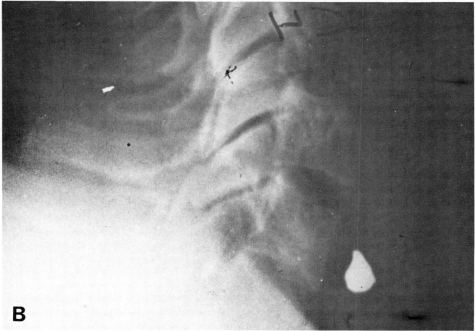

*Fig. 3A.* Bullet at level of C7. Trajectory indicated by fragments. Patient was paralyzed. *B.* Same patient as 3A. Bullet passed anteriorly out of canal.

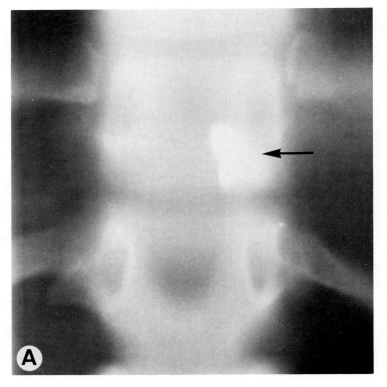

*Fig. 4A.* Laminographic anterior-posterior view of bullet in canal just inferior to pedicle of T11.

lumbar puncture is helpful. Vertebral bony injury, bilateral neurologic findings, sphincter dysfunction, or a lesion proven by surgical exploration also assist in verification.

Kislow[43] has emphasized, as we have,[76] that the level of segmental spinal injury itself may be inaccurate in localizing the actual bony vertebral injury. He found that the level of bone injury differed from the level of the cord lesion in one segment in 15 percent, by two segments in 17.5 percent, by three segments in 6.2 percent, by four segments in 13.7 percent, by five segments in 6.2 percent, and by six or more segments in 41.4 percent of wartime spinal compound fractures.

The familiar signs and symptoms as well as general problems related to acute spinal injury and paraplegia of any cause have been discussed amply and in detail by Guttmann[33] and in many chapters in this volume; hence, they will not be emphasized further in this discussion. Also chronic symptoms and signs as a result of sequelae and complications are essentially identical in all spinal injuries and will not be further discussed here.

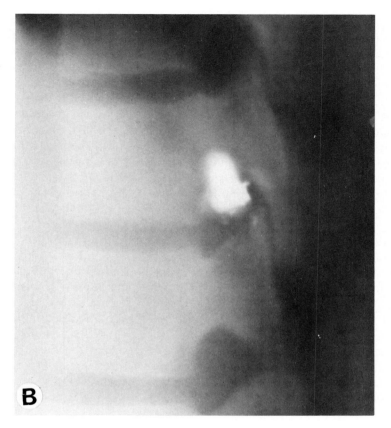

*Fig. 4B.* Laminographic lateral view of same patient as in 4A. Bullet in spinal canal.

## BALLISTICS

Ballistics is the science of motion of projectiles which may be divided into interior ballistics, the motion of bullets within the weapon, and exterior ballistics, the motion of the bullet from the muzzle of the wounding instrument to the target.[26] Wound ballistics can be considered a branch of exterior ballistics in that it concerns movement of a projectile outside of the weapon, but as the movements of missiles in tissues differ markedly from those in air, it is really a separate branch.[8] It may be noted that results of shots from the same lot of ammunition vary, even when equivalent tissues are penetrated. The considerable variation in destructiveness has to do with various minute aspects of construction of bullets and idiosyncrasies of the muzzle of the gun. The energy of the projectile upon hitting a target is not necessarily the only factor with regard to the amount of quantitative damage to the animal tissue. Although the mass of bullets from sidearms and rifles may be similar, energy is much higher in the case of rifles. Velocity is of great importance in determining impact energy. The muzzle velocity of handguns is generally 600 to 1100 ft/sec whereas rifles have initial velocity of 2000 to 4000 ft/sec, and changes in velocity are decidedly more influential than changes in mass in wounding capability.[22-24] In addition to actual energy imparted in the tissue as a factor in causation of wounds, spin of the bullet is also important. This imparts a force that has the property of maintaining a long axis throughout its flight in air, parallel to its position at the time it was launched. Another property of the bullet, namely precession, also functions in exterior ballistics. Precession or wobble is a gyroscopic action invoked by any force tending to displace the axis of rotation and acting at right angles to it. A perfectly balanced bullet has little precession. Thus, forces acting from without, e.g., wind resistance, tissue resistance, dense media, variations in the balance of the bullet, all function in wounding severity. The longitudinal path of the bullet, about a center of gravity, causes the axis of the projectile to rotate in and out of the direct line of flight. This deviation of the axis is called the yaw and is a gentle, almost imperceptible, rhythmic deviation of the bullet throughout its flight, resembling a sine wave. The yaw period is defined as the alteration from the true line of flight and in ordinary flight this is equal, so that as the bullet goes in and out of its direct path, one might speak of a node at each time interval in which the bullet returns to its main line of flight. When a bullet enters a medium denser than air, its motion is retarded so that there is a change in the length of the yaw period. In passing through three inches of water a rifle yaw period of 15 ft in air is reduced to a few inches. Wounds of the spine may vary even at the same missile velocity. If thin bone is encountered, the bullet may pass through leaving a relatively small track. A more resistant, thicker bone impact may cause more extensive destruction by secondary missiles although the primary missile force is blunted. On the other hand, there may be an explosive type of wound as a result of the enormous energy that is imparted. Factors of greatest importance are (1) velocity, (2) tissue density, and (3) bullet wounding, which is a function of shape, mass (including any deformation of the mass), the position of the center of gravity, and spin of the missile.[22] These factors are operative in the bullet that produces injury without serious deformity or dissolution of the missile. In the latter event, multiple secondary missiles are formed and cause additional damage.

The obvious wound track that is present after the bullet has passed through tissue is demonstrable and unmistakable. A less well comprehended aspect of missile damage is the temporary cavity found during instantaneous passage of the projectile. The temporary cavity, particularly in gelatinous nervous tissue is primarily a result of expended kinetic energy, and there is little relationship to bullet shape or composition. It is in effect an explosive cavitational force. All tissue cells lying adjacent to the main track and the temporary cavity become secondary missiles that move outward at enormous speeds to give rise to the expansion cavity. Its size is directly proportional to the energy absorbed by the surrounding tissue.

There are at least three major theories concerning wounding capabilities of bullets.[26] All are directly related to bullet speed and mass. The first is the so-called momentum theory in which the formula is momentum equals mass multiplied by velocity. It has been proposed by those designers of firearms who believe that mass and velocity are of equal importance in wounding and advocate the use of heavy bullets. The heavy bullet is popular in Africa where thick-skinned game is hunted. These are bullets in excess of 250 grains and muzzle velocities seldom exceed 2600 ft/sec. A second and more accepted theory is the kinetic energy theory in which kinetic energy equals the mass/2 multiplied by velocity squared/2. This concept ascribes more importance to velocity than to mass. Doubling mass doubles kinetic energy but doubling velocity quadruples it. The third theory is the power theory in which power equals mass multiplied by velocity cubed. This concept puts a premium on velocity and, as with the kinetic energy theory, small increments in velocity result in enormous changes in wounding potential.

In clinical practice it may not be possible to estimate residual missile velocity in wounds inflicted from a long distance. The large majority of wounds encountered in civilian practice are sustained at shorter distances, usually 50 yards or less, by sidearms. In the latter cases for practical purposes, the published muzzle velocity may be applied to calculations. The published muzzle velocity may also be utilized when considering wounds sustained under 100 yards with high-velocity rifles.

If the terms "missile" and "projectile" are used in reporting, they should be qualified. Finck[26] describes a missile or projectile as implying bullets, pellets from shotguns, or fragments from devices such as grenades and explosive shells. Lagrade,[48] in a monograph on gunshot wounds, stated: "Under the term gunshot wound, the military surgeon includes in his battle return all wounds resulting from the effects of any explosive force." On the other hand, Wallace and Meirowsky[73] utilized the term high-velocity missiles to refer only to bullets from rifles, carbines, machine guns, and other automatic weapons, so that in most military medical literature one cannot be certain if such terms refer to bullets or explosive shells unless explicitly stated. In inflicting injuries the characteristics of the missile itself are of considerable importance, causing different types of injury. The shape of the bullet may be pointed, be round, or have a flat tip. Hollow bullets result in fragmentation and may be encountered in any of the shapes mentioned above. Also, composition of the bullet may be homogeneous, e.g., constructed of one substance such as lead, zinc, magnesium, wood, plastic, or even wax. The composition of the bullet may be described as coated, e.g., a lead bullet covered by a thin layer of copper or brass, and a third category may be a jacketed bullet that has a core of lead or steel partly or totally surrounded by a thicker jacket of copper or steel. Some jacketed bullets have aluminum or bronze tips while armor-piercing ammunition belongs to the jacketed group. Lead bullets are easily deformed and usually expand upon impact. A frequent source of confusion when estimating caliber may occur when a bullet fragments after ricocheting from a bony surface. These fragments can cause multiple wounds that at first may wrongfully be attributed to fragmentation of shrapnel. In addition, damage may be caused by foreign materials either pushed in or due to the suction effect immediately following passage of a high-velocity missile through tissue.

## ASSOCIATED INJURIES

The direct trajectory of the missile may cause associated injuries of blood vessels in the neck and trachea, vital structures within the thorax, as well as abdominal injuries. Such associated injuries as a result of a single missile may take precedence in treatment over the spinal injury. These complications occur in approximately 25 percent of civilian cases, but 77 of 114 military patients (67 percent) had major associated injuries.[40] Chest injuries causing hemopneumothorax are most common, followed by gastrointestinal and renal lesions. Traumatic subarachnoid pleural fistulae resulting from bullet wounding have been described[5] in thoracic injuries but are rare. These are generally self-limited but uncommonly may require thoracentesis and/or later closure of the dural or pleural rent. Sherk et al.[68] reported an arteriovenous fistula of the vertebral artery with a gunshot injury of the atlas.

## INVESTIGATIONS

In all patients, anterior-posterior and lateral x-rays of the appropriate area should be obtained (Figs. 1–4). This is for the purpose of exact localization of the bullet and its fragments as well as for determination of trajectory. Determination of exact trajectory may be inaccurate and mostly academic since deflection by tissues as well as ricocheting from bone may occur. In a few instances, in spite of careful radiographic survey, fractures of vertebral elements cannot be detected although they do exist and may be found at laminectomy. Also, in some patients the trajectory may indicate that the spinal canal has not been transgressed by the missile. In those cases where there is actually no bony disruption, shock waves are presumed to have caused permanent neurologic dysfunction, although it is possible that deflection of the bullet may have occurred and the straight line between radiographic location of the metallic fragment and the area of entrance may not represent the true trajectory.[46] It is also theoretically possible that a bullet has transgressed the spinal canal without injury to bone. Polytomography has enabled us to determine the exact position of the bullet in relation to the spinal canal when this was questionable.

A question exists as to the need for myelography for more accurate localization of the spinal cord lesion prior to laminectomy. The present author has not advised myelography in most patients prior to surgery since the level of laminectomy can be adequately determined in almost all cases from neurologic examination, approximate trajectory, and fracture site as seen on x-ray. The cerebrospinal fluid (CSF) is frequently bloody in spinal missile injuries.[76] It has been said that myelography with bloody CSF may lead to arachnoiditis.

The possibility of arachnoiditis is a lesser argument against myelography. Lumbar puncture is usually unnecessary, in the author's opinion, in acute cases since it adds little information. It has been suggested and is also the author's view that positive or negative Queckenstedt's test does not enable one to predict prognosis and that decision for or against operation should not be based on CSF dynamics.[53]

## PATHOLOGY

The pathology of acute missile injuries to the spinal cord is best described from gross surgical dissections, since few patients' spinal cords with acute missile injuries have been studied histologically.[6,7] The destruction of the spinal cord may vary from complete anatomic severance to a normal gross appearance with or without slight contusion and edema. In the latter case, even with a normal-appearing spinal cord, permanent paralysis may ensue and is in fact a frequent occurrence in civilian practice. Cadwalader[7] emphasized, after studying gunshot injuries to the brain and spinal cord, that even when no actual penetration occurs damage may be severe. In those cases he emphasized the lack of hemorrhage with extensive softening. Bone fragments and foreign material may be found implanted into spinal cord. Small epidural and subdural hematomas may occur. One might surmise the actual histologic appearance of the spinal cord from the nature of acute central nervous system injuries seen and reported in brain. An excellent description of overall spinal pathology is provided by Wolman.[75]

Any discussion of spinal missile injuries must consider the reaction of central nervous system tissue to retained metal fragments, as this has been a central issue in the decision as to extent of surgical therapy. Some maintain that retained metal must be removed under any circumstances. Fischer et al.[27] studied changes in the cat brain after introduction of metallic and insulated wire composed of silver, copper, and stainless steel, or coated with four insulating materials. Silver and copper without insulation caused noticeable histologic damage and necrosis. Stainless steel and insulating materials were well tolerated. Pilcher[61] reported on outcome in an experimental preparation of penetrating wounds of the brain. A total of 54 dogs had metallic foreign bodies introduced into the cerebral substance. These were unsterile and were inserted to varying depths and left in place for different periods of time. Foreign bodies penetrating the ventricle and allowed to remain protruding through the skin invariably produced a fulminating infection involving meninges, brain, and ependyma. Removal of the protruding foreign body within 12 hours after its insertion greatly reduced the incidence of fatal infection as did failure to penetrate the ventricle. Closure of the scalp over the foreign body reduced the incidence of fatal infection and prolonged survival time if infection developed. Deeply inbedded foreign bodies that did not communicate with the skin or subarachnoid space did not cause fatal infection unless the ventricle had been traversed. In the author's experience, metal in the tissues surrounding the spinal cord is well tolerated. Courville[15] has reported on histologic findings in ancient missile wounds of the brain, and his major interest was in scar formation in relation to these defects. In that report bullets were retained in cerebral tissue for 43, 47, and 50 years respectively, and in a fourth patient for several years; the exact time was unknown. These patients died of unrelated extracerebral causes. In that paper, as well as in others cited, few ill effects of the foreign body per se were reported.[30,67]

## TREATMENT

All patients receive large doses of parenteral broad spectrum antibiotics and tetanus prophylaxis. Corticosteroids in large doses have been administered recently without any rise in infection rate, which already had been quite low. The beneficent effects of corticosteroids on severely damaged spinal cords is doubtful.

Although the clinical results[44,45] of all causes of insult to the spinal cord and cauda equina are nearly identical, to accurately assess the effects of operation or any other treatment in a given patient, the various wounding agents as well as elapsed time must be considered independently. In the acute stage, hypovolemia, muscle and sphincter paralysis, respiratory disturbances, anesthesia, ileus, and temperature irregularities occur in varying degrees no matter what the etiology or extent of central nervous system disconnection. In addition, the chronic paraplegic state is characterized by spasticity, urinary tract infection, and bedsores. In missile injuries, shock due to blood loss and other extensive associated injuries often complicate the picture. Thus, although the effects of a fracture dislocation due, e.g., to a fall are exactly those of a bullet injury, the associated pathology varies and considerations leading to proper treatment may also be unrelated. This distinction may possibly apply to injuries from civilian bullets in contrast to those resulting from wartime missiles, which generally either have higher velocities or cause more extensive wounding.[77,78]

The generally poor outcome in civilian cases is surprising.[36,76] Recovery does not seem to depend on the form of therapy; no patient with signs of complete loss of neural function had significant neurologic recovery no matter what therapy was employed. The lack of neurologic return perhaps is related to the low velocity of the civilian sidearm missile with a decreased incidence of concussive-type trajectories, direct hits being necessary for the damage. There is no agreement that surgery is better than no therapy in this situation, even when gross neurologic derangement is present.[32] An argument against surgery is the fact that in some patients subjected to laminectomy the spinal cord appears normal. This is particularly true in combat where higher velocity bullets impart greater energy and can cause significant central nervous system dysfunction as a result of a distant penetration with resultant shock waves. Thus there may be a higher incidence of "concussion" in war wounds. Roussy and Lhermitte[64] found a high incidence of concussive type wounds. This is postulated as the reason for the immediate complete loss of neurologic function with later significant rapid clinical recovery reported in some military publications. Injuries restricted to the area of the bony vertebral column in civilian wounds without depression of fragments and minimal proximal soft tissue explosive effects probably do not cause spinal cord decompensation even of a transient nature. A military high-energy bullet with an identical trajectory could conceivably result in severe neurologic loss due to shock waves in spite of noninvolvement of the central nervous system by the missile.

The sensory level can be utilized to decide the area of laminectomy but variations in sensory loss in relation to wounding occur as emphasized by Kislow.[43] For these reasons, if a normal-appearing cord is encountered at operation, then the laminectomy should be extended. X-ray evaluation of the magnitude of vertebral fracture has been inaccurate compared with direct vision of bony disruption at the time of surgery in judging whether depression of fragments or cramping of spinal contents exist. In many cases no fracture could be identified on x-rays, and none was discerned at the time of surgery because of ventral trajectory. In other cases no fracture is seen on preoperative x-rays, but at surgery extensive bony depression and fragmentation exist. In no case has dislocation been present so that instability has never been encountered in the present author's experience. Stabilization by tongs in cervical fractures has, therefore, been unnecessary and fusion has not been required. In chronic cases having laminectomy, abnormal curvatures have been encountered.

It might appear that the presence of a bullet or a large metallic fragment within the spinal canal is an absolute indication for laminectomy, since it is a contaminated foreign body and, although relatively benign, takes up space within an already full canal. Removal of the bullet in these cases was attended by no gross improvement,[76] although not all patients were operated upon promptly. Infection did not develop in any patient in whom fragments remained, but large doses of antibiotics were administered. Also, contaminated foreign material other than metallic may soil the track leading to the spine so that debridement may be required.

Cauda equina injuries are generally not as severe as spinal cord lesions because of sparing of roots. The intact roots may account for spotty neurologic loss. They are attended by a better overall prognosis compared to spinal cord injuries, but significant neurologic improvement did not occur in severely injured patients.[76,77,78]

In several cord injury patients the initial sensory and motor level fell a few segments (with or without surgery) within the early days following trauma. This has been attributed to higher concussive effects or cephalad circulatory disturbances with a possible relation to transient edema. The level observed in these patients, after dropping slightly, did not fall further and complete loss of function remained but at a slightly lower level. The importance of this observation is that, if the sensory level immediately after injury is used as the sole guide to the site of laminectomy, the operation may be a few segments cephalad to the actual injury. Also such a dermatomal fall should not generate false optimism.

Recently it has been shown in an experimental situation that local cooling can prevent spinal cord damage following trauma.[1] This does not necessarily mean that it will have value in treating spinal cord missile injuries in man, but in view of rather uniform agreement on the lack of benefit of most other forms of treatment to date, such therapy is deserving of a scientific trial. Thus, the author's own tentative guidelines in the management of spinal trauma due to bullet wounds are as follows. In general, patients with complete lesions seen after 24 hours[1] will not be operated upon unless there is gross contamination. Patients seen within 12 hours will have laminectomy and be considered for cooling.[1] There is, however, considerable controversy in this area as is discussed elsewhere. Significant intraspinal foreign bodies will be removed. Finally any management regime must be individualized and at present must be considered arbitrary.

## REVIEW OF PERTINENT LITERATURE

Signs, symptoms, and pathology of spinal injuries in warfare have been elaborated in the three classic papers of Holmes.[37-39] Munro[55-58] has discussed additional aspects of combined civilian injuries to the spinal cord. Claude and Lhermitte,[11,49] Naffziger,[59] Fay,[25] Mayfield and Cazan,[53] Knight,[47] Cohen and Rogers,[12] Botterell et al.,[4] Matson,[50] Davis and Martin,[21] Campbell,[9] Campbell and Meirowsky,[10] Davis,[20] and Meirowsky[54] have contributed to the understanding of operative and late management in combat trauma to the spinal cord. Daniels[18] has reported fractures and dislocations of the spine in warfare. Tinsley[72] discussed compound injuries of the spinal cord in warfare and observed that anatomic damage, including that to bone, is far worse when seen at surgery than as suggested by preoperative x-ray studies. Our experience reinforces that concept.

Taylor et al.[71] discussed general problems in war injuries of the spine, and Ford[28] displayed World War I radiographs in gunshot wounds of the spine. Keith and Hall[41] reported similar studies. Davis and Martin[21] describe spinal cord injuries including various aspects of treatment. Wannamaker[74] describes spinal cord injuries of warfare during the Korean conflict discussing 254 penetrating wounds and 46 closed fracture dislocations. Jacobson and Bors[40] reported on spinal cord injuries in Vietnamese combat as seen in a Veterans Administration Hospital in the continental United States. Of 114 patients, 57 (50 percent) had spinal injuries due to bullets. The remainder were caused by shell fragments (33), blast (13), and miscellaneous injuries; 107 had laminectomies. These were seriously damaged individuals and apparently few had significant neurologic recovery below the level of injury. Thirteen percent had cervical, 22 percent upper thoracic, 32 percent lower thoracic, and 33 percent of patients had lumbosacral injuries; 69 percent had complete and 31 percent had incomplete lesions.

The aforementioned papers report a variety of etiologies for wartime spinal cord injury. In combat many casualties result from fragmentation injuries which are more massive and must be considered seriously contaminated. These are obviously at variance from civilian bullet wounds. Rifle bullet wounds in warfare result from greater impact energy than that from handguns, as in most civilian cases, because of the high velocity of a rifle projectile.

Buckshot injuries to the spinal cord are uncommon. Four spinal injury patients of a total of 24 central nervous system shotgun injuries were reported by Sights.[69] One recovered completely by one year after having been immediately paraplegic. No perforation of dura was seen at laminectomy. Another patient was rendered immediately and permanently paraplegic. A third had damage to the conus medullaris with loss of sphincter function. Progressive improvement in function occurred. The fourth patient had no neurologic deficit. At close range this type of injury causes an enormous explosive force. Seven years after a buckshot pellet lodged in the L2–L3 interspace the patient described by Daniel and Smith[17] developed excruciating pain and hyperesthesia without other signs. Myelography revealed a complete block. With removal of sterile suppurative and metallic material complete recovery ensued.

Many opinions have been expressed regarding the problem of surgical intervention in spinal cord injuries, including those of Covalt et al.,[16] Matson,[52] and Davidoff,[19] who stated when speaking of all causes of spinal cord injury: "Laminectomy for the treatment of spinal cord injury is seldom indicated and when indication exists, should seldom be done as an emergency." Mayfield and Cazan[53] considered laminectomy in compression injuries of the cord only if there was an incomplete lesion and the patient was progressively losing function. This clinical sequence has been extremely uncommon in the present author's[76] as well as Heiden et al.'s[36] bullet injury experience. Scarff,[65] referring to gunshot wounds, stated that all should be explored because of their compound nature and a missile within the spinal canal should always be removed no matter how long after injury. Matson,[50] when speaking of treatment of compound spine injuries at forward army hospitals said:

> When neurological examination reveals a complete physiological transection of the cord at a well-demarcated level and there is a history of instantaneous loss of all motion and sensation from the moment of injury with no subsequent change, an early operation is not indicated. If x-rays demonstrate that a foreign body has transversed the spinal canal or lies across the canal or if bony fragments largely obliterate the canal, in instances of complete physiological transection, the outlook is even more hopeless. . . . In the presence of either complete or incomplete physiological transection of the cord, laminectomy is not indicated in the absence of x-ray evidence of fracture or of foreign body encroaching upon the spinal canal . . . Spinal shock, as a result of trauma in the neighborhood of the spinal column without actual mechanical pressure on the cord or division of its continui-

ty, is a definite entity. Decompression of such a concussed cord is felt to be of no avail.

Matson also stated that injuries to the cauda equina should be explored.[51]

Kennedy et al.[42] advocated more frequent operative intervention in spinal cord injuries not due to subluxation for the following indications: (1) It is impossible to determine clinically whether an apparently complete transverse lesion of the cord is not really a temporary physiological interruption, (2) a CSF block is demonstrable, (3) the disability is progressive, and (4) a CSF leak exists and the dura must be closed. Suwanwela et al.[70] discussed prognosis in spinal cord injury with special reference to patients with motor paralysis and sensory preservation in relation to surgical therapy.

Comarr and Kaufman[14] surveyed neurologic results of 858 spinal cord injuries of combined etiologies; of 579 laminectomized patients, 16 percent had significant postoperative improvement. Of 279 patients not operated upon, 29 percent were improved. Laminectomized patients were felt to represent a group with more severe injuries, and cauda equina lesions improved with greater frequency than spinal cord lesions. Spinal subarachnoid block was an important factor influencing prognosis. Patients with complete block who were not operated upon did not improve. Gross observation of the injured cord at surgery did not afford a reliable indication of prognosis unless the cord was obviously transected. Many patients having normal-appearing cords did not improve, but many with subtotal lesions improved. In that regard Haynes[35] described complete loss of function with normal-appearing cords in several cases of war wounds of the spinal cord.

Concussion of the spinal cord is generally, but not necessarily, understood to imply transient neurologic findings without a gross anatomic lesion. We have not seen such cases in civilian practice resulting from bullet injuries. Baker and Daniels[2] discussed eight military patients in whom a lesion was caused by a perforating bullet that passed transversely near the spinal cord striking or barely missing bone. Paralysis of the extremities persisted from a few hours to a few weeks with complete recovery. In those patients initial bladder disturbances were absent. Groat et al.[31] attempted to clarify the term "uncomplicated spinal cord concussion." They believed this term implies a complete functional block of the spinal cord at the level of application of a force sufficient to cause neural physiologic decompensation. Baldwin[3] provided the histologic descriptions of two cases of spinal concussion. There was a small focus of softening in the posterior and lateral columns and in the ventral horns. Hassin[34] described traumatic degeneration of the spinal cord as spinal concussion because microscopic findings were present. Lhermitte[49] felt that spinal concussion as described above was due to the reaction of the entire spinal cord and the sudden elevation of CSF pressure caused by the bullet energy. Obviously a clear clinical and morphologic definition of the term concussion is necessary and differs in various publications.

In Pool's 57 cases of wartime gunshot wounds of the spine,[62] surgical management was accomplished in 35 (61.4 percent); there were 3 cervical, 16 thoracic, 14 lumbar, and 2 sacral injuries. Of the 35 operative patients, 20 showed appreciable postoperative improvement, 11 showed none, and 4 died (11.4 percent). The highest incidence of improvement was in the group with cauda equina lesions (12 of 14 cases). Pool's patients apparently had bullet and fragmentation injuries.

## PROGNOSIS

Collier[13] emphasized that if pathologic toe signs, reflexes, and spasticity occur prior to the seventh day the lesion is incomplete and some recovery may occur. We have seen several such patients but recovery of neurologic function has been insignificant. In the author's experience the prognosis of a spinal bullet injury with initial severe neurologic deficit is extremely poor, regardless of therapy. Very few patients have recovered significant neurologic function if they had complete loss of motor and sensory function initially. One patient who had severe but incomplete loss of function now ambulates with braces and arm crutches. This dismal outlook is not true judged by reviewing military literature as mentioned earlier in the discussion. Prognostic prediction in the military is complicated by lack of accurate follow-up, resulting from evacuation principles necessitated by warfare, but it would appear that a significant number of the latter group have gross functional improvement.

## REFERENCES

1. Albin MS, White RJ, Acosta-Rua G, Yashon D: Study of functional recovery produced by delayed localized cooling after spinal cord injury in primates. J Neurosurg 29:113-119, 1968
2. Baker GS, Daniels F, Jr: Concussion of the spinal cord in battle casualities. J Neurosurg 3:206-211, 1946
3. Baldwin RS: Spinal concussion. A histologic study of two cases. Arch Neurol Psychiatr (Chicago) 32:493-500, 1934
4. Botterell EH, Jousse AT, Aberhart C, Cluff JW: Paraplegia following war. Can Med Assoc J 55:249-259, 1946
5. Bramwit DN, Schmelka DD: Traumatic subarachnoid-pleural fistula. Radiology 89:737-738, 1967
6. Bucy PC, Ladpli R: Recoverable paraplegia. JAMA 185:685-691, 1963
7. Cadwalader WB: Acute softening of the brain and cord without hemorrhage in non-penetrating gunshot wounds caused by impact contusion. Arch Neurol Psych 2:244-245, 1919
8. Callender GR: Wound ballistics. War Med (Chicago) 3:337-350, 1943
9. Campbell E: Recent notes on wounds of the brain and spinal cord. Symposium on treatment of trauma in the armed forces, VII-1-VII-7 (March 1952). Army Medical Service Graduate School, Walter Reed Army Medical Center, Washington, D.C., 1952
10. Campbell E, Meirowsky A: Penetrating wounds of the spinal cord. In Bowers F (ed): Surgery of Trauma. Philadelphia, Lippincott, 1953, p 605
11. Claude H, Lhermitte J: Formes cliniques de las commotion de la moelle cervicale par projectiles de guerre. Rev Med (Paris) 35:535-554, 1916

12. Cohen H, Rogers L: War injuries of the spine and cord. In Bailey H (ed): Surgery of Modern Warfare, 3rd ed, vol. 2. Baltimore, Williams and Wilkins 636–658, 1944
13. Collier J: Gunshot wounds and injuries of the spinal cord. Lancet 1:711–716, 1916
14. Comarr AE, Kaufman AA: A survey of the neurological results of the 858 spinal cord injuries. A comparison of patients treated with and without laminectomy. J Neurosurg 13:95–106, 1956
15. Courville CB: Old missile wounds of the brain. Bull Los Angeles Neurol Soc 21: 49–74, 1956
16. Covalt DA, Cooper IS, Holen TI, Rusk HA: Early management of patients with spinal cord injury. JAMA 89–94, 1953
17. Daniel EF, Smith GW: Foreign-body granuloma of intervertebral disc and spinal canal. J Neurosurg 17:480–482, 1960
18. Daniels JT: Fractures and dislocations of the spine in warfare. Am J Surg 72: 414–423, 1946
19. Davidoff LM: Spinal cord injuries. Surg Clin North Am 21:433–441, 1941
20. Davis L: Treatment of spinal cord injuries. Arch Surg 69:488–495, 1954
21. Davis L, Martin J: Studies upon spinal cord injuries. II. The nature and treatment of pain. J Neurosurg 4:483–491, 1947
22. Demuth WE, Jr: Bullet velocity and design as determinants of wounding capability: an experimental study. J Trauma 6:222–232, 1966
23. Demuth WE, Jr: Bullet velocity as applied to military rifle wounding capacity. J Trauma 9:27–38, 1969
24. Demuth WE, Jr: Bullet velocity makes the difference. J Trauma 9:642–643, 1969
25. Fay T: Surgical management of spinal cord trauma and the neurogenic bladder. Penn Med J 46:221–227, 1942
26. Finck PA: Ballistic and forensic pathologic aspects of missile wounds. Conversion between Anglo-American and metric-system units. Milit Med 130:545–569, 1965
27. Fisher C, Sayre GP, Bickford RC: Histologic changes in the cat's brain after introduction of metallic and plastic coated wire used in electroencephalography. Proc Mayo Clin 32:14–22, 1957
28. Ford CS: Gunshot roentgenograms. Washington, DC, Government Printing Office, 1916, p 337
29. Fuchs EC: The problems of gunshot injuries of the spinal cord and cauda equina (Report of ten patients). Neurochirurgia (Stuttg) 17:153–162, 1974
30. Greenwood J, Jr: Removal of foreign body (bullet) from the third ventricle. J Neurosurg 7:169–172, 1950
31. Groat RA, Rambach WA, Jr, Windle WF: Concussion of the spinal cord: an experimental study and a critique of the use of the term. Surg Gynecol Obstet 81: 63–74, 1945
32. Guttmann L: Spinal deformities in traumatic paraplegics and tetraplegics following surgical procedure. Paraplegia 7:38–49, 1969
33. Guttmann L: Spinal cord injuries. Oxford, Blackwell Scientific Publishers, 1973
34. Hassin GB: Pathological considerations of contusion of cauda equina. J Neuropathol Exp Neurol 3:172–183, 1944
35. Haynes WG: Acute war wounds of the spinal cord. Am J Surg 72:424–433, 1946
36. Heiden JS, Weiss MH, Rosenberg AW, Kurze T, Apuzzo MLJ: Penetrating gunshot wounds of the cervical spine in civilians: Review of 38 cases. J Neurosurg 42:575–579, 1975
37. Holmes G: Spinal injuries of warfare. I. The pathology of acute spinal injuries. Br Med J 2:769–774, 1915
38. Holmes G: Spinal injuries of warfare. II. The clinical symptoms of gunshot injuries of the spine. Br Med J 2:815–821, 1915
39. Holmes G: Spinal injuries of warfare. III. The sensory disturbance in spinal injuries. Br Med J 2:855–861, 1915

40. Jacobson SA, Bors E: Spinal cord injury in Vietnamese combat. Paraplegia 7:263–281, 1970

41. Keith A, Hall ME: Specimens of gunshot injuries of the face and spine. Br Surg 7:55–71, 1919–1920

42. Kennedy F, Denker PG, Osborne R: Early laminectomy for spinal cord injury not due to subluxation. Am J Surg 60:13–21, 1943

43. Kislow VA: Clinical peculiarities of war wounds of the spinal cord. Bull War Med 4:705, 1944

44. Klemperer WW: Spinal cord injuries in World War II. I. Examination and operative technique in 201 patients. US Armed Forces Med J 10:532–552, 1959

45. Klemperer WW: Spinal cord injuries in World War II. II. Operative findings and results in 201 patients. US Armed Forces Med J 10:701–714, 1959

46. Klemperer WW, Fulton JD, Lamport H, Schorr MC: Indirect spinal cord injuries due to gunshot wounds of the spinal column in animal and man. Milit Surg 114:253–265, 1954

47. Knight G: War injuries of the spine and spinal cord. In Maingot R, Slesinger EG, Fletcher E (eds): War Wounds, and Injuries, 2nd ed. Baltimore, Williams and Wilkins, 1930, p 499

48. Lagarde LA: Gunshot Injuries, 2nd ed. New York, William Wood, 1916, p 457

49. Lhermitte J: Etude des lesions histologiques fines de la commotion de la moelle epiniere. Ann Med (Paris) 4:295–307, 1917

50. Matson DD: Treatment of compound spine injuries in forward army hospitals. J Neurosurg 3:114–119, 1946

51. Matson DD: The treatment of acute compound injuries of the spinal cord due to missiles. Springfield, Ill., Charles C Thomas, 1948, p 64

52. Matson DD: Craniocerebral trauma. In Bowers F (ed): Surgery of Trauma. Philadelphia, Lippincott, 1953, p 605

53. Mayfield FH, Cazan GM: Spinal cord injuries. Analysis of six cases showing subarachnoid block. Am J Surg 55:317–325, 1942

54. Meirowsky AM: Penetrating wounds of the spinal canal. Problems of paraplegia and notes on autonomic hyperreflexia and sympathetic blockade. Clin Orthop 27:90–110, 1963

55. Munro D: Cervical cord injuries. A study of 101 cases. N Engl J Med 229:919–933, 1943

56. Munro D: Thoracic and lumbosacral cord injuries. A study of 40 cases. JAMA 122:1055–1063, 1934

57. Munro D: The rehabilitation of patients totally paralyzed below the waist, with special reference to making them ambulatory and capable of earning their own living. II. Control of urination. N Engl J Med 234:207–216, 1946

58. Munro D: The treatment of injuries to the nervous system. Philadelphia, Saunders, 1952, p 284

59. Naffziger HC: The neurological aspects of injuries to the spine. J Bone Joint Surg 20:444–448, 1938

60. Nagoulitch I, Borne G, Belval J: Spinal cord wounds due to firearms and knives. Comparative study of 50 cases. Lyon Chir 64:424–433, 1968

61. Pilcher C: Penetrating wounds of the brain. Ann Surg 103:173–198, 1936

62. Poer DH: Newer concepts in the treatment of the paralyzed patient to war time injuries of the spinal cord. Ann Surg 123:510–515, 1946

63. Pool JL: Gunshot wounds of the spine. Observations from an evacuation hospital. Surg Gynecol Obstet 81:617–622, 1945

64. Roussy G, Lhermitte J: La forme hemiplegique de la commotion directe de la moelle cervicale avec lesion de la XI paire carnienne. Ann Med (Paris) 4:458–469, 1917

65. Scarff JE: Injuries of the vertebral column and spinal cord. In Brock S (ed): In-

juries of the Brain and Spinal Cord and their Coverings, 4th ed. New York, Springer, 1960, p 739

66. Schneider RC, Webster JE, Lofstrom JE: A follow-up report of spinal cord injuries in a group of World War II patients. J Neurosurg 6:118–126, 1949

67. Schnitker MT: Encasement of foreign body (bullet) in the third ventricle for nine years. J Neurosurg 7:173–174, 1950

68. Sherk HH, Giri N, Nicholson JT: Gunshot wound with fracture of the atlas and arteriovenous fistula of the vertebral artery. Case report. J Bone Joint Surg 56A:1738–1740, 1974

69. Sights WP, Jr: Ballistic analysis of shotgun injuries. J Neurosurg 31:25–33, 1969

70. Suwanwela C, Alexander E, Jr, Davis CH: Prognosis in spinal cord injury with special reference to patients with motor paralysis and sensory preservation. J Neurosurg 19:220–227, 1962

71. Taylor J, Watson-Jones R, Nissen KI: Discussion of war injuries of the spine. Proc R Soc Med 34:447–458, 1941

72. Tinsley M: Compound injuries of the spinal cord. J Neurosurg 3:306–309, 1946

73. Wallace PB, Meirowsky AM: The repair of dural defects by graft. Ann Surg 151: 174–180, 1960

74. Wannamaker GT: Spinal cord injuries. A review of the early treatment of 300 consecutive cases during the Korean conflict. J Neurosurg 11:517–524, 1954

75. Wolman L: The neuropathology of traumatic paraplegia. Paraplegia 1:233–251, 1964

76. Yashon D, Jane JA, White RJ: Prognosis and management of spinal cord and cauda equina bullet injuries in sixty-five civilians. J Neurosurg 32:163–170, 1970

77. Yashon D: Missile injuries of the spinal cord. In: Proceedings of the Nineteenth Veterans Administration Spinal Cord Injury Conference, Scottsdale, Arizona, October 31, 1973. Washington DC, US Government Printing Office, February 1977

78. Yashon D: Missile injuries of the spinal cord. In Vinken PJ, Bruyn GW (eds): Injuries of the Spine and Spinal Cord Handbook of Clinical Neurology. New York, Elsevier, 1976, pp 209–220

# 14

## Stab Wounds
## of the Spinal Cord

### INTRODUCTION

Stab wounds of the spinal cord may be inflicted by knives, ice picks, or other pointed objects (Figs. 1–4).[6,8,10] Weapons such as sharpened bicycle spokes and screwdrivers, for example, have been reported. In some instances the patient does not know what weapon was utilized because he is surprised from the rear. In many thoracic stab injuries the patient was bending over resulting in spreading of the lamina. Usually the weapon is withdrawn by the attacker but occasionally it lodges securely and is not removed. Also, the tip may break off in or near the spinal canal. Stab wounds of the spinal cord are uncommon in most parts of the world. Lipschitz reported on his large experience with these lesions in South Africa. Of all cases of traumatic paraplegia admitted to his unit before 1962, 60 percent were due to stab wounds (130 cases). Of these only 4 patients were females and 83 percent occurred between the ages of 15 and 40.[8,9]

### PATHOLOGY

The lesion consists of a sharp injury through the dura into the spinal cord (Figs. 1, 2). Usually the wound is inflicted between the interface between laminae and rarely is the lamina disturbed. In the thoracic region the direction of the wound must be upwards in most cases, so as to pass between overlapping laminae. A direct anteroposterior stab wound is deflected by the lamina but may fracture the lamina if a large heavy instrument is utilized. The intervertebral foramen is also an avenue by which a thin, pointed in-

239

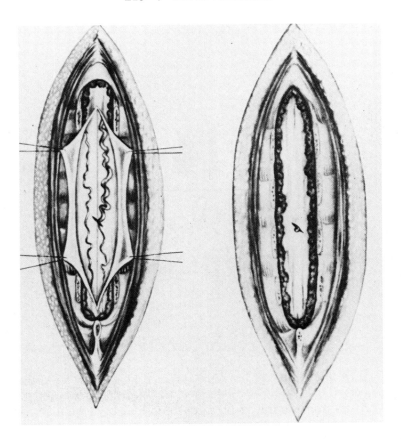

*Fig. 1.* LEFT. Surgical sketch showing small stab wound in dorsal column with open dura. Superior vein is dilated. RIGHT. Surgical sketch showing stab wound as it appeared prior to opening dura. (By permission of Surgery, Gynecology, and Obstetrics 48:659, 1929, Rand and Patterson)

strument may enter. In the cervical canal the direction of injury may be straight anteroposterior or even downwards in the case of the upper cervical spine. In the lumbar region, the wound may be inflicted in an anteroposterior direction.

The weapon may damage the cord or cauda equina directly, but indriven bone fragments also occasionally produce damage. The vascular supply of the cord, either arterial or venous, can also be damaged with resulting sequelae, including ischemic necrosis and edema.

An interesting and sometimes puzzling neurologic syndrome is a contrecoup spinal cord lesion in which the opposite side of the cord to the advancing knife blade is damaged. The pia is quite tough and the cord is forced to the opposite side of the hard bony canal and the impact against the opposite bony canal causes damage. In stab wounds almost any combination of tracts

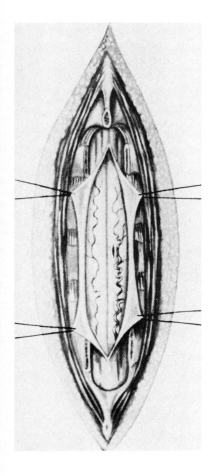

*Fig. 2.* Surgical sketch showing small stab wound in dorsal column. Inferior vein dilated, complete recovery from Brown-Sequard syndrome. (By permission of Surgery, Gynecology, and Obstetrics 48:659, 1929, Rand and Patterson)

may be involved therefore, depending on the sharpness of the blade, its site of introduction, and path.

Subdural hematomas, as well as epidural hematomas, have been described in these injuries. In subacute and chronic patients abscess formation as well as osteomyelitis have occurred. The incidence of infection has diminished with the advent of antibiotic therapy.

## CLINICAL FEATURES

The stab wounds may be isolated or multiple stab wounds may occur. In most cases more than one stab wound is present but only one involves the spinal cord. In many cases a variant of the Brown-Sequard syndrome occurs. Although a true Brown-Sequard syndrome is very uncommon, evidence of partial Brown-Sequard syndromes is quite common. Brown-Sequard's lec-

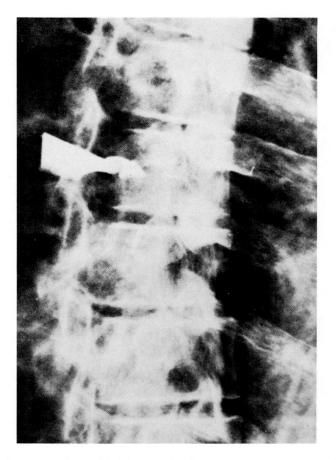

*Fig. 3.* Lateral x-ray of knife blade at T7 level. Spastic paraparesis and diminished sensation to T10. (By permission of International Surgery 57:147, 1972, Adornato and Collis)

tures of 1869,[3] concerning the syndrome that bears his name are of interest. In his discussion he includes five cases of stab wound of the spinal cord, each being described in detail. The first concerned a 35-year-old man who was stabbed in the back of the neck just to the left of the midline. He sustained a wound of the spinal cord which resulted in paralysis of voluntary movement in the right limbs, "hyperaesthesia of the four kinds of sensibility in the right lower limb, with anesthesia of the same kinds of feeling in the left limbs and signs of vasomotor paralysis in the face and eye on the right side." The patient was examined 12 years later by Hughlings Jackson, who found that he had largely recovered the use of his formerly paralyzed right arm and leg. He had married and said that his sexual power was not much diminished, although "the faculty of retaining his water" was still somewhat weak.

Brown-Sequard's second case was that of a 22-year-old woman who was

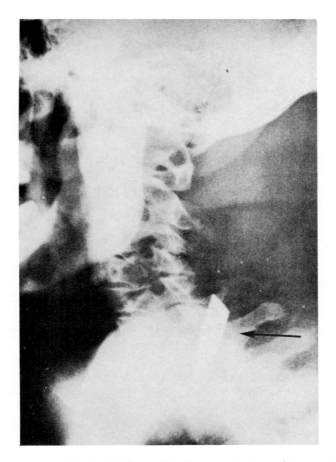

*Fig. 4.* Lateral x-ray of knife blade at C7. (By permission of International Surgery 57:147, 1972, Adornato and Collis)

stabbed by a pocket knife slightly to the left of the seventh cervical vertebra. This resulted in an "incised wound of the right lateral half of the spinal cord, upon or near the roots of the last cervical pair of nerves; paralysis and hyper-aesthesia of the right lower limb, and signs of paralysis of the vasomotor nerves of the face, ear, and eye on the same side; complete anaesthesia to touch, tickling, heat and cold, and painful impressions in the left lower limb, with conservation of voluntary movements and of the muscular sense." The miosis on the right probably indicated a Horner's syndrome. Several months later she had acquired a little movement in the right lower extremity and some return of feeling in the left.

His third case had to do with a 25-year-old man who was stabbed just behind the left ear with a dirk knife; this resulted in a "wound of the cervical region of the spinal cord: paralysis of voluntary movement of the right side, and constriction of the pupil on the same side; anaesthesia on the left side."

Brown-Sequard's fourth instance, a case of Boyer (1831),[2] had previously been reported by Eve (1851).[5] A drummer of the Paris National Guard was wounded in the right posterolateral aspect of the neck by a sabre thrown at him from behind. He suffered immediate paralysis of the right arm and leg and anesthesia of the left side of the body. Subsequently, the right leg recovered, but the paralysis of the right arm and anesthesia of the left side of the body persisted.

Brown-Sequard's fifth case was first published by Begin (1840–41). The patient was wounded in the right side of the neck posteriorly and died four days later. From the first there was "paralysis of motion in the corresponding side, with conservation of sensibility." There is no indication as to whether or not sensation was preserved on the left side of the body. At autopsy "a fragment of a knife was found lodged in the spine, the point entering the posterior part of the pharynx between the sixth and seventh cervical vertebrae, and the base firmly fixed in the right lamina of the sixth vertebra. The right side of the spinal cord had been divided obliquely from the line of origin of the posterior roots to the anterior median sulcus." The above translation was from St. John and Rand.[13] The level of entrance in the back of the knife does not necessarily bear a constant relation to the level of the cord lesion. The cord lesion may, in fact, be above or below the external wound and vascular damage is a factor.

Cerebrospinal fluid leakage occurs uncommonly and in almost all cases ceases spontaneously. If the cerebral spinal fluid leakage persists then open operation is indicated to close the dural rent.

Adornato and Collis[1] summarized two patients with stab wounds of the spinal cord with large retained fragments. Both of these cases were of interest because of the long period of time elapsed before the retained fragments became symptomatic. They felt that the intramedullary extension of the sinus tract and granuloma which occurred after that long period should not be excised because of the possibility of it enhancing the patient's neurologic deficit. These and the following reports indicate the frequency of the delayed onset of symptoms and signs. Castillo and Kahn[4] presented a patient who carried on normal activity for a period of years with his spinal cord transfixed by a knife blade two and one-half inches in length. The knife blade was broken off in the canal in a longitudinal midline direction so that the patient, in effect, had a longitudinal myelotomy. After the knife blade was removed the patient did quite well on long-term follow-up. Wolfe reported the case of a 35-year-old man who was stabbed in the back and suffered only transient paresthesia in one leg but was asymptomatic for 21 years when he began to develop progressive myelopathy. Eight years later he showed a Brown-Sequard syndrome at the T7 level. X-rays showed the tip of a knife blade and with its removal some neurologic recovery occurred.

Brown-Sequard (1869)[3] was quick to notice increased sensitivity to touch or pain in certain cases, describing it as "increased sensibility to touch, tickling, heat and cold, and painful impressions (pricking, pinching, galvanism, etc.)." He believed that this phenomenon was due "in great measure at least to the vasomotor paralysis" caused by the lesion. In our cases hyperesthesia and dysesthesia has been a recurring complaint.

## RADIOLOGIC INVESTIGATION

Anterior-posterior and lateral x-rays need to be taken. Oblique views may better demonstrate bony lesions. Myelography is not indicated under ordinary circumstances. Lumbar puncture need not be done unless infection is suspected. Routine cultures, as well as any special cultures, are then taken. There is almost always no block on jugular compression so that this test need not be done.

In the case of progressive symptoms or suspicion of subdural or epidural hematoma, myelography could be carried out to look for a block. In our experience this has not been required and the incidence of such hematomas is extremely low.

## TREATMENT

The immediate treatment is local wound cleaning, usually minimal suture, and tetanus toxoid or other prophylaxis as indicated. Antibiotics should be given and we preferred to give these in meningitic doses. The exact antibiotic is subject to considerable debate, however. Since the advent of antibiotics sepsis has not been a major problem. All of these patients should be treated with high doses of antibiotics to prevent such infection. If a retained metallic fragment is present in the spinal canal or near it, then the question of surgical intervention becomes more significant. In our view certainly if a fragment is in the spinal canal it should be removed. In the case of progressive paralysis exploration is indicated to rule out abscess or hematoma.

Wright[15] reported an intramedullary spinal cord abscess secondary to a stab wound with good recovery following operative drainage. The patient was treated with chloromycetin and penicillin. Bacterial cultures grew *Klebsiella pneumoniae* and an unidentified Streptococcus species.

Indications for operation include removal of a retained foreign body shown on x-ray, progression of neurologic deficit, depressed bone fragments, sepsis as a persistent sinus or other signs of abscess or granuloma, and persistent cerebrospinal fluid leak. LeBlanc et al.[7] reported on a stab wound of the cauda equina and emphasized that criteria for exploration of cauda equina stab wounds differ from those applied to similar injuries of the spinal cord. They felt that reapproximation of the severed nerve roots by suturing could be carried out in the case of the cauda equina injuries. Their patient, they state, did improve considerably following anastomosis. Rand and Patterson[11] reviewed reports of stab wounds of the spinal cord until 1929. Their attitude toward surgical intervention was similar to that existing at the present time.

## PROGNOSIS

In general, the prognosis is relatively good as there is a high incidence of improvement. On occasion, of course, there is no improvement and the prognosis is similar to other causes of spinal injury. Rosenberg[12] stressed the spontaneous improvement that may occur. There is a high incidence of spontaneous improvement in knife wounds since the initial damage causes considerable edema and therefore there can be some recovery of function. The ultimate prognosis should be guarded since it is almost impossible to tell the permanency of the injury at the time of initial observation.

## ASSOCIATED INJURIES AND COMPLICATIONS

Lipschitz[9] reported on associated injuries and complications of stab wounds of the spinal cord. Some patients also had head injuries in Lipschitz's series. This poses a problem since it is almost impossible to carry out an adequate spinal cord neurologic examination in the presence of an unconscious patient. Lipschitz made the interesting observation that unconscious patients had a "cold nose" and "warm feet" due to vasodilatation of the lower extremities and lack of such above the level of the lesion. One diagnostic difficulty, he pointed out, occurs in patients who have had a vertex skull-brain injury over the sagittal sinus in the region of the motor cortex. Here one may get weakness of both legs simulating paraplegia. This could, in any paraplegic patient, represent a diagnostic difficulty. Fortunately, its occurrence is rare.

Associated with stab injuries to the spinal cord are the cutting of major vessels in the neck, with all types of vascular complications. Injuries to the brachial plexus may occur and, in fact, this may be a route through which the blade travels, so that the patient may have a combined brachial plexus and spinal cord injury. This could be a diagnostic difficulty. Injuries to the trachea, esophagus, thoracic cavity, lymphatic ducts, limbs, and other vertebral column injuries have been reported. Abdominal wounds are common, including renal, liver, and splenic injuries.

## REFERENCES

1.  Adornato DC, Collis JS, Jr: Stab wound of the spinal cord. Int Surg 57:147–150, 1972
2.  Boyer A: Traite des maladies chirurgicales, et des operations qui leur conviennent, 4th ed. Paris, l'auteur (et) Migneret, 1831
3.  Brown-Sequard CE: Lectures on the physiology and pathology of the nervous

system; and on the treatment of organic nervous affections. Lancet 2:593, 659, 755, 821, 1868; 1:1, 219, 703, 873, 1869

4. Castillo R, Kahn EA: Asymptomatic transfixion of spinal cord by a knife blade. J Neurosurg 7:179–184, 1950
5. Eve PF: Three cases of partial paralysis from puncture wounds of the spinal marrow. New Orleans M & SJ, 1851
6. Guttmann L: Spinal cord injuries: Comprehensive management and research. Oxford, Blackwell Scientific Publications, 1973, p 694
7. LeBlanc HJ, Gray LW, Kline DG: Stab wounds of the cauda equina. Case report. J Neurosurg 31:683–685, 1969
8. Lipschitz R, Block J: Stab wounds of the spinal cord. Lancet 2:169–172, 1962
9. Lipschitz R: Associated injuries and complications of stab wounds of the spinal cord. Paraplegia 5:75–82, 1967
10. Nagoulitch I, Borne G, Belval J: Spinal cord wounds due to firearms and knives. Comparative study of 50 cases. Lyon Chir 64:424–433, 1968
11. Rand GW, Patterson GH: Stab wounds of the spinal cord. Surg Gynecol Obstet 48:652–661, 1929
12. Rosenberg AW: Stab wounds of the spinal cord. Bull Los Angeles Neurol Soc 22:79–84, 1957
13. St. John JR, Rand CW: Stab wounds of the spinal cord. Bull Los Angeles Neurol Soc 18:1–24, 1953
14. Wolfe SM: Delayed traumatic myelopathy following transfixion of the spinal cord by a knife blade. A case report. J Neurosurg 38:221–225, 1973
15. Wright RL: Intramedullary spinal cord abscess. Report of a case secondary to stab wound with good recovery following operation. J Neurosurg 23:208–210, 1965

# 15

## Pharmacologic Treatment

Treatment of spinal cord injury with corticosteroids cannot be considered experimental, although clinical benefit has not been absolutely proved. Similarly, mannitol or urea are frequently given in the hope of decreasing edema, but, again, unequivocal proof of their efficacy has not been established experimentally or clinically. Such modes of treatment carry little risk and therefore are used widely and justifiably in patients with severe spinal cord injuries. This chapter outlines various pharmacologic regimens used experimentally in animals with some measure of success. Because the catecholamine hypothesis[35,39] and the possible treatment evolving from this theory are discussed elsewhere, it will not be covered in this chapter.

One rationale for steroid use is based on the fact that anatomic or physiologic complete high thoracic or cervical cord transection results in disruption of corticosteroid feedback pathways, preventing increased endogenous steroid production, which is the usual response to stress in nonspinal injuries. In addition, steroids are said to contribute to membrane stabilization and reduction of edema, therapy benefiting the acutely injured spinal cord.

Mannitol or urea act as an osmotic diuretic, decreasing spinal cord edema in minutes, in contrast to the hours required by steroid therapy. Methylprednisolone sodium succinate is one steroid that may be used. An initial dose of 500 mg can be given intravenously immediately, followed by 125 mg every 6 hours for 7 to 10 days. The dose may then be tapered. Dexamethasone may be given, 10 mg intravenously immediately and 4 mg every 6 hours thereafter, followed by a tapered dose. Lately, dexamethasone in doses as high as 50 to 100 mg intravenously has been given. Mannitol may be given intravenously, 500 cc in 20 percent solution, over a one-hour period and intermittently thereafter. We sometimes continue this regimen for 7 to 10 days, paying close attention to electrolyte balance. Parker et al.[36] suggested that mannitol was beneficial in the treatment of experimental spinal cord edema in dogs, and

Joyner and Freeman,[24] also reporting experiments in dogs, suggested that urea was of some benefit for the same reasons.

Various papers reporting experimental use of combinations of pharmacologic agents will be cited and evaluated one against the other or against no treatment. In the evaluation of experimental drugs, the maxim *aegrescit medendo* (the remedy is worse than the disease) must be considered. Many drugs have side effects that may complicate the disease process. Therefore, side effects, toxicity, and contraindications must be closely examined before any drug is utilized in the treatment of human spinal cord injury.

Dimethyl sulfoxide (DMSO) has been reported to have three highly desirable properties for treatment of spinal cord trauma: it provides a strong diuresis and is said to reduce edema and protect cells from mechanical damage.[5] De la Torre et al.[13,14] suggested that DMSO was beneficial in the treatment of experimental spinal cord injuries. Kajihara et al.[25] also suggested that DMSO was a valuable agent: their DMSO-treated dogs showed significantly more rapid rate of recovery of motor function than did untreated controls and urea-treated and Decadron-treated animals.

Ducker and Hamit,[15,16] as a result of a study in dogs, recommended use of dexamethasone in the treatment of spinal cord injuries, and de la Torre et al.[13] also suggested that dexamethasone aided recovery. Kuchner and Hansebout[29] combined steroids and hypothermia in the treatment of spinal-injured dogs with beneficial results. On the other hand, Lewin et al.[30] suggested that dexamethasone had only minimal effect on edema following experimental spinal cord injury, but did prevent loss of potassium from the injured spinal cord.

Steroid drugs have an anti-inflammatory affect possibly due to direct action on the fibroblastic cell, interfering with elaboration of ground substance and altering permeability of vessels. Ortiz-Galvan[34] investigated the effect of hydrocortisone directly on the exposed experimentally injured spinal cord and found that the inflammatory action was lessened, but edema and necrosis of the spinal cord were not altered. Healing was delayed, and the mesodermal scar was diminished. Degeneration of nerve fiber was generally unaffected, but medium and fine axons seemed to degenerate at a slower rate than in controls, although this was subject to interpretation. Secondary degeneration and myelin changes were delayed but not diminished. Ortiz-Galvan concluded that local steroid treatment would have no effect on spinal injury.[34]

Killen et al.[27] used low molecular weight dextran (LMWD, mean molecular weight, 40,000) to increase red blood cell suspension stability, thereby decreasing sludging, blood viscosity, and coating of the endothelial surface of the vascular system, as well as expanding the volume of the vascular space. The total effect of administration of LMWD is to increase arterial bed perfusion. Although use of this substance for prevention of ischemia in spinal injury is theoretically sound, Killen did not find it helpful. Dawes et al.[12] evaluated the effect of LMWD and heparin on spinal cord ischemic injury incident to a standardized temporary occlusion of the thoracic aorta. The administration of LMWD did not protect the spinal cord; however, a 60 percent reduction in paralysis was demonstrated in animals receiving heparin immediately preceding aortic occlusion. They concluded that heparin significantly decreased the incidence of ischemic damage of the spinal cord.

Blaisdell and Cooley[7] observed that lowering of canine cerebral spinal fluid pressure protected the spinal cord against ischemia caused by temporary occlusion of the thoracic aorta. They lowered cerebrospinal fluid pressure by drainage or by administration of urea. The protection effected was thought to be an increase in the arterial perfusion pressure of the spinal cord by a degree equivalent to the decrease in pressure of cerebrospinal fluid. The small increase in effective perfusion pressure was apparently critical for the prevention of ischemic injury to the spinal cord.

Hyperbaric oxygen has been used experimentally in the treatment of the injured spinal cord. Kelley et al.[26] showed that almost immediately by use of oxygen electrodes, the PO2 of the injured spinal cord was decreased. Maeda[31] treated dog spinal cord injury with hyperbaric oxygen of up to three atmospheres and produced improvement in the PO2 of the injured cord, but did not perform functional studies. Hartzog et al.[22] observed improvement in one of five baboons with spinal injury treated by hyperbaric oxygen therapy.

Hedeman[23] evaluated the experimental therapeutic effects of LMWD, an antiedema agent, catecholamine receptor blockers, and a catecholamine synthesis inhibitor. Results showed a high degree of protection provided by phenoxybenzamine, an alpha-adrenergic receptor blocker, and a lesser degree of protection from haloperidol, a dopaminergic blocker, and low molecular weight Dextran. Alpha-methyltyrosine and steroids given postinjury were of no therapeutic value. Gurden and Feringa[21] tried to establish a connection between long motor tract regeneration and norepinephrine blockers. One group of animals received dibenamine to block the effect of excess norepinephrine on blood vessels but no benefit was demonstrated.

Piromen is a pyrogenic polysaccharide that has been used experimentally to aid in regeneration of transected spinal cords. Windle et al.[44] were the first to investigate this substance. Friedlander and Bailey[19] reviewed published experimental results and treated over 100 patients. In animals, Windle[44] found that some anatomic regeneration of the cord occurred after the use of piromen, provided the separation between severed ends was no greater than 1 mm with growing fibers aligned along a loose reticulin, a circumstance resembling that observed in regenerating peripheral nerve. The absence of massive gliosis and the presence of good vascularization were important. The promptness with which the drug was given after injury, the duration of its use, and the youth of the animal all contributed to and enhanced anatomic regeneration. In the clinical survey, only about 10 percent of patients had beneficial results, but many of these were long-term injured patients.

Brodner et al.[9] investigated antifibrinolytic therapy, using epsilon aminocaproic acid (EACA) in experimental spinal cord injury in cats. They concluded that EACA had no significant therapeutic effect. Campbell et al.[10] reported that intravenous administration of EACA and methylprednisolone in cats appreciably protected injured spinal cord by minimizing hemorrhage and edema. The success of this combined medication regimen was attributed to steroid stabilization of neural cell membranes and lysosomes contained therein. Edema was partially prevented as escape of proteolytic enzymes was inhibited. EACA inhibited the action of proteolytic enzymes that ordinarily lead to propagation of hemorrhages and nervous tissue destruction.

Richardson and Nakamura[37] evaluated spinal cord edema in cats by electron microscopy, using extradural compression as a model of spinal injury. The effects of treatment with mannitol, methylprednisolone, and hypothermia were studied. Mannitol acted primarily on the capillary endothelium and the astrocytic vascular feet. Methylprednisolone prevented many changes in the capillary wall, particularly in the basement membrane, with a lesser affect on astrocytes. Local hypothermia had some effect on basement membrane, but its primary effect was on astrocytic vascular feet. Treatment with combined methylprednisolone and hypothermia produced the most striking affect on spinal cord edema, resulting in almost normal appearance in the capillary, pericapillary, and neuronal elements.

Feringa et al.[18] gave cyclophosphamide to rats after spinal cord transection in an effort to modify the immune response. This immunosuppressive treatment had no effect on regeneration of central nervous system axons. Feringa's theory was that the immune response is important in suppressing regeneration. The proliferation of glial tissue in the area of transection is felt to be an indication of an immune response. In an earlier report, also based on studies of rats, Feringa et al.[17] suggested that immunosuppressive treatment with azathioprine as well as cyclophosphamide might be of value in promoting regeneration. Histologic comparison of treated animals and controls showed no difference in glial scar at the site of transection.

Campbell et al.[11] utilized steroids, myelotomy, hypothermia, and dural decompression to treat spinal injury in cats; 40 percent of animals treated with steroids and dural decompression regained the ability to walk after a 400 g/cm force injury, and 80 percent of animals treated with steroids and myelotomy regained the ability to walk. None of 10 control animals regained motor or sensory function below the level of injury during a 90-day period of observation.

Albin et al.[2,3,4] introduced localized spinal cord hypothermia in the treatment of spinal injury. The rationale was that temperature reduction might decrease metabolic activity, increase tolerance to ischemia and hypoxia, and possibly thus diminish the inflammatory response and edema. In a series of experiments,[1-3] it was shown that hypothermia ameliorated to some extent the devastating effects of spinal injury. In a later report, White[43] reviewed the status of spinal cord cooling. Thienprasit et al.[42] reported that delayed local cooling was effective in minimizing the neurologic deficits of experimental spinal injury. Kuchner and Hansebout[29] treated spinal cord injured dogs with dexamethasone or local hypothermia. A third group of animals received both and, although recovery of function was poor in earlier weeks, these animals eventually surpassed other groups in neurologic function regained.

Zielonka et al.[45] suggested that during local hypothermia in experimental spinal injury, there was less of autoregulation causing increase in spinal cord blood flow. Negrin[33] described methods of inducing hypothermia in cord. Bricolo et al.[8] reported use of spinal cord hypothermia in patients with 50 percent salutory results. They felt that their results justified application of the hypothermic procedure to humans. Koons et al.[28] reported effects of local hypothermia used for treatment of spinal cord injury. Although they could not establish statistically valid results, they were encouraged. Selker[38] found no beneficial effects of hypothermia in eight patients with either spinal injury or chronic spasms. Black and Markowitz[6] did not observe benefit from spinal cord cooling in spinal injured dogs. Tator[40,41] found that normothermic-perfused spinally injured animals responded as well as those having hypothermic perfusion.

Goldsmith et al.[20] revascularized spinal cord tissue by using intact omentum in dogs. They showed that connections can be made between the intact omentum and the spinal cord interface vessels. This has potential usefulness in the treatment of spinal injury by mechanical means. Love[32] transplanted the spinal cord. Severe kyphoscoliosis was the predominant etiologic factor in most cases. In all his patients, he felt the procedure was useful.

## REFERENCES

1. Albin MS, White RJ, MacCarty CS: Effects of sustained perfusion cooling of the subarachnoid space. Anesthesiology 24:72–80, 1963
2. Albin MS, White RJ, Locke GS, Massopust LC, Kretchmer HE: Localized spinal cord hypothermia. J Int Anesthesia Res Soc 46:8–16, 1967
3. Albin MS, White RJ, Acosta-Rua GJ, Yashon, D: Study of functional recovery produced by delayed localized cooling after spinal cord injury in primates. J Neurosurg 24:113–130, 1968
4. Albin MS, White RJ, Yashon D, Harris LS: Effects of localized cooling on spinal cord trauma. J Trauma 9:1000–1008, 1969
5. Ashwood-Smith MJ: Radioprotective and cryoprotective properties of dimethyl sulfoxide in cellular systems. Ann NY Acad Sci 141:45–62, 1967
6. Black P, Markowitz RS: Experimental spinal cord injury in monkeys: Comparison of steroids and local hypothermia. Surg Forum 22:409–411, 1971
7. Blaisdell FW, Cooley DA: The mechanism of paraplegia after temporary thoracic aortic occlusion and its relationship to spinal fluid pressure. Surgery 51:351, 1962
8. Bricolo A, Dalle Ore G, DaPian R, Facciolo F: Local cooling in spinal cord injury. Surg Neurol 6:101–106, 1976
9. Brodner RA, Vangilder JC, Collins WF: The effect of antifibrinolytic therapy in experimental spinal cord trauma. J Trauma 17:48–54, 1977
10. Campbell JB, DeCrescito V, Tomasula JJ, et al: Experimental treatment of spinal cord contusion in the cat. Surg Neurol 1:102–106, 1973
11. Campbell JB, DeCrescito V, Tomasula JJ, et al: Effects of antifibrinolytic and steroid therapy on the contused spinal cord of cats. J Neurosurg 40:726–733, 1974
12. Dawes RB, Lepley D, Jr, Carey L, Ellison EH: Heparin and low molecular weight dextran in thoracic aorta occlusion. Arch Surg 88:699, 1964
13. de la Torre JC, Kawanaga HM, Rowed DW, et al: Dimethyl sulfoxide in central nervous system trauma. Ann NY Acad Sci 243:362–389, 1975
14. de la Torre JC, Johnson CM, Goode DJ, Mullan S: Pharmacologic treatment and

evaluation of permanent experimental spinal cord trauma. Neurology (Minneapolis) 25:508–514, 1975

15. Ducker TB, Hamit HF: Experimental treatments of acute spinal cord injury. J Neurosurg 30:693–697, 1969
16. Ducker TB, Perot PL: Spinal cord oxygen and blood flow in trauma. Surg Forum 22:413–415, 1971
17. Feringa ER, Johnson RD, Wendt JS: Spinal cord regeneration in rats after immunosuppressive treatment. Arch Neurol 32:676–683, 1975
18. Feringa ER, Kinning WK, Britten AG, Vahlsing HL: Recovery in rats after spinal cord injury. Neurology 26:839–843, 1976
19. Friedlander WJ, Bailey P: Clinical use of piromen in spinal cord diseases and injury. Neurology 3:684–690, 1953
20. Goldsmith HS, Duckett S, Chen WF: Spinal cord vascularization by intact omentum. Am J Surg 129:262–265, 1975
21. Gurden GG, Feringa ER: Effects of sympatholytic agents on CNS regeneration, cystic necrosis after spinal cord transection. Neurology (Minneapolis) 24:187–191, 1974
22. Hartzog JT, Risher RG, Snow C: Spinal cord trauma: Effect of hyperbaric oxygen therapy. Proc 17th VA Spinal Cord Injury Conf 70–71, 1969
23. Hedeman LS, Ranajit S: Studies in experimental spinal cord trauma. Part 2. Comparison of treatment with steroids, low molecular weight dextran, and catecholamine blockade. J Neurosurg 40:44–51, 1974
24. Joyner J, Freeman LW: Urea and spinal cord trauma. Neurology 13:69–72, 1963
25. Kajihara K, Kawanaga H, de la Torre JC, Mullan S: Dimethyl sulfoxide in the treatment of experimental acute spinal cord injury. Surg Neurol 1:16–22, 1973
26. Kelly D, Lassiter K, Calogero J, Alexander E: Effects of local hypothermia and tissue oxygen studies in experimental paraplegia. J Neurosurg 33:554–563, 1970
27. Killen DA, Edwards RH, Tinsley EA, Boehm FH: Effect of low molecular weight dextran, heparin, urea, cerebrospinal fluid drainage, and hypothermia on ischemic injury of the spinal cord secondary to mobilization of the thoracic aorta from the posterior parietes. J Thorac Cardiovasc Surg 50:882–886, 1965
28. Koons DD, Gildenberg PL, Dohn DF, Henoch M: Local hypothermia in the treatment of spinal cord injuries. Cleve Clin Q 39:109–117, 1972
29. Kuchner EF, Hansebout RR: Combined steroid and hypothermia treatment of experimental spinal cord injury. Surg Neurol 6:371–376, 1976
30. Lewin MG, Hansebout RR, Pappius HM: Chemical characteristics of traumatic spinal cord edema in cats. J Neurosurg 40:65–75, 1974
31. Maeda N: Experimental studies on the effect of decompression procedures and hyperbaric oxygenation for the treatment of spinal cord injury. J Nara Med Assoc 16:429–447, 1965
32. Love JG: Transplantation of the spinal cord for the relief of paraplegia. Arch Surg 73:757–763, 1956
33. Negrin J: Spinal cord hypothermia: Neurosurgical management of immediate and delayed post-traumatic neurologic sequelae. NY State J Med 75:2387–2392, 1975
34. Ortiz-Galvan A: Action of local hydrocortisone on spinal cord wounds: effect on inflammation, repair, degeneration, and regeneration. Arch Neurol Psychiatr 76:34–41, 1956
35. Osterholm JL, Mathews GJ: Treatment of severe spinal cord injuries by biochemical norepinephrine manipulation. Surg Forum 22:415, 1971
36. Parker AJ, Park RD, Stowater JL: Reduction of trauma-induced edema of spinal cord in dogs given mannitol. Am J Vet Res 34:1355–1357, 1973
37. Richardson HD, Nakamura S: An electron microscopic study of spinal cord edema and the effect of treatment with steroids, mannitol, and hypothermia. Proc VA Spinal Cord Injury Conf 18:10–16, 1971
38. Selker RG: Ice water irradiation of the spinal cord. Surg Forum 22:411–413, 1971

39. Tator CH: Acute spinal cord injury: a review of recent studies of treatment and pathophysiology. Can Med Assoc J 107:143–150, 1972

40. Tator CH: Acute spinal cord injury in primates produced by an inflatable extra-dural cuff. Can J Surg 16:222–231, 1973

41. Tator CH: Acute spinal cord injury: a review of recent studies of treatment and pathophysiology. Can Med Assoc J 107:143–150, 1972

42. Thienprasit P, Bantli H, Bloedel JR, Chou SN: Effect of delayed local cooling on experimental spinal cord injury. J Neurosurg 42:150–154, 1975

43. White RJ: Current status of spinal cord cooling. Clin Neurosurg 20:400–407, 1973

44. Windle WF, Clements CD, Chambers WW: Inhibition of formation of a glial barrier as a means of permitting a peripheral nerve to grow into a brain. J Comp Neurol 96:359, 1972

45. Zielonka JS, Wagner FC, Dohrmann GJ: Alterations in spinal cord blood flow during local hypothermia. Surg Forum 25:434–435, 1974

# 16

# Nerve Root Avulsion

The diagnosis of avulsion of the intraspinal roots of the spinal cord in the cervical and lumbar areas can be made on examination. Cervical injuries, by far the most common, usually result from traction exerted when the face is turned away from the side of injury and the arm on the side of injury is pulled downward, along with the shoulder. This stretch causes the nerve roots to be avulsed either intraspinally or within the intervertebral foramina.

The diagnosis can be made on the presence of segmental motor and sensory deficit involving the fifth, sixth, and sometimes the seventh cervical spinal roots. Paralysis of serratus magnus, levator scapulae, and the rhomboid muscles indicates that the lesion in the nerve roots is medial to the emergence of the nerve supply of the long thoracic and dorsal scapular nerves that innervate these muscles. A lower brachial plexus injury may also result from traction, but more often results from hyperextension of the arm upward. The diagnosis is made by signs of segmental sensory and motor deficit of the eighth cervical, first thoracic, and sometimes the seventh cervical roots in combination with a Horner's syndrome. All the segments from C5 to T1 may be involved in cervical nerve root avulsions.

Myelography is an excellent verifying diagnostic study. If myelograms are normal, a lesion is probably within the brachial plexus extraspinally. Diagnosis is confirmed by demonstration of a pseudomeningocele on myelography (Figs. 1–3). Murphey et al.[10] emphasized the importance of myelographic demonstration for prognostic purposes. Murphey and Kirklin[11] emphasized the importance of differential diagnosis because early suture of components of the brachial plexus may be worthwhile in recovery of some function, although this has been debated. Once the diagnosis of cervical nerve root avulsion is made, the prognosis for recovery of meaningful function is extremely poor.

The first case of cervical root avulsion was reported by Flaubert[6] in 1872;

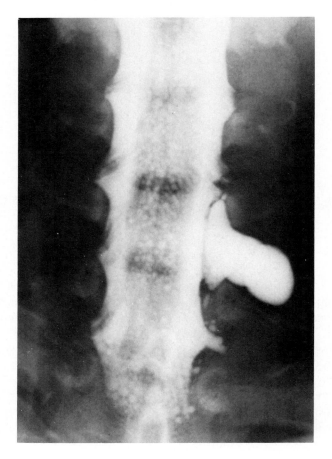

*Fig. 1.* Myelogram showing nerve root pseudocyst indicative of nerve root avulsion (case 1).

Apert[2] recorded another case in 1898. Duchenne,[4] in 1872, provided the first clinical description of a root avulsion occurring in a newborn child. Klumpke,[9] in 1885, described the clinical picture and reported the presence of Horner's syndrome with damage to the first thoracic root or its sympathetic ramus. Erb[5] localized the lesion electrically, and Frazier and Skillern[7] verified the avulsion during laminectomy. Adson[1] and Jefferson[8] made contributions to the literature.

Patients with nerve root avulsions are not uncommon in the trauma practice of neurosurgeons, orthopedists, and physiatrists. We see a few each year, probably owing to the increase in motorcycle accidents and the high number of automobile accidents. This injury can occur in infants during delivery. Zorub et al.[13] discussed 70 patients seen between 1960 and 1972. Of these, 21 were verified on myelography or at surgery as complete avulsion injuries. They emphasized the extremely poor prognosis.

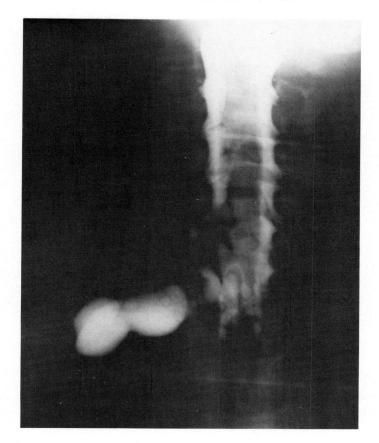

*Fig. 2.* Myelogram showing nerve root pseudocyst indicative of nerve root avulsion (case 2).

In addition to neurologic examination and myelography, electromyography and the axon reflex test may be helpful in diagnosis. The electromyogram may reveal an absent or decreased decruitment pattern immediately after denervation and within the following two to three weeks. Denervation potentials may be present. Evoked motor potentials may be decreased, and if the lesion is preganglionic, the sensory nerve action potential will be normal, since the sensory arc is intact. No response will be noted within one week after interruption if the lesion is postganglionic. Electromyography of the serratus anterior and rhomboid muscles is important in delineating the level of the lesions, since they are innervated by elements of the anterior primary rami of C5–C6–C7 just after they emerge from the vertebral foramina. An abnormal electromyogram of these muscles will indicate not only degeneration, but also the proximity of the lesion to the cord and hence the likelihood of spinal cord avulsion. Electromyography of the posterior cervical triangle will help to distinguish whether the lesion is intraforaminal or extraforaminal,

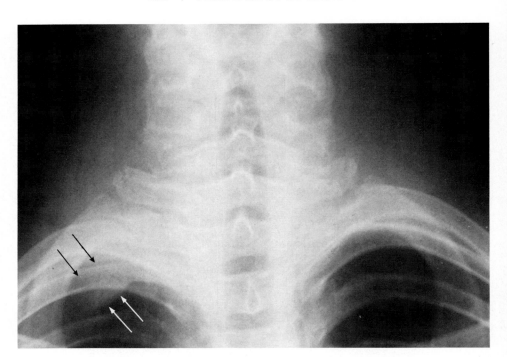

*Fig. 3.* Plain anteroposterior chest x-ray showing pseudocyst (arrows) (case 2).

since the deep muscles of the back of the neck are supplied segmentally by the primary posterior division of the spinal nerve root just lateral to the intravertebral foramina. If motor unit activity potentials are absent, or if fibrillation potentials are observed, damage to the nerve root in question is close to the spinal cord and probably intraforaminal or preganglionic. If the electromyogram is normal, the lesion is distal to the intervertebral foramina and probably postganglionic.

The axonal reflex test is based on the triple response to interdermal histamine injection. This test is not widely used, but does provide a means of distinguishing preganglionic from postganglionic root injury. The flare response to histamine is dependent upon the presence of intact cutaneous axons whose cell bodies are within a dorsal root ganglion. Thus, in ganglionic lesions or when the dorsal and ventral roots are avulsed intraspinally, the triple response of wheal, vasodilation, and flare occurs. When the lesion is distal to the ganglion, the axon is separated from the cell body, and only a wheal and vasodilation occur. If the lesion is distal to the ganglion, it is most likely outside the intervertebral foramina. Absence of the flare thus makes it a negative test and indicates extraspinal cause.

The myelogram shows a traumatic pseudomeningocele and is considered excellent evidence of the presence of a nonrepairable lesion (Figs. 1–3). Laminectomy has been recommended by some, but almost all surgeons feel that it would serve no useful purpose. Exploration of the brachial plexus for other lesions may be indicated, but these lesions are not under consideration here.

One difficult problem associated with this injury is severe and intractable pain. Pain in some cases has been reported to be causalgic in nature, but in our experience this is not common. In those patients responding to stellate blocks, perhaps stellate ganglionectomy will reduce or alleviate pain, but in our experience, stellate blocks have not been helpful. Posterior rhizotomy has been described as unsuccessful, but intramedullary spinothalamic tractotomy followed by excellent results has been reported by White and Sweet.[12] They also reported patients having mesencephalic tractotomy and thalamotomy. Zorub et al.[13] employed stereotactic mesencephalotomy or dorsal column stimulation. Six patients underwent mesencephalic tractotomy, three with excellent results for up to six years. One patient had partial relief, and there were two failures. Seven patients had dorsal column stimulators implanted in the high cervical cord. One of these had an unsuccessful mesencephalotomy and had three years of excellent pain relief. Two patients had pain relief for six months, but experienced recurrence. Four additional patients failed to respond.

In most cases, the patient is functionally one-armed. Early amputation with arthrodesis of the shoulder should be considered, but this is distasteful to physicians as well as patients and families. The patient, however, is better off with a prosthesis in most instances. Patients retaining the useless arm spend much of the time holding that arm with the normal arm, thus becoming incapacitated. A well-planned amputation will at least enable them to be somewhat independent. However, amputation will not relieve pain, and patients should be warned of this in advance. Drug addiction and psychologic impairment should be avoided if possible.

Lumbosacral nerve root avulsions are very uncommon but have been reported.[3] Intradural avulsion of the individual nerve roots forming the lumbosacral plexus can also be demonstrated by myelography with a prognosis equally as poor as that in cervical nerve root avulsions. Diagnosis is frequently difficult to distinguish from that of lumbosacral plexus injury. Patients with lumbosacral nerve root avulsions and lumbosacral plexus injuries frequently have pelvic fractures, and there may be sacral fractures as well. In one case,[3] lesions were bilateral, but most are unilateral. Most patients presenting with these injuries are seriously ill due to the magnitude of associated trauma. Usually the diagnosis of the lesion is postponed because a detailed neurologic examination of the lower extremities cannot be done immediately, owing to the severity of other injuries and the poor condition of the patient. When the patient has flaccid paralysis or sensory loss, the differential diagnosis of peripheral nerve injury, plexus injury, or nerve root avulsion is troublesome. Early persistence of causalgic or other severe pain in an extremity suggests possible root avulsion, according to Barnett and Connolly.[3] Although pain can be a problem, it is not commonly reported, and surgical explorations of the avulsed root have not been carried out. It is conceivable that such unilateral pain might be treated with cordotomy.

## REFERENCES

1. Adson AW: The gross pathology of brachial plexus injuries. Surg Gynecol Obstet 34:351–357, 1922
2. Apert E: Paralysie traumatique radiculaire inferieure du plexus brachial. Bull Soc Med Hop Paris 15:613–619, 1898
3. Barnett HG, Connolly ES: Lumbosacral nerve root avulsion: Report of a case and review of the literature. J Trauma 15:532–535, 1975
4. Duchenne GBA: De l'Electrisation Localisee et de son Application a la Pathologie et a la Therapeutique, 3rd ed. Paris, Bailliere, 1872, pp 357–362
5. Erb W: Uber eine eigenthumliche localisation van lahmungen im plexus brachealis. Verhandl der Naturhist-Med Ver Zu Heidelburg NF 1:130–137, 1874
6. Flaubert M: Memoire sur plusier cas de luxation. Rep Gen Anat Physiol Path Clin Chir 3:55–69, 1872
7. Frazier GH, Skillern PG, Jr: Supraclavicular subcutaneous lesions of the brachial plexus not associated with skeletal injuries. JAMA 57:1957–1963, 1911
8. Jefferson G: Discussion on injuries to the brachial plexus. Proc R Soc Med 23: 1282–1286, 1930
9. Klumpke A: Contribution a l'etude des paralysies radiculaires du plexus brachial paralysies radiculaires totales. Rev de Med 5:591–616, 1885
10. Murphey F, Hartung W, Kirklin JW: Myelographic demonstration of avulsing injury of the brachial plexus. Am J Roentgen 58:102–105, 1947
11. Murphey F, Kirklin J: Myelographic demonstration of avulsing injuries of the nerve roots of the brachial plexus. A method of determining the point of injury and the possibility of repair. Clin Neurosurg 20:18–28, 1973
12. White JC, Sweet WH: Pain and the Neurosurgeon. Springfield, Ill., Charles C Thomas, 1969
13. Zorub DS, Nashold BS, Cook WA: Avulsion of the brachial plexus. I. A review with implications on the therapy of intractable pain. Surg Neurol 2:347–353, 1974

# 17

## Spinal Injuries in Children

Spinal injuries in children are similar to those in adults except that frequently bone injury is not visualized on x-ray. Because of the elasticity of the spine in infants and young children a fracture dislocation may reduce spontaneously leaving residual cord damage but no sign of vertebral injury. White and Albin[24] implicate forward bulging of the ligamentum flavum during forcible extension as a cause of cord damage. Wolman[26] implicates, in addition, sudden injury of the cord in forcible flexion injuries when cervical vertebrae are displaced and result in momentary stretching of the cord over the posterior aspect of the vertebral bodies. Burke[5] stresses stretching of the cord as a frequent pathogenetic mechanism in children.

Many infants and children die or are injured in automobile accidents each year. Psychologically for the mother the most secure location for an infant in an auto is the mother's lap. In fact, however, this position may be the most dangerous, for at impact, the infant may be crushed between the mother's body and the interior of the auto. These unrestrained children are close to the hard surfaces of the interior of the auto and frequently are hurled sideways or upwards resulting in severe injuries. The level of spinal injury is usually cervical or upper thoracic. The rear seat remains safer than the front and proper restraints should be urged for infants and small children.[12]

Many automobile injuries in children may be prevented by the use of proper restraining systems.[3] An infant's basinette may be placed in the rear seat, its long axis parallel to the long axis of the auto, seat belt securing the rear legs of the basinette and the extended front legs secured by the middle front seat belt passed under the seat. The child should be placed feet forward in this type of car bed. To prevent further injury from a rollover, a net or webbing adds to security. Automobile manufacturers have designed car seats for older children which afford some degree of safety during impact.[3]

Cullen[8] described spinal injuries in battered children emphasizing that vertebral lesions may go unrecognized in the absence of neurologic signs or bony deformity. One of his patients with old vertebral injury was erroneously treated for osteomyelitis when physicians misdiagnosed a healing vertebral fracture with callus and new bone formation.

Neurologic responses in infantile spinal paralysis must be interpreted with great caution. For example, crying in response to a painful stimulus applied to the foot usually indicates that sensory pathways are intact. On the other hand such discomfort may be due to mass withdrawal responses sufficient to cause pain originating at a higher level as is sometimes the case in adult paraplegics. Anal sphincter tone and the "wink" reflex are other indices of nervous system function but should be interpreted with caution since in chronic paraplegia both or either may be intact. Absence of sweating below the level of a spinal cord lesion may be significant, but in chronic paraplegia sweating may return and this sign should be interpreted with caution. Glassauer and Cares[13] emphasized that hyperthermia can occur because of the inability to sweat and to thermoregulate.

In the absence of x-ray evidence of bony injury myelography may be useful in demonstrating block or other anatomic lesion causing spinal dysfunction, although in some cases the myelogram is normal.[21,22] Melzak[17] reported that of 29 children with severe spinal injuries, only 13 had x-ray evidence of vertebral injury. Lack of obvious vertebral fracture dislocation in juveniles has been observed by many writers including Burke,[4] who reported seven such cases.

Extensive softening and infarction of the cord has been reported after major and even relatively minor neck injuries, emphasizing the importance of blood flow to the spinal cord. Ahmann et al.[1] described children in whom extensive paralysis due to infarction developed after relatively minor trauma. One child had been pushed off a swing and the second child had suffered a direct blow to the face. The delayed syndrome evolved during several hours beginning with flaccid weakness of both arms and leading to total paralysis. Diagnosis was difficult and pathologic study revealed ischemia resulting from infarction of the cervical spinal cord and medulla. No fracture dislocation was observed. The authors postulated hyperextention of the cervical spine to have occurred in both instances.

Dunlap et al.[9] emphasized the normal appearance of slight subluxation of the second on the third cervical vertebra in children, which is observed on lateral view of a mildly flexed cervical spine. Teng and Papatheodorou[20] emphasized the physiologic movement of C2 on C3 in young children. They reported three cases of actual traumatic anterior subluxation stating that precise diagnosis could be based on persistent displacement in the neutral position or in hyperextension of the cervical spine differentiating the normal physiologic state from traumatic subluxation. Weiss and Kaufman[23] reported a 12-month-old child with "hangman's" fracture (see Chap. 8) and pointed out that although this is a rare lesion in children, the physiologic subluxation observed should not be misleading to the physician. The patient was treated by Hoen's skeletal traction (see Chap. 9) for 23 days with a good result.

Ewald[10] treated an odontoid fracture in a 17-month-old child by halo traction alone.

Traumatic subluxation of C2 on C3 may be differentiated from the physiologic state by (1) a clinical history of flexion injury of the cervical spine, (2) clinical findings including traumatic torticollis, cervical stiffness, and muscular spasm, (3) pain in neck movements, (4) neurologic deficit, (5) local tenderness over the spinous processes, and (6) x-ray evidence of anterior displacement not only in flexion but in neutral and in hyperextension of the cervical spine. The latter movements should be made with some caution.

Cattell[7] found a 24 percent incidence of physiologic subluxation of C2 on C3 in children between the ages of one and seven years. They felt this was due to (1) the high mobility of the cervical spine in children, (2) the location of a fulcrum for cervical movement at C2, and (3) the relatively horizontal position of the C2–C3 articular facets permitting anterior movement. The articular facets in infants and children are oriented in a somewhat more horizontal plane than in the adult; vertical adult orientation is not completely achieved until the eighth year.[2] Sullivan et al.[19] accept up to 4.0 mm anterior subluxation of C2–C3 or C3–C4 as a normal variant. Gaufin and Goodman[11] also emphasize special problems associated with cervical spine injuries in children and stress a certain degree of normal C2–C3 mobility and the absence of radiographic evidence of fracture dislocation in severe cord injury.

Hubbard[15] described injuries of the spine in children and adolescents. None of 28 patients with stable spines had evidence of neural trauma. Of 14 with unstable spine, 6 suffered spinal cord injuries and 2 nerve root injuries. He stressed the high incidence of scoliosis in hyperflexion injuries of the thoracic and lumbar spine persisting months and years after the initial injury. He stressed that the clinical course is generally more benign than that following similar injuries in adults and advised early operative reduction and stabilization of fracture dislocations when indicated. Laminectomy was also advised (see Chap. 12). Campbell and Bonnett[6] also stressed the high incidence of spinal deformity (kyphosis, scoliosis, and/or lordosis) in girls 12 years of age or younger and in boys 14 years of age or younger appearing six months following paraplegia or quadriplegia. Burke[5] stresses the high incidence of kyphoscoliosis in children with or without laminectomy. His data are reproduced in Table 1.

LaBlanc and Nadell[16] emphasized that in spite of severe trauma, no bony lesion may be seen on vertebral x-ray in children with paralysis and spinal cord disruption. In their three patients, laminectomy was carried out. Burke[4,5] stresses the high incidence of normal vertebral x-rays.

Bladder function may pose a problem in management. Burke[4] stressed that it is less difficult to maintain a sterile urine in infants and children. Many do extremely well treated by simple expression of urine at intervals returning very little residual urine, others develop spastic automatic bladders that function well, and still others do well with intermittent catherization. The percent of child patients so treated who maintain sterile urine is certainly higher than that in similar adult patients.

## TABLE 1.*
### INCIDENCE OF KYPHOSCOLIOSIS†

| NO. OF PATIENTS | VERTEBRAL INJURY | CONSERVATIVE MANAGEMENT | ≥1 FUSIONS | TOTAL |
|---|---|---|---|---|
| 16 | No bony injury | 5 (3) | 5 | 10 (3) |
| 7 | Minimal bony injury | 1 (1) | 3 (2) | 3 (3) |
| 6 | Major bony injury | 0 | 2 (2) | 2 (2) |
| TOTAL   29 | | 6 (4) | 10 (4) | 16 (8) |

*After Burke.[5]
†Number of laminectomies in parenthesises.

Both Griffith[14] and Ewald[10] stressed that fractures of the odontoid in children could be managed nonsurgically with traction, halo traction, or casting for from three to six weeks. Griffith[14] commented on the ease of reduction, certainty of union, and lack of complications in children with these fractures as opposed to adults. Griffith[14] used Crutchfield tongs and Burke[4] and Nickel et al.[18] used halo traction. It is noteworthy that neurologic complications are seldom a problem and are usually transitory. Frequently delay in recognizing the neck injury is due to the presence of a severe associated lesion.

Detection of an odontoid fracture requires differentiation of a true fracture caused by significant trauma from congenital nonunion of the odontoid, possibly with displacement caused by minor trauma. The distinction is important because in most children the former can be treated conservatively while the latter usually requires fusion. Sometimes the distinction is impossible but other signs of significant trauma such as a retropharyngeal hematoma are helpful. Failure of a trial of conservative therapy usually mandates a fusion. Wollin's[25] roentgenographic criteria of os odontoideum may be helpful. These include overdevelopment of the anterior arch of the atlas with attenuation of the posterior arch, which may be bifid.

## REFERENCES

1. Ahmann PA, Smith SA, Schwartz JF, Clark DB: Spinal cord infarction due to minor trauma in children. Neurology 25:301–307, 1975
2. Bailey DK: The normal cervical spine in infants and children. Radiology 59:712–719, 1952
3. Burg FD, Douglass JM, Diamond E, et al: Automotive restraint devices for the pediatric patient. Pediatrics 45:49–53, 1970
4. Burke DC: Spinal cord trauma in children. Paraplegia 9:1–14, 1971
5. Burke DC: Traumatic spinal paralysis in children. Paraplegia 11:268–276, 1974
6. Campbell J, Bonnett C: Spinal cord injury in children. Clin Orthop 112:114–123, 1975

7. Cattell HS, Filtzer DL: Pseudosubluxation and other normal variations in the cervical spine in children. J Bone Joint Surg 47A:1295–1309, 1965
8. Cullen JC: Spinal lesions in battered babies. J Bone Joint Surg 57B:364–366, 1975
9. Dunlap JP, Morris M, Thompson RG: Cervical spine injuries in children. J Bone Joint Surg 40A:681–686, 1958
10. Ewald FC: Fracture of the odontoid process in a seventeen-month-old infant treated with a halo. J Bone Joint Surg 53A:1636–1640, 1971
11. Gaufin LM, Goodman SJ: Cervical spine injuries in infants. Problems in management. J Neurosurg 42:179–184, 1975
12. Glasauer FE, Cares HL: Traumatic paraplegia in infancy. JAMA 219:38–41, 1972
13. Glasauer FE, Cares HL: Biomechanical features of traumatic paraplegia in infancy. J Trauma 13:166–970, 1973
14. Griffiths SC: Fracture of odontoid process in children. J Pediatr Surg 7:680–683, 1972
15. Hubbard DD: Injuries of the spine in children and adolescents. Clin Orthop 100: 56–65, 1974
16. LeBlanc HJ, Nadell J: Spinal cord injuries in children. Surg Neurol 2:411–414, 1974
17. Melzak J: Paraplegia among children. Lancet 2:45–48, 1969
18. Nickel VL, Perry J, Garrett A, Heppenstall M: The halo: a spinal skeletal traction fixation device. J Bone Joint Surg 50A:1400–1409, 1968
19. Sullivan CR, Bruwer AJ, Harris LE: Hypermobility of the cervical spine in children: a pitfall in the diagnosis of cervical dislocation. Am J Surg 95:636–640, 1958
20. Teng P, Paptheodorou C: Traumatic subluxation of C2 in young children. Bull Los Angeles Neurol Soc 32:197–202, 1967
21. Vinz H: Frakturen im Bereich von Brust und Lenoenwirbelsaule Bei Kindern. Zentralbl Chir 89:817–827, 1964
22. Vinz H: Wirbelkorperbruche ber Kindern—Ergebnisse einer Nachuntersuchung. Zentralbl Chir 90:626–636, 1965
23. Weiss MH, Kaufman B: Hangman's fracture in an infant. Am J Dis Child 126: 268–269, 1973
24. White RJ, Albin MS: Spine and spinal cord injury. In Gurdjian ES, Lange WA, Patrick LM et al (eds): Impact Injury and Crash Protection. Springfield Ill., Charles C Thomas, 1970, pp 63–83
25. Wollin DG: The os odontoideum. Separate odontoid process. J Bone Joint Surg 45A:1459–1471, 1963
26. Wolman L: The neuropathology of traumatic paraplegia. Paraplegia 1:233–251, 1964

# 18

## Birth Injury

It is possible that spinal cord injury at birth is more common than has been thought.[3,4] Some patients with upper motor lesions attributable to "cerebral palsy" may have had cervical spine injuries. Gordon and Marsden,[9] for example, describe a patient who died as a result of a cervical spine injury but who had been diagnosed as infantile spinal muscular atrophy. Crothers and Putnam[7] emphasized two points distinguishing children with spinal cord injuries from children with cerebral damage: (1) intelligence is likely to be normal and speech unimpaired in spite of severe motor disabilities, and (2) evidence of bulbar palsy may appear as the child grows older and may be due to post-traumatic cyst extension (see Chap. 7). Towbin[19] estimates that evidence of spinal or brain stem injury appears in more than 10 percent of autopsies in the neonatal period. The chief indication of such injury in the neonate is respiratory depression, which leads to hypoxia and secondary brain damage. X-rays of the spine are usually normal, adding to difficulty in diagnosis. This is also true of older children with vertebral injury.

Lesions of the spinal cord at birth can be due to stretch injury or compression. Laceration and hemorrhage of the cord and brain stem may occur, and spinal and cranial nerve roots may be damaged and avulsed concomitantly. Epidural hemorrhage may occur in conjunction with any of these injuries. Such injuries may be due to excessive longitudinal traction, especially when combined with flexion and torsion of the spinal axis, which may occur in breech delivery when traction is applied to the trunk and in manipulating the after-coming head, as well as in vertex delivery when forceps traction is applied. Shoulder presentation with traction on the cord secondary to traction on the brachial plexus and hyperextension of the head is contributory. Other contributing factors include prematurity, primiparity, intrauterine malposition, dystocia, and precipitate delivery. The most common site of spinal cord trauma at delivery is the low cervical region and the cervical thoracic junction.

Jellinger and Schwingshackl[13] reported two neonates with birth injury of the spinal cord who survived several weeks. Both had breech delivery and manual extraction. Clinical signs were flaccid tetraparesis and generalized muscle atrophy with hyperreflexia of the lower limbs and presence of breathing disorders. Postmortem examination in both infants showed destruction of the cord over several segments. The authors stressed that the differential diagnosis includes infantile spinal muscular atrophy. They also suggested that pathology in findings in the late stages of spinal cord birth injury does not differ significantly from those in the adult. Hellstrom and Sallmander[12] recommended caesarean section when the fetus is in the transverse position to avoid spinal injury since the incidence of spinal injury increases in that position.

Shulman et al.[18] reported complete transection of the spinal cord occurring in a cephalic delivery following a midforceps rotation. The infant presented with apnea, anesthesia below the level of the midneck, and flaccid quadriplegia. At necropsy transection of the cord and atlantoaxial dislocation were found. This is unusual in that the cord was injured following cephalic presentation because cord injury usually follows breech presentation. The authors felt that the injury was caused by rotational forces on the head and neck. In their review of the spinal injury literature they observe that while shoulder dystocia was common and forceps delivery was used in most, five patients had uneventful cephalic deliveries. Pridmore et al.[17] reported a similar case in which the membranes had been ruptured and delivery was accomplished under general anesthesia. Kielland's forceps rotation was carried out uneventfully and no amniotic fluid was seen during labor and delivery. He stressed that spinal injury should be considered in the presence of neonatal distress, apnea, and flaccidity.

Although severe spinal cord injury following cephalic delivery is extremely uncommon, it occurs not infrequently following breech delivery. However, its true incidence is unknown since most neonatal autopsies do not routinely include an examination of the spinal cord. In over 10 percent of 600 fetal and neonatal autopsies in which brain and cord were examined, Towbin[20] found evidence of significant spinal or brain stem injury. Lesions included spinal epidural hemorrhage, meningeal laceration, trauma to nerve roots, arteries, ligaments, and vertebral bodies. In breech presentation the mechanism of injury is most likely related to stretch. Injury during cephalic delivery may occur during difficult or prolonged labor usually accompanied by rotational manipulation that results in excessive torsion rather than traction or stretch. If forceps are used stretch force may also be involved. All such injuries most commonly occur in the cervical spine. Fetal malpositions such as face or brow presentation or in utero opisthotonos may render the fetus vulnerable to spine injuries. X-rays in utero can provide a clue as to malposition with possible consequent spinal damage.

Hellstrom and Sallmander[12] as well as Abrams et al.[1] stressed the significance of hyperextension of the fetal head. In breech presentations and transverse lies, which were more common, they suggested that spinal injury could be avoided by caesarean section.[1] Bhagwanani et al.[5] confirmed these observations.

Reduction in fetal muscular tone due to hypoxia is a predisposing factor to spinal cord injury during delivery. De Souza and Davis[8] describe a neonate in which prolapse of a nonpulsating umbilical cord during breech delivery was followed by an increase in heart rate and discharge of meconium. A rapid breech extraction followed. Transection of the midcervical spinal cord was found at autopsy. In such a case the obstetrician must decide between rapid delivery with risk of trauma to the baby and delayed delivery with possible ischemic nervous system complications. Apnea is the most common symptom of spinal injury in the newborn. Flaccidity and anesthesia below the level of transection occurs. Flaccidity is usually the rule but reflexes may subsequently become hyperactive.

Leventhal[14] pointed out that the vertebral bodies of the infant are a series of elastic cartilages surrounded by inelastic connective tissue. He showed, in autopsy specimens, that the vertebral column could be stretched two inches and the spinal cord considerably less. The disparity between the pliable bony ligamentous column and the less elastic spinal cord and meninges may explain the occurrence of severe cord stretch paralysis without evidence of bone injury.

The mechanism of spinal injury remains unclear in many cases. Since actual fracture dislocation is unusual on postpartum x-ray, it may be postulated that it does not occur at all or that it may be only temporary and may be a consequence of the elasticity of the newborn vertebral column.

Clinical symptoms vary according to the level of injury. The obstetrician may report a loud snap from within the birth canal during extraction. Postnatal shock and respiratory distress are common. Flaccidity is the rule during the early stages. The infant exhibits lack of response to pin prick and lack of motion below the level of the lesion. Bladder function is lost but suprapubic pressure is efficacious and catheterization is seldom necessary. Automatic bladder develops rapidly in infants.

Treatment is conservative and supportive. According to most authorities, myelography and surgery are seldom required but our position possibly leads to a more aggressive approach. If myelography were to demonstrate a block perhaps immediate laminectomy with or without myelotomy would be justified. This is a minority opinion, but neither the conservative nor the aggressive approach has been conclusively demonstrated to be superior.

Harris and Adelson[10] examined 19 consecutive sudden and unexpected infant deaths (crib deaths). Although none of these revealed a mechanical injury to the cervical thoracic vertebral column, spinal epidural venous congestion frequently accompanied by foci of epidural hemorrhage was present in nearly every child. Similar findings were observed in infants dying of acute inflammatory disease as well as in children who were victims of the classical sudden death syndrome. They concluded that physical trauma does not play a significant role in the pathogenesis of the sudden death syndrome in infants. This is in contradistinction to Towbin's opinion[19] that spinal injury does play a role in unexplained neonatal deaths even in the absence of evidence of actual trauma.

In an analysis of postmortem findings in the spinal cord, Byers[6] and Norman and Wedderburn[16] found scattered hemorrhages to be the principal intraspinal lesions. Extensive scar formation with fusion of the spinal cord and meninges occurs. Some hemorrhage outside the spinal cord may be found in acute cases. Damage to the vertebral arteries was also described by Byers.[6] Lindberg et al.[15] reported, as did Towbin,[19,20] other pathologic findings including laceration of the cord, edema, congestion, neuronal damage, and necrosis.

Walter and Tedeschi[21] found that in six of eight consecutive sudden and unexpected infant deaths, subarachnoid hemorrhage and concurrent spinal cord and brain stem injury were present at postmortem examination. In each, the trauma had been so mild that it escaped recognition. They felt that prenatal factors as well as physiologic neonatal hypoxia might contribute to and enhance effects of minor trauma. The associated findings of visceral congestion, pulmonary edema, atelectasis and hyaline membrane disease were felt to be secondary manifestations of cardiorespiratory distress of central origin. Hedley-Whyte and Gilles[11] described delayed or decreased myelination of axons proximal and distal to transection in paralyzed infants compared to normal controls. They attributed this lack of normal myelination to absence of peripheral axon connections.

Allen et al.[2] analyzed 31 children initially classified as having infantile spinal muscular atrophy or amyotonia congenita; 18 cases were found to have a clinically nonprogressive, nonfamilial neurologic disorder from birth. They felt that the most likely pathologic finding in these cases was spinal cord injury related to delivery. In addition, 5 cases of probable spinal cord injury occurring at the time of delivery were found in 127 consecutive breech deliveries. They believed that spinal injury in the newborn was frequently misdiagnosed.

Allen et al.[2] demonstrated by myelography laceration of the spinal cord related to breech delivery in three infants. They emphasized the prominent protuberant abdominal configuration and intercostal paralysis observed in the presence of spinal lesions. Their patients underwent laminectomy. Spinal cord injury in the newborn is frequently difficult to diagnose and thus the obstetrician, pediatrician, and pediatric neurologist should be cognizant of it as a possibility in any infant who suffers from paralysis or respiratory distress.

## REFERENCES

1.  Abrams IF, Bresnan MJ, Zuckerman JE, Fischer EG, Strand R: Cervical cord injuries secondary to hyperextension of the head in breech presentation. Obstet Gynecol 41:369–378, 1973
2.  Allen JP, Myers CG, Condon VR: Laceration of the spinal cord related to breech delivery. JAMA 208:1019–1022, 1969

3. Allen JP: Birth injury to the spinal cord. Northwest Med 69:323–326, 1970
4. Bresnan MJ, Abrams IF: Neonatal spinal cord transection secondary to intra-uterine hyperextension of the neck in breech presentation. J Pediatr 84:734–737, 1974
5. Bhagwanani SG, Price HV, Laurence KM, Ginz G: Risks and prevention of cervical cord injury in the management of breech presentation with hyperextension of the fetal head. Am J Obstet Gynecol 115:1159–1161, 1973
6. Byers RK: Spinal-cord injuries during birth. Develop Med Child Neurol 17:103–110, 1975
7. Crothers B, Putnam MC: Obstetrical injuries of the spinal cord. Medicine 6:41–126, 1927
8. De Souza SW, Davis JA: Spinal cord damage in a new-born infant. Arch Dis Child 49:70–71, 1974
9. Gordon N, Marsden B: Spinal cord injury at birth. Neuropaediatrie 2:112–118, 1970
10. Harris LS, Adelson L: "Spinal injury" and sudden infant death. A second look. Am J Clin Pathol 52:289–295, 1969
11. Hedley-Whyte ET, Gilles FH: Observations on myelination of human spinal cord and some effects of parturitional transection. J Neuropathol Exp Neurol 33:436–445, 1974
12. Hellstrom B, Sallmander U: Prevention of spinal cord injury in hyperextension of the fetal head. JAMA 204:107, 1968
13. Jellinger K, Schwingshackl A: Birth injury of the spinal cord. Neuropaediatrie 4:111–123, 1973
14. Leventhal HR: Birth injuries of the spinal cord. J Pediatr 56:447–453, 1960
15. Lindberg U, Hagberg B, Olsson Y, Sourander P: Injury of the spinal cord at birth. A report of two cases. Acta Paediatr Scand 64:546, 1975
16. Norman MG, Wedderburn LCW: Fetal spinal cord injury with cephalic delivery. Obstet Gynecol 42:355–358, 1973
17. Pridmore BR, Hey EN, Aherne WA: Spinal cord injury of the fetus during delivery with Kielland's forceps. J Obstet Gynaecol Br Commonw 81:168–172, 1974
18. Shulman ST, Madden JD, Esterly JR, Shanklin DR: Transection of spinal cord. Arch Dis Child 46:291–294, 1971
19. Towbin A: Latent spinal cord and brain stem injury in newborn infants. Develop Med Child Neurol 11:54–68, 1969
20. Towbin A: Neonatal damage of the central nervous system. In Tedeschi CG (ed): Neuropathology: Methods and Diagnosis. New York, Little, Brown, 1970, pp 609–653
21. Walter CE, Tedeschi LG: Spinal injury and neonatal death. Report of six cases. Am J Obstet Gynecol 106:272–278, 1970

# 19

# Associated Injuries

In many patients, trauma to the spinal cord is accompanied by injuries involving other organ systems. Guttmann[7] found that in a series of 396 patients paralyzed as a result of trauma, 113 (28 percent) had major associated injuries involving the skull and brain, long bones, pelvis, ribs, thoracic cavity, sternum, scapula, and clavicle, as well as injuries to internal organs. These injuries associated with injury to the spinal cord may be of such magnitude and severity that their treatment takes precedence over management of the spinal injury. For example, a patient with a ruptured spleen urgently requires surgery as a lifesaving measure. Certain other chest, abdominal, and great vessel injuries take precedence in a similar manner.

Lipschitz,[12] in an evaluation of injuries associated with stab wounds of the spinal cord, reported 86 separate injuries accompanying 252 spinal stab wounds. Major associated injuries occurred in the cervical arteries, brachial plexus, trachea, esophagus, thoracic cage, limbs, and abdomen. As might be anticipated, he stressed the difficulty in diagnosing spinal cord injuries in the unconscious patient. In unconscious patients with paralysis due to spinal cord injury, he noted that a "cold nose" and "warm feet" due to vasodilation below the paralytic lesion may be present. This is not found in isolated head injuries. Conversely, Lipschitz reported three unconscious patients with isolated bilateral midline injuries over the sagittal sinus and motor cortex in whom the erroneous diagnosis of spinal injury was made. In stab wounds the diagnosis is even more difficult as x-rays of the spine are usually negative.

Bricker et al.[3] described 18 patients with major injuries to the chest, thoracic outlet, or abdomen associated with spinal cord injuries. They stressed that appropriate management of such patients was as it would have been without the spinal cord injury, the surgeon and anesthesiologist keeping foremost in mind the importance of proper positioning to avoid further neurologic damage. They also stressed the labile nature of cardiac and vasomotor responses of the neurologically damaged patient. They felt in general that neurosurgical intervention should be secondary in life-threatening conditions that require urgent thoracic and abdominal surgical procedures.

Meinecke[14] reported that in 340 (57.1 percent) associated injuries in 595 traumatic cord lesions, 42 percent were cranial injuries, 31 percent thoracic injuries, and 37 percent limb injuries. Tricot and Halbot[22] report only 28 associated injuries among 250 patients with cord damage. Jacobson and Bors[9] reported 67 percent major associated injuries in 114 traumatic Vietnam War spinal injuries, 43 involving the chest and 26 the abdominal organs. Acute associated injuries frequently take precedence in treatment (see Chap. 5). Other authors reporting on associated injuries are Bénassy,[2] Frankel,[5] Harris,[8] McSweeney,[13] and Silver.[18]

Injury to the neck may indirectly cause cerebral signs and symptoms. Simeone and Goldberg[19] reported a patient who, as a result of hyperextension injury of the neck, suffered thrombosis of her vertebral artery. This led to death from hindbrain ischemia. That the vertebral artery was occluded was documented both by arteriography and surgical removal of the clot. Bell[1] described a patient in whom basilar artery insufficiency was directly related to atlanto-occipital instability and transient compression of the vertebral arteries. Lewin[11] has documented several patients with cerebral ill effects caused by injury to one or both vertebral arteries.

Keggi et al.[10] reported vertebral artery insufficiency secondary to trauma and osteoarthritis of the cervical spine. Other authors including Coburn,[4] Gosch et al.,[6] Suechting and French,[20] Thomas et al.,[21] and Schneider et al.[16,17] have contributed to the understanding of vascular insufficiency of the brain stem and spinal cord in spinal trauma. Signs and symptoms of vertebral artery sufficiency are clinically manifested by neurologic sequelae of reduced basilar artery blood flow. Standard neurologic texts[5] describe more completely the numerous hindbrain syndromes that may result. Osteoarthritis of the cervical spine may be contributory. On occasion the neurologic status improves with reduction of the cervical fracture dislocation.

## REFERENCES

1. Bell HS: Basilar artery insufficiency due to atlanto-occipital instability. Am Surg 35:695–700, 1969
2. Bénassy J: Associated fractures of the limbs in traumatic paraplegia and tetraplegia. Paraplegia 5:209–211, 1968
3. Bricker DL, Waltz TA, Telford RJ, Beall AC, Jr: Major abdominal and thoracic trauma associated with spinal cord injury: problems in management. J Trauma 11:63–75, 1971
4. Coburn DF: Vertebral artery involvement in cervical trauma. Clin Orthop 24:61–63, 1962
5. Frankel H: Associated chest injuries. Paraplegia 5:221–225, 1968
6. Gosch HH, Gooding E, Schneider RC: Cervical spinal cord hemorrhages in experimental head injuries. J Neurosurg 33:640–645, 1970
7. Guttmann L: Spinal Cord Injuries: Comprehensive Management and Research. Oxford, Blackwell Scientific Publications, 1973, pp 175–177

8. Harris P: Associated injuries in traumatic paraplegia and tetraplegia. Paraplegia 5:215–220, 1968
9. Jacobson SA, Bors E: Spinal cord injury in Vietnamese combat. Paraplegia 7:263–281, 1970
10. Keggi KJ, Granger DP, Southwick WO: Vertebral arterial insufficiency secondary to trauma and osteoarthritis of the cervical spine. Yale J Biol Med 38:471–478, 1966
11. Lewin W: Cerebral effects of injury to the vertebral artery. Br J Surg 52:223–225, 1965
12. Lipschitz R: Associated injuries and complications of stab wounds of the spinal cord. Paraplegia 5:75–82, 1967
13. McSweeney: The early management of associated injuries in the presence of co-incidental damage to the spinal cord. Paraplegia 5:189–196, 1968
14. Meinecke FW: Frequency and distribution of associated injuries in traumatic paraplegia and tetraplegia. Paraplegia 5:196–211, 1968
15. Murray DS: Post-traumatic thrombosis of the internal carotid and vertebral arteries after non-penetrating injuries of the neck. Br J Surg 44:556–561, 1957
16. Schneider RC, Crosby EC: Vascular insufficiency of brain stem and spinal cord in spinal trauma. Neurology 9:643–656, 1959
17. Schneider RC, Schemm GW: Vertebral artery insufficiency in acute and chronic spinal trauma. J Neurosurg 18:348, 1961
18. Silver J: Chest injuries and complications in the early stages of spinal cord injury. Paraplegia 5:226–243, 1968
19. Simeone FA, Goldberg HI: Thrombosis of vertebral artery from hyperextension injury to the neck. J Neurosurg 29:540–544, 1968
20. Suechting RL, French LA: Posterior inferior cerebellar artery syndrome following a fracture of the cervical vertebra. J Neurosurg 12:187–189, 1955
21. Thomas LM, Hardy WG, Lindner DW, Gurdjian ES: Carotic and vertebral artery involvement in cervical-cranial trauma. Clin Orthop 27:127–134, 1963
22. Tricot A, Halbot R: Traumatic paraplegia and associated fractures. Paraplegia 5:211–215, 1968

# 20

## Abdominal Complications

Undiagnosed abdominal disease accounts for approximately 10 percent of all fatalities among patients with spinal cord injuries, and a perforated viscus with peritonitis is most common.[5] Corticosteroid treatment of acute spinal injury is now more or less routine so that associated gastrointestinal complications are more frequent. Because of the quadriplegic's inability to perceive painful abdominal stimuli (Fig. 1) and because many signs of a surgically significant abdominal condition are absent, appropriate treatment may be delayed.[8,9] A high index of suspicion must be maintained by the individual caring for these patients.

Ileus is common in the acute quadriplegic so that bowel obstruction, partial or complete from whatever etiology, may be obscured.[4] Fortunately, the commonest cause of lower bowel obstruction with constipation is fecal impaction and this can be diagnosed and remedied by rectal examination. Increasing girth and tightness of the abdomen may be an early sign. Thus daily abdominal girth measurements are indicated. Constipation is common in these patients and may be overlooked as an early sign. Auscultation of the abdomen can aid in establishing the diagnosis of obstruction of ileus, although peristalsis can be hypoactive in recent spinal injuries. X-ray of the abdomen will show dilated loops of bowel and fluid levels later in obstruction. Loss of appetite, nausea, and vomiting occur. Nasogastric suction may produce a large volume of aspirate. Seizures, presumably due to electrolyte disturbance, have been reported.[4] Stool should be examined for gross or microscopic blood. Adhesions, carcinoma, volvulus, as well as other causes of intestinal obstruction, have been observed in quadriplegic patients.[2,7]

Signs of dysfunction of autonomic reflexes, such as sweating, elevated pulse rate, and elevated blood pressure, may be present but some patients with chronic disease such as chronic cholecystitis can be asymptomatic. Patients may develop aversion to food and others may be aware of diffuse dis-

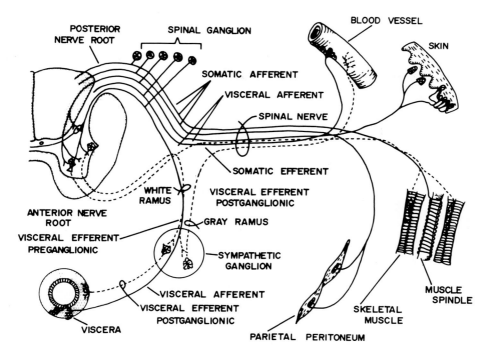

*Fig. 1.* Conduction of pain stimuli from abdominal viscera and peritoneum to the spinal cord. (Modified from Gray's Anatomy, 29th ed., Fig. 12-73)

comfort or exhibit restlessness with a feeling that something is wrong that cannot be localized.[1]

Signs of a more severe abdominal condition with either perforation or bowel necrosis may be masked by lack of pain. Persistent nausea and vomiting affords a clue. Miller et al.[6] describe such a patient and in addition present a patient with severe abdominal signs with merely a viral enteritis. Occasionally pain is felt in the supraclavicular area owing to referral of the pain of diaphragmatic irritation by means of common dermatomal C4–C5 innervation of the diaphragm and the skin of the shoulder.[8] The pulse of a quadriplegic patient may be elevated for many reasons not related to abdominal illness and thus may not be taken seriously. Pulse elevation, however, or bradycardia in some cases are important signs[1] particularly when this is a change from the stable condition. Change in spasticity from extensor to flexor muscles teleologically to protect the abdomen has also been noted.[2] Conduction of pain stimuli from abdominal viscera to the cord may be by way of the thoracic sympathetic, splanchnic, hypogastric, or pelvic nerves and then to the dorsal root ganglion (Fig. 1).[3,5] Therefore, in some patients even with a cervical cord lesion discomfort may be felt but is usually not well localized.

Very often not only quadriplegic patients but also paraplegic patients[2] have temperature elevations, raised white counts, loss of appetite, etc., so it is sometimes difficult to depend on these signs for identification of abdominal diseases. X-rays are helpful and lateral decubitus or upright films may reveal free air in the case of perforation. Localized tenderness or generalized abdominal tenderness is unusual but muscle guarding and rigidity may or may not be present even with peritonitis. Unexplained shock has occasionally been the first alerting sign, although in retrospect other clues were always present. Other reported causes of surgically significant abdominal conditions that may result in perforation or necrosis include appendicitis, peptic ulcer, and gallbladder disease. Abscesses, kidney and bladder disturbances, or ruptured spleen[3,5] will also cause acute abdominal conditions.

Greenfield[2] extensively discussed problems in diagnosis encountered in patients with chronic paraplegia. He reported two cases involving the appendix, two cases of cholelithiasis, one of perisigmoid abscess, and one of a traumatic spleen injury complicated by postoperative subphrenic abscess. He felt, based on his experience, that patients with chronic paraplegia withstand abdominal operations well and heal as quickly as normal individuals. This has also been our experience, so that abdominal exploration should not be delayed.

Pollock and Finkelman[8] emphasized that in patients with chronic spinal cord injuries the motor function of the gastrointestinal tract is within normal limits except for possibly a sluggish colon. However, no pain is felt when gastrointestinal structures are compromised. They stated that hunger, appetite, satisfaction, and repletion are normal but thirst seems increased. Hoen and Cooper[3] stressed the existence of a nonneurologic problem when abdominal pain occurs in the paraplegic patient. They emphasized the importance of establishing baselines of physical findings as well as laboratory data. They felt that surgical exploration is justified when a definite cause of abdominal pain in paraplegia and quadriplegic patients cannot be established.

## REFERENCES

1. Charney KJ, Juler GL, Comarr AE: General surgery problems in patients with spinal cord injuries. Arch Surg 110:1083–1088, 1975
2. Greenfield J: Abdominal operations on patients with chronic paraplegia, report of cases. Arch Surg 59:1077–1087, 1949
3. Hoen TI, Cooper IS: Acute abdominal emergencies in paraplegics. Am J Surg 75:19–24, 1948
4. Holden EM: Intestinal obstruction in spinal cord injury patients. Proc Ann Clin Spinal Cord Injury Conf 15:110–112, 1966
5. Ingberg HO, Prust FW: The diagnosis of abdominal emergencies in patients with spinal cord lesions. Arch Phys Med Rehabil 49:343–348, 1968
6. Miller LS, Staas WE, Jr, Herbison GJ: Abdominal problems in patients with spinal cord lesions. Arch Phys Med Rehabil 56:405–408, 1975
7. O'Hare JM: The acute abdomen in spinal cord injury patients. Proc Ann Clin Spinal Cord Injury Conf 15:113–117, 1966
8. Pollock LJ, Finkelman I: The digestive apparatus in injuries to the spinal cord. Surg Clin North Am 34:259–268, 1954
9. Wolff HG, Wolf S: Pain. Springfield, Ill., Charles C Thomas, 1948, pp 56–60

# 21

# Pulmonary Complications

## INTRODUCTION

Incidence of early morbidity and mortality from pulmonary causes is high among patients with high spinal injury. The cause of death in many instances is bronchopneumonia or pulmonary embolism. Pathologic changes in the lungs may be due to paralysis of respiratory musculature, particularly the diaphragmatic, intercostal, and abdominal muscles, which combine with loss of vasomotor control and enforced recumbency to increase possibilities of pulmonary complications. Paralysis of abdominal musculature makes clearing of bronchial and pharyngeal secretions difficult since coughing is diminished. Paralysis of abdominal, diaphragmatic, and intercostal muscles decreases ventilatory excursion of the chest and results in inadequate ventilation of certain pulmonary segments and greater liability to collapse and infection. Enforced recumbency increases likelihood of aspiration and hypostatic pneumonia as well as deep femoral and pelvic vein thrombosis. Therapy may include use of antibiotics, anticoagulants, oxygen, suction, assisted ventilation, and tracheotomy. Silver[15] has provided an excellent review of chest complications occurring in early stages following spinal cord injury.

## PARALYSIS OF RESPIRATORY FUNCTION

Chest complications in quadriplegics are largely related to impairment of normal breathing mechanisms and the patient's inability to cough as a result of paralysis of intercostal and abdominal musculature. Phrenic nerve dysfunction may contribute in part to loss of diaphragmatic tone and further lessen ventilatory capacity. Occasionally loss of diaphragmatic function is unilateral. With a lesion at C4 or higher apnea occurs. Paralytic ileus so common in acute spinal injuries further lessens diaphragmatic breathing efficacy. Early aspiration of gastric or pharyngeal contents following injury occurs commonly but can be prevented by proper suctioning and toilet. Head injuries and fractured ribs increase the incidence of pulmonary complications in tetraplegics.

During the period immediately following a cervical or high thoracic spinal injury pneumonitic complications are most common. These include atelectasis, pneumothorax, bronchopneumonia, lung collapse, lung abscess, and pleural effusion. Two rare causes of pleural effusion are chylothorax from direct damage to the thoracic duct and subarachnoid-pleural fistula. In the latter, cerebrospinal fluid accumulates in the chest cavity. Bramwit and Schmelka[3] reported a case secondary to a gunshot wound. Campos et al.[5] reported a patient injured in an auto accident in whom the diagnosis of cerebrospinal fluid (CSF) fistula was made by myelographic detection of contrast material in the chest. The patient was a child of five who was treated by thoracotomy and laminectomy. In almost all other reported patients only pleural aspiration of fluid has been required.

Early symptoms of pneumonia include cough, chest discomfort, chest pain, and dyspnea. Tachycardia, tachypnea, and fever can be present. Rales may be heard but auscultatory examination of the chest may reveal only diminished breath sounds. Sputum should be obtained for culture and sensitivity, but is frequently difficult to obtain because of difficulty coughing, and test results are nonspecific or fail to demonstrate a predominant pathogen.

Repeated chest x-rays are probably the most effective means of diagnosing pneumonitic complications. Lateral x-ray views should be considered so that the posterior dependent portion of the lungs can be visualized. Even in some patients with no symptoms and signs there is x-ray evidence of pathologic pneumonitic processes.

Smoking should be discouraged in the first weeks following injury since it increases bronchial and pulmonary secretion and damages cilia. Treatment of any respiratory complication includes proper suctioning, deep breathing, postural drainage, chest percussion, positive pressure respiration, tracheostomy, and appropriate antibiotics. Blood gas determinations may be required to assess the need for supportive oxygen therapy.

The lower the spinal injury the less the incidence of pulmonary complications but pulmonary complications can occur even in lumbar cauda equina injuries. Muscles of respiration include the intercostals, diaphragm, and abdominals. The sternocleidomatoid and trapezius are the most important auxiliary respiratory muscles. Guttmann's[7] suggestion that 0.3 to 0.5 mg Prostigmine be given every four to five hours to patients with ileus has proved invaluable and even a "life-saving" measure to aid in returning bowel function earlier, thus lessening respiratory distress. He also stresses that edema of the lungs can be due in part to the fluid overload resulting from disturbed fluid balance presumably occurring in the paralyzed patient.

When vital capacity becomes adequate (500 to 800 cc) the patient can be weaned from the respirator. Hitchcock and Leece[8] presented evidence that automatic respiration in man is mediated through the reticulospinal pathways lying in the anterolateral column of the cervical spinal cord. Belmusto et al.[2] and Nathan[12] concluded that fibers concerned with respiration in man occupied an area from C1 to C3 between 3 and 5.5 mm from the lateral margin of the cord. Belmusto et al.[2] are of the opinion that the spinothalamic and respiratory pathways are intermingled. Hitchcock and Leese[8] believe that this intermingling of fibers is limited. There seems little doubt that the reticulospinal tract, just medial to the lateral spinothalamic tract, is concerned with respiration and there seems good evidence for a combination of voluntary and automatic respiration. If reticulospinal pathways are damaged, only voluntary respiration, dependent on consciousness, is possible; cessation of breathing during sleep may occur. The voluntary control of respiration is presumably accomplished through the corticospinal tract and the final common pathway for both voluntary and involuntary control is through the anterior horn cell.

Roncoroni[14] described a nine-year-old boy with traumatic complete spinal cord transection at C2 who did not feel breathless during apnea. Studies conducted during diffusion respiration tended to show that neither chemical stimuli due to hydrogen ion or $PaCO_2$ nor pulmonary vagal receptor activity was capable of inducing respiratory distress. Complete loss of thoracic motor activity and proprioceptive information may explain the absence of the sensation of breathlessness when ventilation was suddenly arrested. He proposed that absence of distress during apnea was due to the high-level spinal section that prevented any respiratory muscle activity or transmission of proprioceptive information.

Jennett[9] found that development of hypoxic tachycardia in man does not depend on central stimulation in the brain stem and increased sympathetic impulse traffic from medulla to thoracic spinal cord. She suggested that in quadriplegic patients hypoxia caused an identical increase and reoxygenation cause a similar decrease in heart rate, as it does in normal persons. She suggested, however, that if medullary and spinal centers were involved the efferent pathway must be vagal.

Moulton and Silver[10] studied patients with traumatic tetraplegia and found that chest movements were reduced with paradoxical sucking in of the lateral wall of the rib cage. When the head was tilted 30 percent up and 30 percent down postural effects were observed in apical and sternochondral regions. Paradoxical movements appear to be due to both a loss of action of the paralyzed intercostal muscles and impairment of the diaphragm secondary to paralysis of intercostal and abdominal muscles.

Brisman et al.[4] found that pulmonary edema is a frequent autopsy finding in patients with acute injuries of the cervical spine. They found that when central venous pressure had been measured it usually has been normal, and postulated that possibly an elevation in the left heart pressure not reflected in the right heart circulation explained normal central venous pressure. They had no explanation for the disparity in left and right heart function.

## PULMONARY EMBOLISM

Respiratory complications in quadriplegics are common and all too often such a complication is diagnosed as pneumonitis when in fact pulmonary embolization has occurred. Chest pain, hemoptysis, dyspnea, swelling of the leg, and hypotension may be significant. However, many quadriplegic patients have such symptoms in the absence of pulmonary embolism. A lung scan may be diagnostic and laboratory data such as elevation of lactic dehydrogenase (LDH), serum glutamic oxalacetic transaminase (SGOT), and abnormal blood gases may be significant. In our practice although respiratory problems are common, pulmonary complications from embolization are uncommon and do not seem to warrant prophylactic anticoagulation.

There is considerable controversy as to whether prophylactic anticoagulation should be carried out in paraplegics and quadriplegics. All agree, however, that after three months of paralysis pulmonary embolization is rare so that anticoagulation is no longer necessary.

Phillips[13] investigated 25 paraplegics by venogram to ascertain the incidence of deep vein thrombosis. Only 4 percent showed evidence of *prior* deep vein thrombosis. The most important factor producing deep leg or pelvic vein thrombosis seems to be venous stasis due to absent muscle pumping associated with prolonged recumbency. Guttmann[6] cautiously advises routine anticoagulant therapy utilizing oral medication. Under emergency circumstances heparin is administered intravenously.

Watson,[19] in an analysis of 234 paraplegics over a five-year period, found a 2.5 percent mortality from pulmonary embolus. Anticoagulant treatment was administered only at the earliest sign of deep vein thrombosis or pulmonary embolus. He concluded prophylactic anticoagulation to be unwarranted.

Naso[11] studied 4 patients who suffered pulmonary embolism among 26 having acute spinal cord injury. Of 17 additional patients having chronic spinal injury, none had any problem with thromboembolic phenomena. Three months was used as the dividing line between acute and chronic injury. The diagnosis of pulmonary embolus was made if findings on the history, examination, and lung scan supported it. Physical signs and symptoms included those previously mentioned and laboratory data were also considered to be significant. Of 6 patients having an additional study of coagulation factors 3 were found to be abnormal.

Tribe and Silver[18] found that the incidence of death due to pulmonary embolism in acute paraplegia was 37 percent and in 1969, they expanded the earlier series and found the incidence increased to 45 percent. This contrasted with findings of others in which no case of embolism was noted in chronic paraplegics. In the acute spinal cord-injured patient certain features are present that are known to predispose to the "hypercoagulable state." Amundsen and associates[1] found that malignancy and the postoperative state predispose to clotting, and fibrinogen levels and factor VIII (AHG) are increased. Trauma has also been found to be associated with hypercoagulability and is characterized by thrombocytosis and decreased fibrinolysis in the early days and weeks following injury.

Silver and Moulton[17] advised prophylactic anticoagulant therapy to forestall pulmonary emboli in acute paraplegia. They contrasted 42 patients given anticoagulants only in accordance wth accepted medical indications when clinical deep venous thrombosis or pulmonary embolus developed. Another with a group of 35 patients were given prophylactic anticoagulants. They concluded that pulmonary embolus is a significant cause of death within 14 days following a traumatic spinal injury and that prophylactic anticoagulant therapy given within a few days of admission appears to offer advantages in preventing pulmonary emboli while not hindering the patient's progress.

Silver,[16] in 1974, stated that pulmonary embolism is the major cause of death in the first few weeks after an acute spinal injury. He reported that anticoagulant therapy was administered to 68 consecutive eligible males prophylactically; 32 patients were deemed ineligible. A period of at least 24 hours was allowed to elapse before commencing therapy and presence of bowel sounds and ability to ingest solid food were mandatory. He felt that ileus is associated with increased gastrointestinal bleeding possibly precipitated by anticoagulants. Severe associated injuries mitigated against anticoagulation therapy as did a history of peptic ulcers. Of the 68 patients, 6 developed nonfatal complications including gastrointestinal hemorrhages. The incidence of pulmonary embolus was higher in the group not receiving anticoagulants. Silver[16] appeared to stop short of recommending general use of anticoagulants.

## REFERENCES

1. Amundsen MA, Spittell JA, Jr, Thompson JH, Jr, et al: Hypercoagulability associated with malignant disease and with postoperative state: evidence for elevated levels of antihemophilic globulin. Ann Int Med 58:608–616, 1962
2. Belmusto L, Brown E, Owens G: Clinical observations on respiratory and vasomotor disturbances as related to cervical cordotomies. J Neurosurg 20:225–232, 1963
3. Bramwit DN, Schmelka DD: Traumatic subarachnoid pleural fistula. Radiology 89:737–738, 1967
4. Brisman R, Kovach RM, Johnson DO, Roberts CR, Ward GS: Pulmonary edema in acute transection of the cervical spinal cord. Surg Gynecol Obstet 139:363–366, 1974
5. Campos BAR, Silva LB, Ballalai N, Negrao MM: Traumatic subarachnoid pleural fistula. J Neurol Neurosurg Psychiatr 37:269–270, 1974
6. Guttmann L: Spinal Cord Injuries: Comprehensive Management and Research. Oxford, Blackwell Scientific Publications, 1973, chap 16, pp 178–181
7. Guttmann L: Spinal Cord Injuries: Comprehensive Management and Research. Oxford, Blackwell Scientific Publications, 1973, chap 17, pp 193–199
8. Hitchcock E, Leece B: Somatotopic representation of the respiratory pathways in the cervical cord of man. J Neurosurg 27:320–329, 1967
9. Jennett S: The effect of brief moderate hypoxia and abrupt re-oxygenation on the

heart rate in human subjects with cervical spinal transection. J Physiol (London) 205:35–36, 1969

10. Moulton A, Silver JR: Chest movements in patients with traumatic injuries of the cervical cord. Clin Sci 39:407–422, 1970

11. Naso F: Pulmonary embolism in acute spinal cord injury. Arch Phys Med Rehabil 55:275–278, 1974

12. Nathan PW: The descending respiratory pathway in man. J Neurol Neurosurg Psychiatr 26:487–499, 1963

13. Phillipps RS: Incidence of deep venous thrombosis in paraplegics. Paraplegia 1: 116–130, 1963

14. Roncoroni AJ: Lack of breathlessness during apnea in a patient with high spinal cord transection. Chest 62:514–515, 1972

15. Silver JR: Chest injuries and complications in the early stages of spinal cord injury. Paraplegia 5:226–245, 1968

16. Silver JR: The prophylactic use of anticoagulant therapy in the prevention of pulmonary emboli in 100 consecutive spinal injury patients. Paraplegia 12:188–196, 1974

17. Silver JR, Moulton A: Prophylactic anticoagulant therapy against pulmonary emboli in acute paraplegia. Br Med J 2:338–340, 1970

18. Tribe CR, Silver JR: Renal Failure in Paraplegia. London, Pitman, 1969

19. Watson N: Anticoagulant therapy in the treatment of venous thrombosis and pulmonary embolism in acute spinal injury. Paraplegia 12:197–201, 1974

# 22

# Cardiovascular Complications

It has been observed that in traumatic quadriplegia blood pressure is lowered within the first few hours or days, although hypotension is difficult to document because the patient's blood pressure prior to the accident is usually unknown. In animal studies such hypotension seems to occur but almost all experimental injuries are situated in the mid- or lower thoracic levels, not interfering with sympathetic outflow. Rosenbluth and Meirowsky[14] describe lowered blood pressure encountered in acute quadriplegia and interpret this as part of a generalized sympathetic blockade. Whether this observed arterial hypotension can significantly contribute to ischemia at the level of the injured spinal cord is problematic but if it does, potentially reversible spinal cord damage could become permanent. Elevating blood pressure somewhat, or as soon as possible, could conceivably prevent or diminish damage. On the other hand, elevated blood pressure may carry risk in infarcted nervous tissue because with breakdown of the blood-brain barrier hemorrhage into the ischemic area could occur.

Silver[18] studied 15 patients in spinal shock with complete functional loss between C3 and T4 who had loss of those efferent spinal vascular reflex pathways from medullary and other cerebral centers. He found that during the stage of spinal shock, when tendon reflexes are abolished, the autonomic reflexes of inspiratory vasoconstriction and autonomic hyperreflexia are preserved.[17] Tilting of a paraplegic patient can result in trapping of venous blood in the legs with insufficient cerebral circulation due to venous blood in the legs.[3] However, compensatory mechanisms, probably due to spinal reflexes, are considerable and tend to maintain circulation soon after injury.

Meinecke[12] noted that in 28 acute paralyzed patients both systolic and diastolic pressures rose 20 mm Hg or more after approximately one week of hospitalization. The lower the spinal lesion the less was the initial depression of blood pressure. He also studied orthostatic blood pressure responses in chronic quadriplegics and found that patients with upper thoracic and cervical cord lesions show a fall in blood pressure and an increase in pulse rate on assuming the upright position, especially more pronounced and prolonged in patients with upper thoracic spinal lesions. Patients with cervical cord injury display adaptive mechanisms earlier. Freyschuss and Knutsson[4] stated that interruption of the spinal cord at cervical levels can be expected to deprive the individual of control from higher centers since no physiologic evidence of sympathetic outflow above the first thoracic segment exists. They speculated that circulatory adjustments elicited in cerebral vasomotor centers are mediated by changes in vagal tone only in quadriplegics. Impairment in vasomotor tone to head up tilt and loss of ordinary blood pressure increase during exercise has been observed in these patients. With time, in many quadriplegics, vasomotor tone returns.

In the acute patient sympathetic blockade is described by Cole et al.[3] to be characterized by disorientation, unresponsiveness, hypotension, bradycardia, and hypothermia. Sherrington[16] and Clark[2] observed that shivering and piloerection occurred only in innervated regions above the level of cord section.

Kunin[9] studied the blood pressure in 152 adult male paraplegic and quadriplegic patients known to have chronic urinary tract infection. Many had x-ray film evidence of renal involvement but few had elevated serum creatinine levels. Elevated blood pressure was rare in that group of patients. In his review of the literature this finding was confirmed, but he emphasized that hypertension and pyelonephritis play a highly significant role in patients who die as a result of spinal cord injury. He states that control of hypertension remains an important goal for patients with recurrent or persistent urinary tract infection.

Thompson and Witham[19] describe paroxysmal systemic arterial hypertension in patients with spinal cord injury. This, they observed, is part of the mass sympathetic discharge or "mass reflex,"[15] described by Head and Riddoch,[7] which includes hypertension, sweating, flushing of the face, congestion of nasal passages, pilomotor erection, shivering, headache, blurring of vision, and changes in pulse rate and quality. All are consistent with the effects of sympathetic discharge. Trigger mechanisms may include almost any somatic stimulus as well as distention of the bladder and rectum.[15] Blood pressures have been found to be more labile when lesions are above the fifth dorsal segment.

Severe intermittent headache accompanying high cord lesions should make one suspicious of this type of sympathetic autonomic discharge, also known as autonomic hyperreflexia. Attention should be directed to the bladder and/or bowel. Blocking of a urinary catheter and distention of the rectum are frequent causes. Instability of blood pressure during surgical procedures may also be of importance. Hypertension can cause excessive bleeding presenting difficulty in accomplishing hemostasis. Cerebrovascular accidents have occurred, possibly as a result of this mechanism, intraoperatively as well as operatively.

Johnson et al.[8] stated, and most agree, that autonomic hyperreflexia is manifest by complaints of sweating, ascending sensations in the chest and neck, flushing, nasal obstruction, headaches, nausea and vomiting, difficulty breathing, shivering, and blurring of vision. On examination, paroxysmal hypertension, bradycardia, arrhythmias, sweating, cutaneous vasodilatation above and vasoconstriction below the lesion, cutis anserina ("goose flesh"), changes in skin and rectal temperature,[11,15] changes in level of consciousness, convulsions, visual field defects, temporary cessation of respiration, EKG changes, and x-ray evidence of enlargement of the heart may be seen. Autonomic hyperreflexia occurs in a high percentage of quadriplegics and is a generalized abnormal sympathetic discharge which in most intact people would cause only a minor physiologic alteration.

Autonomic hyperreflexia can be triggered by many endogenous and exogenous stimuli, occurring below the level of transection. Distention of a hollow viscus is most common. Morbidity and mortality are usually related to central nervous system disorders and usually due to paroxysmal systemic hypertension. Retinal and cerebral hemorrhages account for most problems.

Therapy of autonomic hyperreflexia is difficult. Prevention of the stimulus that causes the syndrome is important particularly during anesthesia. Extensive posterior rhizotomy,[1] cordotomy, and alcohol blocks have been advocated but are not practiced widely. During cystoscopy and other procedures topical and local anesthesia are advocated. Alpha-adrenergic blocking drugs such as phentolamine have been tried with equivocal results. Ganglionic blocking agents have been utilized for temporary periods.

Greenhoot et al.[5,6] showed that with experimental spinal cord injury in dogs alterations of the electrocardiogram, blood pressure, and myocardial histologic changes were produced. They felt that sympathetic discharges occurred within seconds of the injury and were manifested by hypertension and tachycardia. Fuchsinophilic degeneration of myocardial cells was seen in the injured animals.

LaBan et al.[10] found in 14 chronic spinal cord-injured patients that blood volume was significantly elevated utilizing a radioiodinated serum tracer method. Patients with cauda equina injury demonstrated the largest increase while patients with higher lesions had less marked defects. They attributed the blood volume increase to increase in venous capacity, alteration in muscle/fat ratio, and strenuous physical therapy.

Pledger[13] emphasized disorders of temperature regulation in acute traumatic tetraplegia. He stated that the acute cord lesion deprives the patient of almost all means of compensating for changes in environmental temperatures. He emphasized that fever may or may not be a sign of infection and that the latter should be defined by clinical and bacteriologic evidence.

For further discussion on vasomotor control and temperature regulation, see Chapter 3.

## REFERENCES

1. Bors E, French JD: Management of paroxysmal hypertension following injuries to cervical and upper thoracic segments of the spinal cord. Arch Surg 64:803–812, 1952
2. Clark G: Temperature regulation in chronic cervical cats. Am J Physiol 130:712–722, 1940
3. Cole TM, Kottke FJ, Olson M: Alterations of cardiovascular control in high spinal myelomalacia. Arch Phys Med 48:359–368, 1967
4. Freyschuss U, Knutsson E: Cardiovascular control in man with transverse cervical cord lesions. Life Sci 8:421–424, 1969
5. Greenhoot JH, Mauck HP, Jr: The effect of cervical cord injury on cardiac rhythm and conduction. Am Heart J 83:659–662, 1972
6. Greenhoot JH, Shiel F, Mauck HP, Jr: Experimental spinal cord injury. Electrocardiographic abnormalities and fuchsinophilic myocardial degeneration. Arch Neurol 26:524–529, 1972
7. Head H, Riddoch G: Automatic bladder, excessive sweating and some other reflex conditions, in gross injuries of spinal cord. Brain 40:188–263, 1917
8. Johnson B, Thomason R, Pallares V, Sadove M: Autonomic hyperreflexia: A review. Milit Med 140:345–349, 1975
9. Kunin CM: Blood pressure in patients with spinal cord injury. Arch Intern Med 127:285–287, 1971
10. LaBan MM, Johnson HE, Verdon TA, Jr, Grant AE: Blood volume following spinal cord injury. Arch Phys Med 50:439–441, 1969
11. List CG, Pimenta AD: Sweat secretion in man. VI. Spinal reflex sweating. Arch Neurol Psychiatr 51:501–507, 1944
12. Meinecke FW: Regulation of the cardiovascular system in patients with fresh injuries to the spinal cord—preliminary report. Paraplegia 9:109–112, 1971
13. Pledger HG: Disorders of temperature regulation in acute traumatic tetraplegia. J Bone Joint Surg 44B:110–113, 1962
14. Rosenbluth PR, Meirowsky AM: Sympathetic blockade, an acute cervical cord syndrome. J Neurosurg 10:107–112, 1953
15. Sahs AL, Fulton JF: Somatic and autonomic reflexes in spinal monkeys. J Neurophysiol 3:258–268, 1940
16. Sherrington CB: Notes on temperature after spinal transection with some observations on shivering. J Physiol 58:405–424, 1924
17. Silver JR: Circulatory reflexes in spinal man. Paraplegia 2:235–246, 1965
18. Silver JR: Vascular reflexes in spinal shock. Paraplegia 8:231–242, 1971
19. Thompson CE, Witham AC: Paroxysmal hypertension in spinal-cord injuries. N Engl J Med 239:291–294, 1948

# 23

## Chronic Associated Conditions

### TREATMENT OF SEVERE SPASTICITY

Spasticity may occur following cervical and thoracic spinal cord injuries. Sometimes the slightest stimulus can set off a mass spasm. Spasticity accompanying even hopeless paraplegic states should be relieved because it may progress, condemning the patient to a bedridden existence with all the inherent problems of nursing care, as well as to accompanying demoralization. Decubitus ulcer formation, urinary stasis, infection, and stone formation are all too common in these patients. Even if the patient does not have a functional shoulder girdle and is therefore not a candidate for ambulation, it makes a remarkable difference to him if proper positioning in a chair can be accomplished, and perineal care is simplified if adductor spasticity can be relieved.

To these reasons of partial function and psychologic recovery must be added relief of pain. Pain may, in fact, be the overriding consideration to the patient. Pain most commonly occurs in paraplegics who have a "mass reflex"[69] but may also occur in flexor spasms per se without the classic mass reflex. The relationship of pain to spasticity is well established but its exact nature is not wholly understood.[51] The best way to relieve paraplegic spasticity is not well agreed upon, and many methods have been advanced.[31,32,34] Chemical treatments[74] and surgical possibilities[64] were discussed in a symposium on spasticity in 1962.

Nonsurgical therapy revolved around the use of curare and muscle relaxing agents. Although successful use of curare in the treatment of muscular spasticity in paraplegia was reported in the 1940s,[22,49] it was later reported to fail to appreciably alleviate spasm.[20,56] Muscle relaxing drugs, such as the short-acting mephenesin[3] and the somewhat longer-acting diazepam (Valium)[53] and many similar drugs, have had clinical trials with varying degrees of success. Levine[59] advocated Prazepam.

Recently, chemical therapy has centered around intrathecal injection of alcohol[95] or phenol.[55] The use of intrathecal alcohol for the relief of intractable pain was first described in 1931.[23] Its use in paraplegics to relieve muscular spasms was first described and advocated in the 1940s[21,37,82] and has had several proponents since.[10,27] The intrathecal deposition of phenol has been used since 1955 for the relief of pain[63] and, since 1959, to effect a chemical rhizotomy in cases of paraplegia with severe degrees of spasticity.[55,71] It was reported that the majority of patients so treated were benefited,[52] but more recent reports are less convincing.[71] Chemical agents have several undesirable characteristics. They frequently give only transient relief of symptoms[32] and their involvement of nerve fibers is indiscriminate, nonselective, and unpredictable.[71] They reduce bladder function in patients who still maintain a spinal reflex[53] and may destroy sensation, rendering the anesthetic skin more liable to injury. In addition, these agents have the potential of producing severe degenerative and reactive changes such as arachnoiditis, meningitis, vascular thrombosis, and demyelination.[94] Subsequent surgical therapy is thus made more difficult.

Surgical approaches to paraplegic spasticity have been varied, including peripheral nerve section, obturator nerve section,[42] cordotomy with section of the anterior[80] and/or posterior[30] columns, longitudinal myelotomy,[92] and cordectomy,[60] posterior root section,[76,88] and even electrocoagulation of the cord.[34] The approach yielding the best results for extensive spasticity with the least amount of anatomic destruction has been bilateral dorsolumbar anterior rhizotomy first reported by Munro.[69]

In 1933, Munro performed a dorsolumbar anterior rhizotomy to convert spastic paraplegia to flaccid paralysis.[69] Since then, this procedure has been incorporated into the neurosurgeon's armamentarium but has seen a more limited application than it possibly deserves. The majority of early reported cases were patients with traumatic spinal cord transections. Although recent reports have included additional spinal lesions, there appears to be further application of this procedure to nontraumatic paraplegic states not only for the purpose of relieving spasm but also, in certain individuals, for relieving associated pain while preserving sensation and bladder innervation.

A dorsolumbar laminectomy of T11 through L2 is carried out under general anesthesia. The dura is incised, the conus and cauda equina are visualized, and the last slip of the dentate ligament is identified and marked. The ligament is then severed and the cord rotated so that the anterior roots are visualized. The root at the level of the marked dentate ligament is considered L1. Each anterior root from T11 through S2 may then be encircled with a silk ligature, utilizing a ligature carrier. These are tied but no root cut until all anterior roots are so marked bilaterally, and then all roots encircled with silk ligatures are severed. This technical innovation gives good assurance that all intended roots are cut but that no unnecessary ones are included. This more elaborate procedure is not necessary in most cases. A peripheral nerve stimulator is used for identification of questionable anterior roots. Following the transections, the dura is closed as are the fascia, muscle, and skin in turn.

Most authors agree that the rhizotomy should include roots T10 or T11 through S1, sparing the lower sacral segments because of bladder innervation,[32,69] although Kerr[54] has advocated sparing of T10 and T11 to allow reflex tone in the abdominal musculature as a possible aid to micturition.

The major reported difficulty of the procedure has been accurate identification of the roots. It was formerly stated that the last dentate ligament attaches to the twelfth dorsal vertebra and the first lumbar posterior root rides in the fork of this dentate ligament.[26,69] Anatomic evidence has since shown this to be only a fairly constant relationship and that the root lying on the lowest slip of the dentate ligament may vary from T12 to L2.[23,61] Nonetheless, use of the last "firm" dentate as a point of orientation has proved a fairly reliable method of identifying the L1 root.[32]

Another method advanced for root identification states that the first sacral root is the lowest large root to leave the conus medullaris.[61] However, this has also been shown to be inconstant,[32] and S2[94] and S3[31,36] have each been said to be the last large root and useful as a point of orientation.

Since the crux of accurate root identification revolves around the accurate identification of the detrusor nerves so as not to severe the roots that postoperatively might give the patient a reflex bladder, a method has been reported[57] for the use of a cystometrogram apparatus in the operating room to locate the roots responsible for detrusor activity by direct stimulation. In a series of 22 patients, S3 and S4 were found to give maximal detrusor activity. Even if this method is not used, a peripheral nerve stimulator should be available so that, if need be, a given root may be stimulated for identification purposes prior to severance.[54] If the preoperative cystometrogram reveals an atonic, flaccid (neurogenic) bladder, then the preservation of its spinal innervation is of less importance. We have successfully employed a water manometer with a three-way stopcock attached to an indwelling catheter. We can then merely observe the rise in the fluid column with detrusor nerve root stimulation.

In contrast to this concept of leaving intact those nerves innervating the bladder, two groups have advocated denervating the entire sacral cord from T12 through S5.[12,67,68,70] In their opinion, this will not impede the development of good bladder function, but the patient will have an "automatic" bladder instead of a "reflex" bladder. This concept has not been generally accepted. In any event, the patient should be warned that urinary function and ability to have an erection may be altered. Muscle wasting may occur.

Once the roots are identified to the operator's satisfaction and are severed, he may expect good results. Munro[69] analyzed 59 such paraplegics in 1945, and operated on 10 of 19 who had a "mass reflex." In 1950, he reported 39 patients subjected to surgery with disappearance of the spasm in 36.[70] Freeman and Heimburger[33] reported results of anterior rhizotomy in 18 of 230 spastic paraplegics and 5 of 103 patients in a Canadian series[8] were operated on. The majority of these patients were significantly benefited.

These early reports were largely based on patients with traumatic spinal cord transections, but more recent reports have included nontraumatic paraplegic lesions. In Kerr's[54] series of 30 patients undergoing a dorsolumbar anterior rhizotomy for spasticity, 8 had demyelinating disease. Smolik et al.[83] advocated spinal chordectomy in the management of spastic paraplegia with complete sensory loss. This will reduce spasticity to flaccidity but seems an unnecessarily extensive surgical procedure.

Pedersen[75] advocated subarachnoid phenol in the treatment of spasticity. Likewise, Yeo[95] advocated intrathecal alcohol injection for treatment of spasticity. In our experience and that of Hansebout and Cosgrove[41] results of these injections are only temporary, lasting for six months to two to three years. Furthermore, when the patient finally comes to an open surgical procedure, there is considerable scarring, making the procedure more difficult.

Tenotomy has been utilized in the treatment of spastic paraplegia. Peterson[77] preferred tenotomy of the iliopsoas. In our experience this is generally ineffective in the treatment of severe spasticity associated with spinal paralysis since the spasticity involves all muscle groups below the level of the lesion.

## MYELOTOMY

Ivan[48] and Ivan and Wiley[47] advocate myelotomy in the management of spasticity. In 1951 Bischof[5] described longitudinal myelotomy, a procedure which has been promising as an effective method of relieving spasticity while retaining certain spinal cord function. The procedure involves a laminectomy from T10 to L1 and the longitudinal division of the spinal cord into anterior (ventral) and posterior (dorsal) halves from T12 to S1. This procedure avoids all long tracts yet interrupts both the monosynaptic and polysynaptic reflex arcs. Consequently spasticity and flexor spasms are relieved while bladder function, touch, and vibration sense, and in some cases certain motor functions are preserved. In our experience myelotomy has not provided long lasting relief of spasticity. We have had to repeat the procedure using anterior rhizotomy in several cases.

Figure 1 indicates modifications of Ivan and Wiley's[47] techniques of myelotomy. Because the effective part or target of the lesion is the midzone of the gray matter, attempts have been made by Ivan and Wiley to produce a lesion confined only to this area (griseotomy). Ivan and Wiley state, and our own experience verifies, that results of myelotomy are uncertain, both as to preservation of remaining function and long-lasting relief of spasticity. The original myelotomy of Bischof[5] remains the only clinically useful method, although radio frequency and focused ultrasound lesions may be practical sometimes. Virozub[90] reports, in the Russian literature, a 10-year experience with 60 Bischof myelotomies with satisfactory results.

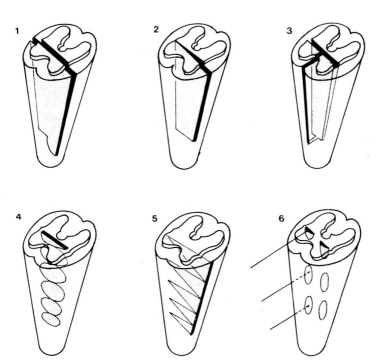

*Fig. 1.* Techniques for myelotomy (see text): (1) original Bischof's myelotomy; (2) modification of Bischof's myelotomy; (3) modification of Bischof's myelotomy; (4) circular griseotomy; (5) triangular myelotomy; (6) stereotaxic selective radiofrequency griseotomy. (Modified from Ivan LP, Wiley JJ: Clin Orthop 108:52, 1975)

## AMYLOIDOSIS

Secondary amyloidosis has been reported frequently in patients dying with spinal cord injury. Premortem coexisting conditions include hypertension, heart failure, severe renal disease, and in some cases, severe chronic decubiti.[62] Amyloidosis has also been reported to follow other chronic diseases such as tuberculosis, rheumatoid arthritis, lymphomas, and chronic neoplasms. Primary amyloidosis is an uncommon disease unassociated with any other systemic affliction. Organs and tissues severely involved in secondary amyloidosis such as spleen, kidneys, adrenals, liver, intestinal mucosa, and salivary glands are almost completely spared in primary amyloidosis. Organs that are spared or involved to only a slight degree in secondary amyloidosis, namely heart, lungs, smooth and striated muscles, skin, and serous membranes, are selectively affected in primary amyloidosis.

Amyloid is mucopolysaccharide-protein complex that stains selectively by various histochemical methods. Albuminuria is usually the first sign of secondary amyloidosis. Examination of the abdomen may reveal hepatosplenomegaly. Other signs include emaciation, anasarca, abnormal serum proteins, anemia, and vital organ failure. The Congo red absorption test can be of value in detecting amyloidosis because of the great affinity of amyloid substance for Congo red. However, in the presence of marked albuminuria a large amount of the dye can be lost in the urine and this should be taken into account. When the one-hour specimen reveals a 60 percent loss of the dye from the serum, amyloidosis may be suspected. A 90 percent or more absorption is unequivocally positive. A biopsy is useful in making a diagnosis but is of academic interest only, since only the basic condition, e.g., renal disease or decubiti,[38] can be treated. For further details, see papers by Maglio,[62] Box,[9] Comarr,[17] Newman and Jacobson,[72] and Thompson and Rice.[89]

## VASCULAR COMPLICATIONS

Paroxysmal hypertension in spinal cord injuries can occur in conjunction with the syndrome of autonomic hyperreflexia,[24] which is the term applied to the clinical picture of uninhibited mass autonomic reflexes due to a spinal lesion above T4 to T6. More than 85 percent of quadriplegics exhibit this syndrome, and the most prominent symptom is related to paroxysmal hypertension. The major splanchnic outflow of the sympathetic system is from T5 to L2 and lesions of the spinal cord above this level prevent normal reflex inhibition of this system by higher centers, thus permitting mass outpouring of autonomic sympathetic stimuli. The afferent for this reflex may arise from many structures, somatic or visceral, below the level of the lesion. Thus pain, temperature variation, muscular movement, or visceral alteration may initiate an afferent stimulus that may provoke the autonomic outflow. Stimuli from the genitourinary tract or rectum are quite important. When autonomic hyperreflexia occurs, attention should be paid primarily to these two organ systems. During intense sympathetic stimulation splanchnic vasoconstriction results in diminished circulation to the lower extremities. Headache, bradycardia, profuse sweating, piloerection, and flushing of the skin may all develop. Flushing of the skin and piloerection develop in areas above the level of the lesion. Other symptoms are congestion of nasal mucosa and mydriasis. On occasion, patients have become dyspneic due to bronchospasm. In an anesthetized patient this syndrome may be masked and cerebral hemorrhage can occur.

Deep venous thrombosis with secondary pulmonary emboli is a decided problem in paraplegic patients. Of great significance in venous stasis is a weakened or absent calf muscle pump, which is common in paraplegic patients, so that clots may form and be propagated to the lungs. The paraplegic patient who spends much time in a wheelchair allows the action of gravity to enhance the possibility of venous thrombosis. Negative intrathoracic pressure aids venous flow to the heart. Patients with high cervical lesions have, at least initially, flaccid paralysis of the intercostal muscles with diminution of or negative suction force. Only the youth of most quadriplegic patients mitigates against greater frequency of deep venous thrombosis and pulmonary emboli. Diagnosis can be verified by venogram.[78] Watson[91] found a 1.5 percent mortality and a 5 percent incidence of pulmonary embolism in 431 paraplegic and quadriplegic patients. There was a 12.5 percent incidence of venous thrombosis. Though most patients had deep vein thrombosis in the lower extremities, in one fatal case, the pelvic veins were found to be the site of thrombosis. Onset of venous thrombosis occurs within one month of injury in almost three-quarters of the patients. Pulmonary embolism occurs in about half the patients at the same time as thrombosis. Diagnosis and treatment of pulmonary embolism are similar to those in patients not having paraplegia.

Hachen et al.[40] noted moderate to severe deficiency within the extrinsic prothrombin activator system in 82 percent of 94 patients with acute spinal cord injury. The clotting defect could be shown to be related to subnormal levels of vitamin K-dependent plasma factors VII and X. In 25 patients, they felt that drug interference, irregular administration of vitamin K substances, and intercurrent disease might have been etiologic. In 36 patients, none of the common etiologic factors of acquired hypoprothrombinemia could be incriminated, e.g., poor intestinal resorption due to lack of bowel salts, hepatobiliary disease, broad spectrum oral antibiotics, drug reactions, hyperpyrexia, and prolonged parenteral feeding. In 25 percent of patients, total correction of factors VII and X was achieved after oral administration of synthetic vitamin K. Of the remaining patients who proved to be resistant to oral vitamin K, all but 2 demonstrated normal levels after intervenous administration of vitamin K. Hachen et al.[40] felt that in acute spinal cord injury intestinal uptake of liposoluble substances may be temporarily impaired.

## PAIN FOLLOWING SPINAL INJURY

Pain is frequently a problem in chronic quadriplegic and paraplegic patients. It is usually due to root compression either in the cervical area or in the cauda equina when the latter has been injured. It should be handled conservatively if possible, and a narcotic analgesic should not be used lest the patient become addicted. Among drugs advocated in the past are carbamazepine (Tegretol, Geigy) or diphenylhydantoin (Dilantin, Parke-Davis). These drugs should be given on a schedule rather than as necessary for pain. The mechanism of pain relief is obscure. Nonnarcotic analgesics and physical therapy including cervical traction, active and passive exercises, heat, massage, ultrasound, etc., usually suffice.

Transcutaneous neurostimulators have been utilized recently with fair results in some cases. Dorsal column-implanted stimulators on the spinal cord rarely give lasting pain relief, and complications such as meningitis do occur. Finally, pain may be relieved by cordotomy. Porter et al.[79] reported that from a total of 637 patients with lower motor neuron lesions, 41 patients required surgical treatment for uncontrollable pain. Spinal rhizotomy in the thoracic and cervical area has been utilized for pain relief. In our experience, this operation has been relatively unsuccessful for pain relief.

Approximately half of the patients had satisfactory pain relief 18 months following cordotomy.[79] Psychiatric therapy is sometimes indicated. In our patients, when pain is intractable, and root impingement is demonstrated by myelography, laminotomy with freeing of the root is sometimes of value. Surgical procedures are a last resort and should be undertaken only after a long period of conservative treatment.

Pain below the level of spinal injury includes various dysesthesias in addition to root pain. These may be perceived as typical phantom limb pain or may be described as numbness, burning, tingling, and dull aching. Carbamazepine and diphenylhydantoin have been useful.

## PRESSURE SORES

Decubitus ulcerations may occur over pressure points or bony prominences in paraplegic patients.[11] These occur in the sacrum, ischial tuberosities, greater trochanters, and malleoli as well as heels and posterior thighs. Such ulcerations can appear very rapidly, even in a few hours, in a paralyzed patient. Exton-Smith[29] differentiates two types of bed sores. The first is a deep or malignant sore which begins with necrosis of underlying tissues and breaks through the skin, the second is the less serious superficial sore with tissue damage confined to the skin. Pressure is a significant cause of both types of decubiti, although contact of excrement with skin may be important. Hypoproteinemia, debilitation, and concurrent infections may contribute to skin breakdown. Battle[1] indicts a loss of vasomotor control in paraplegia as a partial cause of decubiti. Other culpable factors, he states, are anatomic, such as the distance of bony weight-bearing prominences of skin and the thickness of the padding tissues such as fat and muscles between bone and skin. Spasms may be responsible for development of sores in atypical areas, such as inner surfaces of knees and inner ankles. Kahn[50] considers avitaminosis C to be a contributing factor, as well as negative nitrogen balance and dependent edema.

Once the skin is broken, a contaminated ulcer is present. There is no known medication that will rid a chronic open wound of bacteria. Most open decubiti harbor coagulase-positive *Staphylococcus aureus* but almost any other type of organism may be present. Mixed infections thrive on necrotic tissues and blood serum present in the ulcer and antibiotic ointments have proved ineffective in treatment. Prevention is vital in the paralyzed patient. A high-protein, high-calorie, high-vitamin diet should be offered. Anemia and hypoproteinemia should be avoided. Some physiatrists advocate testosterone (25 to 50 mg daily) for a few weeks for its anabolic effect in overcoming negative nitrogen balance.

Positioning to prevent pressure is the key to avoiding decubitus sores and often requires ingenuity. Sheets should be smooth, and foam rubber rings, donuts, pillows, and air mattresses have been employed. Clark[15] advocated skeletal suspension, which has not been used widely. Silicone sprays have been advocated in the prevention and treatment of decubiti by Hughes and Wigley.[46] Kahn[50] also advocates silicone spray but does not use it directly on an established ulcer. Such treatment has been sporadic. The Keane roto-rest turning bed has been utilized recently. It has an oscillatory mechanism and its basic function is to prevent pressure on any area for long periods. The alternating pressure mattress advocated by Bedford[2] serves a similar purpose. Sheepskin is widely used and may be of some aid in preventing bedsores.[11,28] The Stryker and Foster turning frames, circular beds, and various other devices serve the same purpose to prevent pressure on any area for extended periods.

Pressure points should be examined daily for the earliest signs of ulceration. Local edema, or slight reddening, or blanching of intact skin are danger signals. Light massage to improve local circulation and tissue tone and ultraviolet light to reduce the number of local bacteria have been utilized. Many established decubitus ulcers will heal spontaneously if such preventive measures are employed. Debridement of obviously dead tissues should be carried out with sterile forceps and scissors. Ordinary wet dressings without medications will aid in spontaneous debridement. Normal saline can be used as a wet dressing. Antibacterial agents may be of some short-term value but have been generally disappointing. Clark and Rusk[16] advocated use of dried blood plasma in 1953, but this has not been used widely. Oral zinc sulphate for healing of decubitus ulcers was advocated by Brewer et al.[13] but this also has not received wide acceptance.

Most wet dressings aid removal of necrotic tissue by causing maceration of the tissue and debridement when the dressing is removed. Debridement can be accomplished more rapidly with forceps and scissors, but not as smoothly, and viable tissue may be damaged. Accordingly, many physicians turn to agents that produce debridement by digestion or chemical reaction, such as trypsin, vegetable enzymes, phosphoric acid gel, Dakin's solution, and others. These may injure normal tissues or cause pain if the ulcer is not in an anesthetic area. Streptokinase-streptodornase enzymatic mixtures have been helpful. Many other preparations have been used but none have achieved general acceptance.

Shea[81] classified pressure sores into five groups. Grade 1 involves the dermis only and grade 2 involves subcutaneous fat. For both, he advocates local wound care. In grade 3 the deep fascia is involved and surgical correction should be carried out. In grade 4, which involves tissues underlying the fascia, radical surgery is advocated. The 5th grade, also the closed type, should also be treated surgically. The last type is uncommon in our experience, but Shea describes it as possibly involving bone and other deep tissues. It may be deceivingly extensive and may be diagnosed by x-ray of bone for identification and sinography for accurate delineation.

Decubitus ulcers are self perpetuating if left untreated. A thick fibrous bursal-like sac develops with a heavy, grayish, dense, sometimes calcified, wall containing chronically infected granulation tissue. This superficial layer effectively prevents healing. If after a trial of nonsurgical therapy, the decubitus persists and does not show definite progress to healing, surgical repair should be considered.

If spasticity causes severe spasms, these should be overcome by neurosurgical intervention. Otherwise, any surgical procedure for closure of decubiti will be ineffective and a graft will break down.

The purpose of definitive surgery is to remove the ulcer, its contents, surrounding unsatisfactory tissues, infected bursae, and the underlying often devitalized bony prominence. This should be carried out en bloc. The defect is then resurfaced with a transplanted pad of skin and fat. The transposed flap should have a broad pedicle to carry a plentiful blood supply, should be of sufficient size to permit it to lie loosely, without tension, and should have sufficient bulk to eliminate dead space and to withstand weight bearing and friction. Free partial-thickness skin grafts may take on a clean decubitus ulcer but will not hold up well for long periods. They should be used only as temporary measures.

The preferred operative procedure usually employs a delayed flap, which is incised for only a portion of its border, partially elevated, and then resutured in its bed for about three weeks before transfer. This allows for development of better blood supply. Some flaps may have sufficient vascularity to permit immediate transfer. If an error in judgment is made and the flap is lost, a near catastrophic situation results, because it is difficult to provide other tissue coverage of the same decubitus. It is sometimes possible to close a decubitus defect by the transfer of adjacent tissue by undermining and advancement, but if there is tension on such a flap it will probably be unsuccessful.

Sacral ulcers are treated with a flap from the lumbar area and not the buttock, since removal of padding from buttock will cause problems in the ischial area. Ischial ulcers are treated by buttock or thigh flaps. Ostectomy is sometimes required for extensive decubitus ulcers and in rare instances, disarticulation[86] has been carried out as in the case reported by Berkas.[4] Bors'[7] patients required resection of the os calcis for decubitus ulcer of the heel. Conway and Griffith[19] describe experience in over 1000 patients, and Campbell[14] describes extensive experience with operative and postoperative care.

Broad spectrum antibiotics are usually administered after operation and all pressure to the operative site is avoided. The patient is placed on a constipating diet and excess movement is avoided. Drains are removed in 48 to 72 hours and skin sutures removed in 10 to 14 days. The patient is kept at rest for 14 to 21 days and then can assume more varied positions. Prolonged periods of pressure on the surgical site must be avoided. Lanolin ointment has been used to massage the incisional areas after the stitches have been removed.

If extensive cyanosis of the flap is noted, the patient should be returned to the operating room where all sutures should be removed and the flap resutured in its original bed. The dressing routine is reinstituted and in about two weeks the flap transfer is repeated. If only the distal sutured tip of the flap is cyanotic, sutures may be removed and butterfly adhesive tapes may be used to assist in restoring flow.

## ECTOPIC BONE FORMATION

Ectopic bone (extra osseous bone) formation occurs in up to 49 percent of patients with spinal cord injuries. It forms below the level of the lesion characteristically at the hips, knees, shoulders, and elbows. The bone is distinguished histologically from soft tissue calcification in that it consists of cancellous bone, complete with marrow and often with cortex. The bone is formed within muscle and other connective tissue structures. In many cases such bone formation causes no harm. In other patients it is so extensive that limitation of passive or active joint motion and even bony ankylosis can occur. Thus, other complications of restricted motion may occur, such as pressure sores and limitation of activities of daily living.

Nicholas[73] recognized four clinical stages of ectopic bone formation. The first, characterized by negative x-ray findings, soft tissue swelling, and elevated serum and alkaline phosphatase levels, can be confused with infection. This stage progresses to the second in which alkaline phosphatase levels are elevated and swelling is present with positive x-ray findings. By the third stage, x-ray findings are positive and serum alkaline elevated, but swelling has subsided. The most advanced stage is manifested only by extensive positive x-ray signs. In the early stages diagnoses of thrombophlebitis, cellulitis, septic arthritis, and bone tumor may be erroneously considered.

Ectopic bone formation has been observed as early as three weeks after injury but more commonly it occurs months to years later. The alkaline phosphatase, although an excellent indicator of abnormal bone formation, may not necessarily be abnormal even in early stages. In most cases it is slightly elevated but may be elevated up to four to five times normal levels. Hussard[44] described a syndrome consisting of a unilateral decubital pressure ulcer associated with heterotopic bone formation about the hip. With reduction of movement of the hip, the ischial tuberosity sustains increased pressure during sitting. In the presence of a unilateral pressure ulcer, he suggests looking for heterotopic bone formation. Hsu et al.[45] describe the use of radionuclide technetium diphosphonate scan in the diagnosis of heterotopic bone formation. In all of their patients this technique established the diagnosis.

Wharton,[93] in a discussion of management of this syndrome, stated that no treatment is known to prevent the onset of heterotopic ossification or even to halt its progress. Indication for surgery is severe restriction of movement around the joint. Even then, surgery must await maturity of bone. Surgery is quite difficult and complications of hemorrhage, sepsis, and reankylosing have been frequently encountered. A limited wedge resection is probably the most successful approach to the restoration of hip motion. This is useful in the case that is most common in which heterotopic bone extends from pelvis to shaft of the femur anterior to the hip joint, thus restricting movement. Postoperative management consists of antibiotic therapy and flexion of the hip and knee to 90 degrees. A vigorous program of daily active and passive range of motion exercises is initiated after two weeks.

Patients whose hips are ankylosed in a flexed position may require resection of the head and neck of the femur as well as resection of a wedge of heterotopic bone in order to restore a satisfactory range of joint motion. Stewart and Comarr[87] reported approximately 48 resections of the neck of the femur during a 25-year period. They also reported 20 disarticulations of the lower extremity in 2800 spinal cord-injury patients over a 25-year period. Most disarticulations were performed for ectopic ossifications and severe extensive decubitus ulcers. They stated that although these are occasionally required, indications are less frequent as more moderate techniques are employed in the care of paraplegic patients.

Solovay[84] calls attention to neuropathic articular and periarticular changes in the lower extremities of paraplegics and quadriplegics, which constitute examples of Charcot's neuroarthropathy. In the classic Charcot's joint, there may be intra-articular destructive changes with extra-articular soft tissue ossification of the hypertrophic variety. There may be erosion and absorption of the articular surfaces with relaxation of capsular ligaments. Extensive or minimal periarticular ossification may occur in either type of arthropathy. The mechanism producing paraplegic neuroarthropathy is believed to be long-standing continued pressure over anesthetic bony prominences with absence of the warning sensations that prevent continued minimal trauma in a normal individual. Charcot's joint is seen in other conditions where a joint is rendered anesthetic, such as syphilis and syringomyelia.

## LONG BONE FRACTURES

Spinal cord-injured patients have a high incidence of long bone fractures. McMaster and Stauffer[65] separated patients into three groups. The first are those with acute fracture suffered in the same accident that caused the spinal cord injury. The pathophysiology and anatomic location of these fractures do not differ from those seen in nonparalyzed patients. Group 2 is comprised of pathologic fractures in an osteoporotic extremity in the chronic paralyzed patient. These are usually low-energy injuries and classically involve the proximal tibia or distal femur. The injury usually occurs during a minor activity such as during range of motion exercises or positioning in bed. The third group is comprised of traumatic fractures in chronic spinal cord-injured patients involved in another violent accident. These are high-energy injuries that may occur in normal bone above the injury level or in the osteoporotic bones below the level of injury. Eichenholtz[25] and Comarr et al.[18] also described extremity fractures in patients with spinal cord injuries.

Although one cannot be dogmatic in caring for such fractures, most open class 1 fractures were treated surgically, while about one-half the closed fractures were treated by open methods. A few class 2 patients were treated by a variety of internal fixation methods, but most were managed by nonoperative means including pillow splints, casts, and padded plaster splints. A plaster splint to a paralytic extremity should be changed frequently so that pressure ulcers will not occur. In class 3 patients, there was no uniformity of treatment. Exhuberant callus formation is frequently observed in spinal cord-injury patients, particularly in those with poorly aligned fractures. In spinal cord injuries it is not absolutely essential to obtain ideal alignment. The main issue is to retain function after fracture healing. Circular casts must be carefully watched and generally are not used in these patients. Skin traction is dangerous because of possible breakdown. Whenever possible, closed methods are recommended.

Comarr et al.[18] reported that the incidence of renal calculosis among 156 paralyzed patients with fractures was twice as high (14 percent) as that in 1485 similar patients without fractures (6.8 percent). Stones are formed in patients with lower motor neuron lesions more often than in those with upper motor neuron lesions. Nonunion occurred in 16 percent of patients.

Stepanek and Stepanek[85] reported that in 90 paraplegics and quadriplegics studied by radiography, osteoporosis was demonstrated in 65, and myositis ossificans was present in 35. Griffiths and Zimmerman[35] used photon densitometry to evaluate bone lesions and osteoporosis in patients with spinal cord injury. Using ordinary x-ray, it is impossible to demonstrate osteoporosis radiologically until 40 percent of bone mineral has been lost, but photon densitometry made it possible to more accurately assess osteoporosis. Early changes of loss of trabecular bone with preservation of cortical bone in spinal cord injury patients was demonstrated. This type of osteoporosis is different from idiopathic osteoporosis in which they believed that a hormonal mechanism was probably at work. The disuse osteoporosis of spinal injury may be neuronally mediated. Many paraplegic patients had loss of trabecular bone in the normal upper extremities without explanation.

## SPINAL DEFORMITY

Spinal vertebral deformities are not infrequent after a spinal cord injury, and usually occur gradually after long periods of time. Leidholt et al.[58] divided their patients into three categories: the thoracic group from T1 to T10, the thoracolumbar group from D11 to L1 and the lumbar group from L2 to L5. Of 204 patients, 58 had deformities. There were 25 in the thoracic group, 26 in the thoracolumbar group, and 7 in the lumbar group. Severe angulation at a fracture site was judged a deformity. They concluded that deformities of even 30 degrees or more did not significantly affect function. Back pain was not a major complaint. Most of the patients having deformities did not have fusions. Harris and Whatmore[43] discussed the problems in diagnosis of cervical deformities. They urged that tomography be employed when necessary and that the lower cervical vertebrae should always be visualized. This necessitates pulling the shoulders down and out of the way. McSweeney[66] emphasized the lack of tone in spinal muscles as a causative factor in vertebral deformity.

Guttmann[39] concentrated on spinal deformities in traumatic paraplegics and tetraplegics following surgical procedures. In a tirade against surgical intervention under almost any circumstance, he concluded that the deformity of the fractured spine can, in the majority of patients, be successfully reduced by conservative postural reduction and that deformity of the spine can either be prevented or reduced. He stated that operative procedures in the acute and early stages following traumatic paraplegia are indicated only in highly selected cases, if at all. In our experience deformities occur in the vertebral column of spinal injured patients occasionally whether or not they have surgery but less often with fusion. Fusion does not completely prevent deformities but has alleviated the pain and suffering we have observed when angulated vertebral columns cause radicular pain from nerve root pressure.

## REFERENCES

1. Battle R: Pressure sores in paraplegic patients. Br J Plast Surg 1:268–273, 1949
2. Bedford PD: Alternating pressure mattress. Gerontol Clin 3:68–82, 1961
3. Berger FM, Bradley W: The pharmacological properites of a:B dihydroxy-g-(2 methylphenoxy)-propane (Myanesin). Br J Pharmacol 1:265–272, 1946
4. Berkas EM: Multiple decubitus ulcer treatment of hip disarticulation by soft tissue flaps from the lower limbs. Plast Reconstr Surg 27:618–619, 1961
5. Bischof W: Die longitudinale myelotomie erst malig zervikal durchgefuhrt. Zentralbl Neurochir 11:205–210, 1952
6. Bischof W: Zur dorsalen longitudinalen myelotomie. Zentralbl Neurochir 28:123–126, 1967
7. Bors E: Decubitus ulcer of the heel. Report of two cases requiring partial resection of the os calcis. Paraplegia 1:48–54, 1963
8. Botterell EH, Aberhart C, Cluff JW: Paraplegia following war. Can Med Assoc J 55:249–259, 1956
9. Box TRH: Amyloidosis secondary to paraplegia. Can Serv Med J 13:713–718, 1957
10. Bradford FK: The use of a caudal air bubble in the control of alcohol injection to relieve flexion reflexes. J Neurosurg 16:468–470, 1959
11. Breck LW, Gonzalez S: Sheepskins in the prevention of decubitus ulcers. Clin Orthop 21:235–237, 1961
12. Brendler H, Krueger EG, Lerman P: Spinal root section in treatment of advanced paraplegic bladder. J Urol 70:223–229, 1953
13. Brewer RD, Mihaldzic N, Dietz A: The effect of oral zinc sulfate on the healing of decubitus ulcers in spinal cord injured patients. Proc Ann Clin Spinal Cord Injury Conf 17:70–72, 1967
14. Campbell RM: The surgical management of pressure sores. Surg Clin North Am 39:509–530, 1959
15. Clark AG: Skeletal suspension in the treatment of decubiti. Calif Med 72:447–449, 1950
16. Clark AB, Rusk HA: Decubitus ulcers treated with dried blood plasma. JAMA 153:787–788, 1953
17. Comarr AE: Secondary amyloidosis in injuries to the spinal cord. Am J Surg 95:843–844, 1958

18. Comarr AE, Hutchinson RH, Bors E: Extremity fractures of patients with spinal cord injuries. Am J Surg 103:732–739, 1962
19. Conway H, Griffith BH: Plastic surgery for closure of decubitus ulcers in patients with paraplegia. Am J Surg 91:946–975, 1956
20. Cooper IS, Hoen TI: Curare in spastic paraplegia. J Neurosurg 5:464–465, 1948
21. Cooper IS, Hoen TI: Intrathecal alcohol in the treatment of spastic paraplegia. J Neurosurg 5:385–391, 1948
22. Denhoff E, Bradley C: Curare treatment of spastic children. Preliminary report. N Engl J Med 226:411–416, 1942
23. Dogliotti AM: Nouvelle methode therapeutique pour les algies peripheriques. Injection d'alcool dans l'espace sous arachnoidien. Rev Neurol 2:485–486, 1931
24. Ead MN: Paroxysmal hypertension in spinal cord injuries (autonomic hyperreflexia). NZ Med J 63:574–580, 1964
25. Eichenholtz SN: Management of long-bone fractures in paraplegic patients. J Bone Joint Surg 45A:299–300, 1962
26. Elsberg CA: Some features of the gross anatomy of the spinal cord and nerve roots and their bearing on the symptomatology and surgical treatment of spinal disease. Am J Med Sci 144:799–803, 1912
27. Evangelous M, Adraiani J: Chemical rhizotomy (intrathecal alcohol) for paraplegic clonus. Anesthesiology 16:594–597, 1955
28. Ewing MR, Garrow C, McHugh N: Sheepskin as a nursing aid. Lancet 2:1447–1448, 1961
29. Exton-Smith AN: Prevention of pressure sores. Lancet 2:1364, 1961
30. Feld M, Pecker J: Essais de Cordotomie posterieure dans les paraplegies spasmodiques. Application au syndrome paraplegique de Little. Rev Neurol 85:542–543, 1951
31. Frazier CH, Allen AR: Surgery of the Spine and Spinal Cord. New York, Appleton, 1918, p 971
32. Freeman LW, Heimburger RF: The surgical relief of spasticity in paraplegic patients. II. Peripheral nerve section, posterior rhizotomy and other procedures. J Neurosurg 5:556–561, 1948
33. Freeman LW, Heimburger RF: The surgical relief of spasticity in paraplegic patients. I. Anterior rhizotomy. J Neurosurg 4:435–443, 1947
34. Gol A, Dossman WF: Electrocoagulation of the cord and nerve roots in the treatment of spasms of the bladder and lower limbs. J Neurosurg 22:352–353, 1965
35. Griffiths HJ, Zimmerman RE: The use of photon densitometry to evaluate bone mineral in a group of patients with spinal cord injury. Paraplegia 10:279–284, 1973
36. Groves EWH: On the division of the posterior spinal nerve roots: (I) for pain; (II) for visceral crises; (III) for spasm. Lancet 2:79–85, 1911
37. Guttmann L: Discussion on the treatment and prognosis of traumatic paraplegia. Proc R Soc Med 40:219–225, 1946
38. Guttmann L: The problem of treatment of pressure sores in spinal paraplegics. Br J Plast Surg 8:196–213, 1955
39. Guttmann L: Spinal deformities in traumatic paraplegics and tetraplegics following surgical procedures. Paraplegia 7:38–58, 1969
40. Hachen HJ, Rossier AB, Bouvier CA, Ritschard J: Deficiency within the extrinsic prothrombin activator system in patients with acute spinal cord injury. Paraplegia 12:132–138, 1974
41. Hansebout RR, Cosgrove JBR: Effects of intrathecal phenol in man. Neurology (Minneapolis) 16:277–282, 1966
42. Harmon PH: Transabdominal extraperitoneal section of the obturator nerve trunk. J Neurosurg 7:233–235, 1950
43. Harris P, Whatmore WJ: Spinal deformity after spinal cord injury. Paraplegia 6:232–238, 1969

44. Hussard GH: Heterotopic bone formation about the hip and unilateral decubitus ulcers in spinal cord injury. Arch Phys Med Rehabil 56:355–358, 1975
45. Hsu JD, Sakimura I, Stauffer ES: Heterotopic ossification around the hip joint in spinal cord injured patients. Clin Orthop 112:165–169, 1975
46. Hughes JPW, Wigley GS: Silicone sprays in prevention and treatment of decubitus skin disorders in domiciliary nursing. Br Med J 2:153–156, 1962
47. Ivan LP, Wiley JJ: Myelotomy in the management of spasticity. Clin Orthop 108:52–56, 1975
48. Ivan LP: Experience with Bischof's myelotomy. Can J Surg 10:191–195, 1967
49. James DF, Braden S: The use of curare in the treatment of spastic paralysis. J Neurosurg 3:74–80, 1946
50. Kahn S: Guide to the treatment of decubitus (pressure) ulcers in paraplegia. Surg Clin North Am 40:1657–1675, 1960
51. Kaplan LI, Grynbaum BB, Lloyd KE, Rusk HA: Pain and spasticity in patients with spinal cord dysfunction. Results of a follow-up study. JAMA 182:918–925, 1962
52. Kelly RE, Gautier-Smith PC: Intrathecal phenol in the treatment of reflex spasms and spasticity. Lancet 2:1102–1105, 1959
53. Kerr WG: The use of diazepam (Valium) in the relief of spasticity. Paraplegia 4: 149–154, 1966
54. Kerr AS: Anterior rhizotomy for the relief of spasticity. Paraplegia 4:154–162, 1966
55. Koppang K: Intrathecal phenol in the treatment of spastic conditions. Acta Neurol Scand 38:63–68, 1962
56. Kuhn RA, Bickers DS: An evaluation of curare in spasticity due to spinal cord injuries. N Engl J Med 238:615–622, 1948
57. Kuhn RA: A note on identification of the motor supply to the detrusor during anterior dorsolumbar rhizotomy. J Neurosurg 6:320–323, 1949
58. Leidholt JD, Young JJ, Hahn HR, Jackson RE: Evaluation of late spinal deformities with fracture-dislocations of the dorsal and lumbar spine in paraplegics. Paraplegia 7:16–28, 1969
59. Levine IM: Prazepam in the treatment of spasticity. A quantitative double-blind evaluation. Neurology 19:510–516, 1969
60. MacCarty CS: The treatment of spastic paraplegia by selective spinal cordectomy. J Neurosurg 11:539–545, 1954
61. MacDonald IB, McKenzie KG, Botterell EH: Anterior rhizotomy; the accurate identification of motor roots at the lower end of the spinal cord. J Neurosurg 3:421–425, 1946
62. Maglio A, Potenza P: Amyloidosis in paraplegia. Paraplegia 1:131–136, 1963
63. Maher RM: Relief of pain in incurable cancer. Lancet 268:18–20, 1955
64. Malmros R: Neurosurgical possibilities in the treatment of spasticity. A survey. Acta Neurol Scand 38:103–109, 1962
65. McMaster WC, Stauffer ES: The management of long bone fracture in the spinal cord injured patient. 112:44–52, 1975
66. McSweeney T: Spinal deformity after spinal cord injury. Paraplegia 6:212–221, 1969
67. Meirowsky AM, Scheibert CK, Hinchey TR: Studies on the sacral reflex arc in paraplegia. I. Response of the bladder to surgical elimination of sacral nerve impulses by rhizotomy. J Neurosurg 7:33–38, 1950
68. Meirowsky AM, Scheibert CD, Rose DK: Indications for the neurosurgical establishment of bladder automaticity in paraplegia. J Urol 67:192–196, 1952
69. Munro D: The rehabilitation of patients totally paralyzed below the waist: with special reference to making them ambulatory and capable of earning their living. I. Anterior rhizotomy for spastic paraplegia. N Engl J Med 233:453–461, 1945 Correction in 233:731, 1945

70. Munro D: Two year end-results in total rehabilitation of veterans with spinal cord and cauda equina injuries. N Engl J Med 242:1–16, 1950
71. Nathan PW: Chemical rhizotomy for relief of spasticity in ambulant patients. Br Med J 1:1096–1100, 1965
72. Newman W, Jacobson AS: Paraplegia and secondary amyloidosis. Am J Med 15:216–222, 1953
73. Nicholas JJ: Ectopic bone formation in patients with spinal cord injury. Arch Phys Med Rehabil 54:354–359, 1973
74. Pedersen E (ed): Spasticity and neurological bladder disturbances. Acta Neurol Scand 38:156, 1962
75. Pedersen E: Treatment of spasticity by subarachnoid phenolyglycerin. Neurology (Minneapolis) 15:256–262, 1965
76. Penzholz H: Chirurgische eingriffe am nervensystem bei spastischen lahmungen. Zentralbl Neurochir 15:331–342, 1956
77. Peterson LT: Tenotomy in the treatment of spastic paraplegia with special reference to tenotomy of the iliopsoas. J Bone Joint Surg 32A:875–886, 1950
78. Phillips RS: The incidence of deep venous thrombosis in paraplegics. Paraplegia 1:116–130, 1963
79. Porter RW, Hohmann GW, Bors E, French JD: Cordotomy for pain following cauda equina injury. Arch Surg 92:765–770, 1966
80. Schurmann K: Über das spatergebnis der chirurgischen behandlung extrapyramidaler bewegungsstorungen und paraplegischer zustande. Nervenarzt 24:252, 1953
81. Shea JD: Pressure sores. Classification and management. Clin Orthop 112:89–100, 1975
82. Shelden CH, Bors E: Subarachnoid alcohol block in paraplegia; its beneficial effect on mass reflexes and bladder dysfunction. J Neurosurg 5:385–391, 1948
83. Smolik EA, Nash FP, Machek O: Spinal cordectomy in the management of spastic paraplegia. Am Surg 26:639–645, 1960
84. Solovay J: Paraplegic neuroarthropathy. Am J Roentgenol Radium Ther Nucl Med 61:475–481, 1949
85. Stepanek V, Stepanek P: Changes in the bones and joints of paraplegics. Radiol Clin 29:28–36, 1960
86. Stewart JC, Comarr AE: Disarticulation of lower extremity in spinal cord injury patients, a 25-year review, 2,800 patients. Proc VA Spinal Cord Injury Conf 18:70, 1971
87. Stewart JC, Comarr AE: Resection of head and neck of femur in spinal cord injury patients, a 25-year review. Proc VA Spinal Cord Injury Conf 18:66–69, 1971
88. Tarlov JM: Deafferentiation to relieve spasticity or rigidity: reasons for failure in some cases of paraplegia. J Neurosurg 24:270–274, 1966
89. Thompson CE, Rice ML: Secondary amyloidosis in spinal cord injury. Ann Intern Med 31:1057–1065, 1949
90. Virozub ID: Experience with 60 frontal myelotomies in treatment of spastic manifestations in patients with injuries of the spine and spinal cord. Vopr Neirokhir 2:21–26, 1975
91. Watson N: Venous thrombosis and pulmonary embolism in spinal cord injury. Paraplegia 6:113–121, 1968
92. Weber W: Die behandlung der spinalen paraspastik unter besonderer berucksichtingung der lingitudinalen myelotomie (Bischof). Med Mschr 9:510–513, 1955
93. Wharton GW: Heterotopic ossification. Clin Orthop 112:142–149, 1975
94. Wolman L: The neuropathological effects resulting from the intrathecal injection of chemical substances. Paraplegia 4:97–115, 1966
95. Yeo JD: Results of intrathecal injection of alcohol in spinal cord injuries. Med J Aust 1:474–480, 1967

# 24

## Genitourinary Tract
in Spinal Injury

### EARLY STAGES

The syndrome of spinal shock following injury to the spinal cord or cauda equina is reflected early in the bladder and urinary sphincter by a state of atonicity.[42] The smooth muscle of the bladder loses its normal tone, and, should a cystometrogram be recorded at this stage, no normal vesical contractions would be discernible. Atonicity of the bladder is complicated by the fact that the external urethral sphincter is paralyzed and cannot be relaxed, thereby causing outlet obstruction. Thus, the bladder must be emptied by contrived means or dangerous overdistention will occur. Suprapubic cystostomy is no longer routinely used, nor is initial manual compression of the bladder.

### INDWELLING URETHRAL CATHETERS

Use of an indwelling catheter avoids bladder distention but may lead to a host of complications. Infection frequently occurs after as little as 48 or 96 hours[29,36] and is very difficult to treat because of the indwelling catheter. Kass[29] found that 98 percent of patients with indwelling catheters for more than 96 hours had bacteremia despite prophylactic antibiotic therapy. When indwelling catheters are used for a week or more, male patients tend to develop urethritis and prostatitis, and chronic relapsing prostatitis is a common cause of relapsing bladder infection. Long-term use of an indwelling catheter is accompanied by a high incidence of penoscrotal urethral abscesses, diverticulae, fistulae, strictures, epididymitis, and orchitis. When use of a Foley-type balloon indwelling catheter is chronic, crusts form around the balloon and may separate to become bladder calculi. The Gibbon polyvinyl chloride catheter[23] has a narrow diameter, is nonirritant, and has definite advantages over the Foley rubber and other indwelling catheters.

## INTERMITTENT URETHRAL CATHETERIZATION

Guttmann[25,26] introduced intermittent urethral catheterization with a nontouch technic. Guttmann and Frankel[26] in 1966, reviewed their data on 476 spinal injury patients admitted to the Stoke-Mandeville facility within the first 14 days after injury who were managed by intermittent catheterization. On admission, 77.7 percent had sterile urine; on discharge, 62.2 percent had sterile urine. There was a low incidence of chronic sequelae, such as hydronephrosis, vesicoureteral reflux, and calculosis. There were no cases of urethral fistulae. Intermittent catheterization permits some distention of the bladder thereby assisting in restoring tone, which both acts as a physiologic stimulus for micturition and promotes an early return of detrusor muscle activity in some cases.[46,48] Guttmann and Frankel[26] reported return of automatic micturition within 8 to 14 days, refuting the old dogma that automatic reflex micturition occurs only after six to eight weeks following injury.

The nontouch intermittent catheterization technique is employed with full aseptic precautions. The catheter, an 8 or 10 French size, is handled with a sterile hemostat.[48] Patients initially are catheterized every 4 hours until they begin to pass urine either voluntarily, automatically, or by manual abdominal expression. Care must be taken to insure that the bladder is not overdistended. Each catheterization should yield no more than 500 to 600 ml. In recumbent patients with flaccid bladders the lowest point of the bladder may not be emptied, so abdominal expression is used toward the end of the procedure to prevent residual urine.

When automatic voiding or manual expression yields less than 500 ml of residual urine, frequency of catheterization is decreased progressively and fluid intake is increased to produce a 3000 to 4000 cc per 24-hour output. When residual volume is consistently less than 100 cc, intermittent catheterization is decreased to once daily, once weekly, and then stopped. The residual urine is checked monthly for several months, and cystography and cystometrography are employed to ascertain the functional state of the bladder. In Guttmann and Frankel's[26] patients the average time between injury and complete cessation of catheterization was six to seven weeks.

During the initial phase of this program, a urine specimen for bacterial culture and sensitivity is collected at least once weekly. If infection is suspected on the basis of appearance and verified by microscopic examination of cells, administration of a systemic antibiotic is begun while awaiting results of culture and sensitivity. Indwelling catheters are used only when there is a severe urinary infection. Results at discharge are assessed by a midstream rather than a catheterized specimen. Guttmann and Frankel[26] regarded the urine as sterile if, without antibiotics, it contained fewer than four white blood cells per cubic millimeter and revealed no growth on culture.

Intermittent catheterization is accompanied by a risk that the bladder will become overdistended, but if fluid intake is restricted to 1500 ml per day, evenly spaced, and catheterization carried out at 4- or 6-hour intervals, the volume of urine will usually be less than 500 ml. Fluid intake may be increased with proper attention given to the intervals between intermittent catheterizations. Urethral mucosal injury can be prevented by using a narrow caliber (14 French) polyvinyl chloride catheter. The catheter should not be passed while an erection is present.

Bacteria are normally present in the distal urethra, and a small number are carried into the bladder with passage of any catheter despite employment of meticulous technique. Some urologists recommend antibiotic solution instillation. Pearman and England[47] recommend that in addition to liberal lubrication of the catheter a sterile lubricant containing 0.02 percent chlorhexidine digluconate be injected into the male urethra and held for three minutes. After the bladder has been drained, they recommend that 150 mg of kanamycin and 30 mg of colistin in 25 ml of sterile water be placed in the bladder immediately prior to withdrawal of the catheter. They also recommend quantitative bacterial colony counts at each catheterization. Vivian and Bors[62] recommend benzalkonium or a cleansing agent and instillation of one ounce of 1 percent neomycin solution.

Fluid restriction during the period of intermittent catheterization is generally advocated. For example, one maximum recommended is 400 ml of fluid by mouth between bladder catheterizations. Fluid intake can be adjusted for each patient depending on output, and the optimum level may require considerable persuasion of the patient who has had an indwelling Foley catheter and who has been urged to drink large volumes of fluid.

Tidal drainage[14] is no longer used at most centers in the care of spinal-injured patients. This is a technique requiring the bladder to be kept at a reasonable level of fullness by infusion of sterile fluid and to be emptied at intervals. It was in use during and after the second World War but, due to its complexity and the fact that newer methods give equal or better results, has been discontinued.

Pearman[46] recommends long-term prophylaxis for renal and lower tract infection when intermittent catheterization is terminated. He uses methanamine mandelate and ammonium chloride, the latter to acidify the urine, provided the drugs do not cause stomach upset. Burr and Silver[9] use 250 mg of hexamine mandelate and 250 mg methionine in a single tablet for the prevention of urinary tract infection. Hexamine decomposes into formaldehyde and ammonia at a pH of 5.5 or less and possesses broad-spectrum antibacterial activity without implementing the development of resistant strains.[21] Long-term therapy with the latter agents, however, increases bone loss in paralyzed patients and is contraindicated when there is infection with urea-splitting organisms[9] because of the probability of stone formation in the resulting alkaline urine. This combination of alkalinity and hypercalciuria favors stone formation.

In Vivian and Bors'[62] series 76 percent of 64 patients were admitted with indwelling catheters and only 21 percent were discharged with one; 24 percent were admitted without catheters and 79 percent were discharged without one. Similar success has been demonstrated by others;[3,18,22,38,59,63] however, Comarr[15] stressed that patients who are catheter-free still bear close watching, as many become insidiously or acutely infected. Other aspects of early treatment have been reviewed by Band[1] and O'Flynn.[12]

Perkash[49] has had great success with pharmacologic treatment using 30 to 40 mg of bethanechol chloride three times daily for two to three weeks. Patients recovered reflex activity in almost half the average time (32 days compared to 79 days). He also performed modified sphincterotomy of the bladder neck on 10 of 111 patients, increasing the total catheter free to 98 percent. Sphincterotomies were performed on patients who required intermittent catheterization for long periods of time (6 to 12 months).

On the other hand Marosszeky et al.[35] reviewed 77 patients managed initially with indwelling catheters. They found no increased incidence of complications even in patients who required permanent catheterization, and they concluded that there was no major advantage in the use of intermittent catheterization.

### Drugs Useful in Establishing Automatic Function in Upper Motor Neuron Bladder

When the detrusor muscle is hypoactive, the administration of bethanechol chloride subcutaneously or carbachol by intramuscular injection every six hours is recommended. If this treatment is effective, bethanechol chloride can be given orally four times daily. The drug can be gradually tapered as automatic voiding becomes more effective.

Phenoxybenzamine has been advocated when spasticity or hypertonus of the internal sphincter causes urinary retention in the patient with neurogenic bladder.[31,37] This alpha-sympatholytic agent resulted in restoration of micturition in a large number of patients otherwise unresponsive to treatment. McGuire et al.,[37] in addition, found it effective in the treatment of autonomic dysreflexia. Hyperactivity of the bladder causing incontinence can be treated with anticholinergic drugs such as methantheline 50 to 150 mg orally or propantheline bromide 15 to 30 mg orally four times daily. A spastic sphincter can be relieved by diazepam 10 to 20 mg four times daily in some instances.

### Neurologic Examination to Assess Return of Reflex Activity

Three tests may be of value in assessing return of muscular and sphincter function following spinal injury. The first is testing the anal reflex by pricking the mucocutaneous junction with a pin. If a normal reflex arc is present, the anus will contract immediately. The second is testing the bulbocavernosus reflex by inserting a gloved lubricated finger into the rectum, and squeezing gently the glans penis or clitoris at five-second intervals. If the reflex is intact, the anal sphincter muscle contracts briskly. The same response may be elicited by pulling gently on an indwelling Foley catheter. Bors[2] suggested a third reflex action to determine whether bladder function exists. The bladder is catheterized and emptied, and 60 ml of sterile iced antibiotic solution is instilled through the catheter, which is clamped and immediately withdrawn. If the iced solution is expelled within one minute, function (albeit involuntary) is present. In lesions of the cauda equina, such tests will be permanently negative, and only manual compression will cause emptying of the bladder.

Trigger techniques can be used to initiate a spontaneous micturition reflex. Such maneuvers as suprapubic tapping, pulling pubic hair, pinching the glans penis or thighs, or anal sphincter stimulation may cause spontaneous voiding. These techniques greatly aid in the successful application of the intermittent catheterization program.

### Investigation to Assist in Assessment of Returning Bladder and Sphincter Function

The sacral segments of the spinal cord located in the conus medullaris (S2, S3, S4) containing the parasympathetic upper motor neurons to the urinary tract musculature lie at about the level of the first lumbar vertebra. Spinal transections above this level and not involving the parasympathetic outflow result in development of reflex micturition. With damage to the sacral segments, cauda equina, or more distal nerves, the bladder will remain an inert sac which must be emptied by catheterization or manual pressure. It should be remembered that even with lesions above the sacral outflow, rostral infarction and damage can occur resulting in a lower neuron, flaccid bladder. When automatic voiding is delayed (three to six months) further investigations are occasionally helpful. Comarr and Peha[20] stress the large number of false positives and false negatives that occur with various test procedures and conclude that simple clinical capacity—residual urine tests performed at the bedside—is of greatest help. None of the procedures described below is sufficient in itself; each must be interpreted in context.

*Cystometry.* Cystometry is a procedure designed to graphically record vesical activity during introduction of fluid or gases into the bladder. Many varieties of apparatus have been designed, but a water manometer is as simple and satisfactory as any. A graduated reservoir is equipped with a drip bulb. A manometer consisting of a straight glass tube is affixed to a meter stick. A catheter, a Y-tube, and appropriate tubing with appropriate connection complete the equipment. Sterile water or antibiotic solution is allowed to drip into the previously emptied bladder in a slow continuous flow via an indwelling catheter, or in rare cases, through a fine percutaneous needle or catheter inserted suprapubically. Manometric pressure levels are recorded after each 25 cc fluid increment. Reflex contractile waves are noted and recorded in graphic form. The point at which the patient first feels the desire to void and the onset of pain from vesical distention are also recorded. If the patient has neither expelled the catheter nor voided around it after instillation of 400 cc of fluid, he is requested to strain as if voiding. This final reading is designated as the maximum voluntary pressure.

The automatic bladder usually demonstrates a variable pressure curve, forceful contractions, no recognition of the normal urge to void, vague sensations of bladder fullness, and, in higher lesions, an automatic hyperreflexic reaction with flushing, sweating, and possibly increase in blood pressure when the bladder reflex is about to act. Increased tone may be present in patients with lower neuron bladders, and there may be minor reflex detrusor contractions.

*Cystourethrography.* Radiopaque dye is instilled into the bladder employing gravity flow at a height of 15 cm. When the flow of dye ceases or backs up, the bladder is assumed to have reached its capacity. The catheter is then clamped and the amount of instilled dye recorded. Anteroposterior and oblique films are taken and the cystogram produced may show changes such as trabeculations, saccules, and diverticuli. These procedures may be observed by cinefluoroscopy under image intensification and the radiologist should compress the bladder to detect vesicoureteric reflux.

Urethrograms are taken with the catheter removed by gently injecting the contrast medium through the urethra from a syringe at the external urethral meatus. Urethrograms reveal the condition of the vesical neck and posterior urethra as well as demonstrate strictures and diverticuli in the anterior portion of the urethra. Spasm of the external sphincter may be indicated by failure to dilate the posterior urethra with injection of the radiopaque dye.

Voiding films should be taken. If there is significant bacteriuria and infected urine is refluxed up the ureters to the kidneys by the instillation of contrast material, acute pyelonephritis may result. Cystography should not be done in patients who harbor significant bacteriuria. Infection should first be eliminated by an appropriate antibiotic.

*Cystoscopy.* A cystoscopic examination is of value in ruling out an organic obstructive lesion such as urethral strictures or prostatic hypertrophy. During insertion of the cystoscope, sphincteric resistance may be recognized. Bladder calculi may be visualized and extracted during the procedure. The physician also can estimate the degree of bladder infection.

*Tests to Assess Renal Function.* Many tests have been described to assess renal function, and it is outside the scope of this text to discuss them in detail. Only the most useful tests will be discussed.

*Plasma Urea and Creatinine Clearance.* Plasma urea and creatinine may become elevated when there is a diminution in glomerular filtration rate, and urine creatinine clearance has been found to be a reliable renal function test.

The creatinine clearance is calculated by multiplying concentration of creatinine in urine by the volume and dividing the result by the concentration of creatinine in plasma. Urine is collected for 24 hours, and one blood sample is taken during that time. Normal creatinine clearance in men is 120 ml per minute, and in women 85 to 100 ml per minute.

*Intravenous Pyelography.*  Intravenous urograms provide information on both the anatomy of the upper portion of the urinary tract and the function of the kidney. Back pressure from the bladder is demonstrated by ureteral and pelvic dilatation. Impairment of renal function may be manifested by a delay or nonappearance of the dye indicating diminished renal concentration. Tomograms of the kidneys are now taken, when indicated, to better assess cortical scarring.

*Average Flow Rate.*  Iwatsubo et al.[28] advocate the simple evaluation of urinary flow by means of a stopwatch and cup. The volume and velocity of the flow indicate the state of the urine excretory tracts. The normal average flow rate was 15.7 ml per second ± 3.1. In 60 paraplegics the flow rate averaged less and, in general, the worse the condition of the bladder and urethra, the worse the flow rate.

*Renal Scans.*  The use of labeled compounds and renal scan techniques have greatly aided in the assessment of renal function. These tests are simple to perform and avoid the occasional allergic reactions seen with urographic studies. The newest techniques are so exact that not only can function be accurately assessed but anatomy can be photographed so as to produce pictures similar to urographs.

## LATER STAGES

The long-term survival of a patient with a complete spinal cord transection depends primarily on prevention of urologic complications which arise because of alterations in urologic excretory function.

*Vesicoureteric Reflux.*  Vesicoureteric reflux in the paraplegic patient is caused by the combination of obstruction, infection, and possibly, neurogenic ureteral dysfunction. Valadka et al.[61] found the incidence in paraplegics to be 16 percent. Reflux is accompanied by poor drainage of the upper urinary tract and enhanced vulnerability of the kidney to infection. The cystogram is the standard method of demonstrating vesicoureteric reflux,[13] but its appearance is notably capricious. Marked trabeculation of the bladder was not necessarily present, since it was exhibited in only half the patients. A normal intravenous pyelogram does not exclude the possibility of vesicoureteral reflux.[13]

A patient exhibiting vesicoureteral reflux should be carefully observed, and cystograms and intravenous pyelograms should be made at intervals of six months. Reflux without upper urinary tract dilatation can be conservatively treated with antibiotics if bacteriuria is demonstrated. If upper urinary tract dilatation occurs,[27] attempts to alleviate obstruction and eliminate residual urine via transurethral means, e.g., prostatectomy, sphincterotomy, should be made. Urinary diversion into an ileal conduit may be indicated when reflux is associated with advancing dilatation of the upper urinary tract.[4,8]

*Obstruction at the Bladder Neck.* Obstruction at the bladder neck can occur with both upper and lower motor lesions of the spinal cord and may be diagnosed by a voiding cystourethrogram. It may be due to inappropriate action of the detrusor muscle or in some instances, to fibrosis and contracture of the bladder neck due to chronic infection. Transurethral resection of the bladder neck when carried out is associated with good results in only two-thirds of patients, and the benefit is often only transient.

*Obstruction at the External Sphincter.* The external sphincter in the male patient is located just distal to the prostate. Obstruction may be due to a true fibrotic stricture or to overactivity of the striated sphincter muscle owing to spasticity. If the obstruction is due to spasm, it may be relieved by topical anesthesia to the mucosa of the bladder, urethra, and anus, or certain orally administered drugs. If this fails, pudenal nerve infiltration and sacral root anesthesia may be tried. Lately, sphincterotomy has been advocated[41,43,50,53] and the diagnosis may be made by voiding cystourethrogram, the retrograde urethrogram[52] and urethroscopy has demonstrated lasting results in a large number of patients.

Some authors[24] do not advocate sacral rhizotomy or subarachnoid alcohol block for urologic indications only. Similarly, bilateral pudenal neurectomy[60] has been found ineffective or at best temporary in a large number of patients (23 of 39),[24] and the additional disadvantage of loss of ability to have erection makes it even less desirable. For a review of early surgical procedures, see Bors.[2]

*Periscrotal Diverticula and Fistulas.* The presence of a diverticulum and/or fistula itself may not be an indication for urinary diversion. An abscess requires incision and drainage, and the indwelling catheter may act as a wick so that irrigation can be performed. A diverticulum can be emptied manually as urination occurs. Only if the diverticulum reaches a large size or there is recurrent infection does operative intervention become necessary.

If a penoscrotal fistula requires therapy because of recurrent infection or incessant drainage of urine, the method of therapy chosen depends upon whether the patient has a balanced or imbalanced bladder. For the balanced bladder, Comarr[14] recommends bedrest in the supine or side position. The prone position is avoided because of pressure on the urethra. The penis should be free of any pressure, and the area should be well padded to catch urine. Healing time is one to three weeks. If the fistula is large, surgical correction may be required.

If the patient does not have a well-balanced bladder, efforts should be made to heal the fistula without urinary diversion. Electrofulguration of the entire tract with incision and drainage of any abscess may suffice. Occasionally a fistula may heal spontaneously, and achievement of a balanced bladder facilitates spontaneous fistula closure. The fistula may be closed surgically, but, if this fails three times, Comarr[14] recommends urinary diversion.

*Alterations in the Upper Urinary Tract Secondary to Spinal Injury.* Decrease in renal function is a major cause of death in patients with spinal cord injuries. Postmortem examination of such patients often shows gross and microscopic evidence of severe renal damage,[54] the usual changes being hydronephrosis[27] and chronic pyelonephritis. Chronic urinary tract infection, stones, and vesicoureteric reflux are predisposing factors. Intravenous pyelography and voiding cystourethrography usually demonstrate these changes as they occur. In the presence of hydronephrosis, dilatation of the calyces and renal pelvis occurs, and nephrotomography may be required to demonstrate renal outlines.

In 100 patients with spinal injury, Scher[54] found a 20 percent incidence of hydronephrosis; 8 patients had unilateral and 12 had bilateral hydronephrosis. Chronic pyelonephritis was evidenced in 12 patients by scarring of the renal outlines and dilatation and deformity of the calyces; disease was bilateral in 3 patients, and unilateral in 9. Thirteen patients had vesicoureteral reflux, but six showed no trace of upper urinary tract disease.

Amyloidosis is found commonly in association with chronic renal failure and is not uncommon at postmortem examination in paraplegics.[24] Prolonged suppurative disease is the most common underlying factor. Renal stones (calculi) are found less often but may occur due to stasis.[24] Kregzde et al.[32] found a correlation between renal calculosis and lysozymuria but did not explain the causal relation. Comarr et al.[19] found renal calculi to be composed of calcium mangesium ammonium phosphate.

## Other Complications

Lower urinary tract complications such as epididymitis[17] urethral abscess, various fistulae, and diverticuli still occur. Epididymitis was found in 22 percent of 2123 patients.[16] Epididymitis may result from extension of prostatic and urethral infection through the vas deferens or perivasal lymphatics.[17] Trauma from inadvertent pressure on testicles during various maneuvers has been implicated. Vasoresections and epididymo-orchiectomies have been recommended in severe cases.

Vesical calculi may prove troublesome, particularly in patients with long-term balloon catheters. Frequent catheter changes accompanied by vigorous irrigations through a larger catheter to remove debris may help to alleviate the problem. Cystoscopic evaluation and cystolithopaxy at frequent intervals are important in patients with indwelling catheters. The etiology of these stones is unclear. Claus-Walker et al.[12] found bladder calculi in 13 percent of 356 quadriplegic and 336 paraplegic patients. The only definite urinary aberration in these patients was a lowered urinary sodium and potassium thought to be due to the large fluids intake. Another reported complication is an increase in incidence of carcinoma of the bladder.[24,33,39]

## Urinary Tract Infection

Urinary tract infection is an almost constant concomitant of the paraplegic state. Certainly the primary goal should be prevention, and this is the purpose in intermittent catheterization and the achievement of the so-called balanced bladder. Use of the indwelling catheter and presence of residual urine are the primary factors in the cause and persistence of urinary tract infection. In spite of the best efforts, either chronic or acute infection remains uncontrolled in a large number of paralyzed patients and probably is the main reason for the observed high incidence of pyelonephritis, renal insufficiency, and related conditions.[44] However, many recommend use of antibiotics for only an exacerbation of pyelonephritis (clinical sepsis) with chills, fever, and possibly positive blood cultures.[56]

Long-term maintenance of prophylactic chemotherapy is ineffective as long as catheter drainage or significant residual urine persists. The organisms quickly become resistant to prolonged use of antibiotics, or resistant strains become dominant. Sterile urine is encountered only in the patient who has not had a urethral catheter for some time. Persistence of bacteriuria after the catheter has been removed generally is treated with antibiotics, but the choice of the proper drug is controversial. It should be based on the organism found on culture and to its sensitivity.

Herr[25] states that acute hydronephrosis or pyonephrosis is one of the more common acute urologic emergencies seen in the spinal injury patient. The patient has high fever, nausea, vomiting, abdominal spasms, and flank pain if the spinal level is below the eighth thoracic segment. Autonomic dysreflexia may be the first sign in quadriplegics. Treatment consists of draining the 40 to 100 cc of purulent material and stagnant urine from the renal pelvis and ureter with a ureteral catheter and administration of appropriate antibiotics.

The bacteriology of urinary infections in paraplegia has been investigated over the years.[2,40,53] Coliform organisms are primarily responsible, but *Streptococcus fecalis* and various Proteus species also account for a large number of infections. In at least one-third of urine specimens, more than one type of organism is present, but cultured specimens from the bloodstream during sepsis are most likely to show only one organism.

## Other Surgical Procedures

A small contracted bladder occurs less frequently now than in the past, but nevertheless it is sometimes a problem in the management of the urinary tract in patients with spinal injury. Prevention is preferable to treatment as very often reversal is not possible, the bladder wall having become fixed at a small capacity because of thickening and fibrotic change. This is most common in patients with spastic bladders drained for long periods of time by urethral or suprapubic catheters, but the small contracted bladder can also result from atonicity. It should be suspected when urine drains around the catheter or when the patient experiences recurrent cystitis or pyelonephritis.

In upper motor neuron lesions, various methods of treatment have been used, and the simplest measures should be employed initially. Cystometry before and after spinal anesthesia will demonstrate a significant increase in bladder capacity after anesthesia if contracture is not fixed. The next approach might be to block sacral roots 2 and 3 bilaterally via a posterior approach and to instill a local anesthetic. Cystometry should be performed as each nerve is blocked to determine the extent of relief. Sometimes enough relaxation can be obtained by blocking of only two or three roots. S4 might have to be included on occasion, but it is accompanied by diminished or lost anal tone. Having obtained the desired effect, and with the needles in place, 2 ml of absolute alcohol may be injected to render the lesion permanent. The effect may last for months or years if it is initially successful.

Selective sacral neurotomy (rhizotomy) has been advocated for relief of spasticity in the small contracted bladder.[31,34,41,45] The operation is performed by doing a low lumbosacral laminectomy and sectioning appropriate anterior roots bilaterally. The roots chosen are determined by electrical stimulation with a cystometer in place. The motor roots to the bladder will respond by a distinct elevation in pressure. An adjunctive localizing method is to identify the nerves at the appropriate sacral foramina. Brendler et al.[7] had success with such a procedure but also noted an increase in bladder capacity after the more extensive operation of anterior rhizotomy performed mainly for relief of spasticity. Sacral rhizotomy also has been performed for ureteral reflux. However, Cashion and Moeller[10] found tht only 3 of 11 patients benefited from the operation on long-term follow-up and concluded that sacral rhizotomy was not indicated for reflux.

Extensive anterior rhizotomy (T10–T12 to S5 bilaterally) will relieve spasticity and increase the size of a spastic bladder. The same is true of intrathecal alcohol injection (15 to 20 ml), although the latter is nonspecific and accompanied by a high incidence of return of spasticity. It is obvious that these extensive procedures are not recommended for treatment of urologic complications alone.

Evacuation of a spastic bladder by electrical stimulation via electrodes implanted on the bladder has been achieved experimentally in some patients,[5,6,52] but this method remains experimental and is used infrequently at present.

Scott et al.[54,55,57,58] advocate implantation of a prosthetic urethral sphincter in patients with urinary incontinence of various etiologies including spinal injury. This is an expensive procedure involving a complicated mechanical device. However, in certain selected patients it has shown encouraging results.

Urinary diversion in paraplegia is reserved for the patient who fails to respond to more conservative management. This technique is in a constant state of flux, and there are numerous diversionary procedures that can be performed. At present, bilateral cutaneous ureteroileostomy is used most widely. A significant complicaton rate[30] and postoperative deterioration of some normal renal units have caused physicians to perform these procedures less frequently now than several years ago.[20] The patient with severe hydronephrosis and uremia initially should undergo bilateral upper tract diversion with ileal diversion reserved for future consideration depending on return of ureteral and renal function.

Urinary diversion into a bowel segment might be considered in several types of spinal injury patients. There are those who experience such unsatisfactory reflex bladder function that it is impossible to keep them dry. Others, usually those with lower motor neuron lesions, develop reflux and upper urinary complications including pyelonephritis, calculi, and hydronephrosis, and should be diverted. Female patients present a special problem if there is constant leakage, as there is no good collection device for women.[33]

Other methods of supravesical diversion[11,51] are used but have inherent problems. Ureteroenterostomy to the intact sigmoid is out of the question for these patients because of constant retrograde infections and subsequent renal deterioration. Cutaneous ureterostomy cannot be used when normal ureters exist but may be considered in the patient with hydroureters. Nephrostomy has been found to be fraught with problems of infection, stone, and loss of renal function, not to mention the oft-encountered frustrations of changing the catheter.

There are many forms of urinary diversion that can be offered the spinal injury patient. Individualization of the patient is the most important aspect of choosing which type to recommend.[11,51] Close follow-up of the patient is important in timing the procedure to be used. If ureteroileal cutaneous (Bricker) diversion is chosen, it is vital to perform this before there is upper tract drainage in order to obtain the best long-term results.

## REFERENCES

1. Band D: Urological management during the initial phase of traumatic paraplegia. Br J Urol 33:361–369, 1961
2. Bors E: Neurogenic bladder. Urol Surv 7:177–250, 1957
3. Bors E: Intermittent catheterization in paraplegic patients. Urol Int 22:236–249, 1967
4. Bradley WE: Experimental study of the treatment of the neurogenic bladder. J Urol 90:575–582, 1963

5. Bradley WE, Wittmers LE, Chou SN, French LA: A radio transmitter receiver for the treatment of neurogenic bladder. J Neurosurg 19:782–786, 1962

6. Bradley WE, Chou SN, French LA: Further experience with the radio transmitter receiver unit for the neurogenic bladder. J Neurosurg 20:953–960, 1963

7. Brendler H, Krueger EG, Lerman P, et al: Spinal root section in treatment of advanced paraplegic bladder. J Urol 70:223–229, 1953

8. Bricker EM: Symposium on clinical surgery: Bladder substitution after pelvic evisceration. Surg Clin North Am 30:1511–1521, 1950

9. Burr RG, Silver JR: The effect of an antibacterial drug on urinary calcium, magnesium and phosphorus excretion in patients with neurogenic bladder. Br J Urol 47:425–432, 1975

10. Cashion EL, Moeller BA: Long-term results of rhizotomy for ureteral reflux in the spinal cord injured. Paraplegia 13:153–156, 1975

11. Clark K: Ileal conduit urinary diversion in adults with acquired neurogenic bladder. J Trauma 2:142–146, 1962

12. Claus-Walker J, Campos RJ, Carter RE, Chapman M: Electrolytes in urinary calculi and urine of patients with spinal cord injuries. Arch Phys Med Rahabil 54:109–114, 1973

13. Cobb OE, Talbot HS: Radiological findings in early vesico-ureteral reflux among spinal cord injury patients. Paraplegia 9:243–251, 1971

14. Comarr AE: Further observations on tidal drainage. J Urol 79:1024–1026, 1958

15. Comarr AE: Management of penoscrotal fistulas and/or diverticula. J Urol 84:490–492, 1960

16. Comarr AE: Does the catheter-free state bear watching among patients with spinal cord injury? J Urol 86:403–408, 1961

17. Comarr AE: Vasoresection following epididymitis among patients with spinal cord injury. Proc Ann Clin Spinal Cord Injury Conf 15:47–52, 1966

18. Comarr AE: Intermittent catheterization for the traumatic cord bladder patient. J Urol 108:79–81, 1972

19. Comarr AE, Kawaichi GK, Bors E: Renal calculosis of patients with traumatic cord lesions. J Urol 87:647–656, 1962

20. Comarr AE, Peha LJ: Further cinecystourethrography studies among spinal cord injury patients. Urol Int 29:34–37, 1974

21. DePalma JR (ed): Drill's Pharmacology in Medicine, 4th ed. New York, McGraw-Hill, 1971, p 1650

22. Firlit CF, Canning JR, Lloyd FA, Cross RR, Brewer R, Jr: Experience with intermittent catheterization in chronic spinal cord injury patient. J Urol 114:234–236, 1975

23. Gibbon NOK: A new type of catheter for urethral drainage of the bladder. Br J Urol 30:1–7, 1958

24. Gibbon NOK: Neurogenic bladder in spinal cord injury. Urol Clin North Am 1:147–154, 1974

25. Guttman L: Management of paralysis. Br Surg Pract 6:445, 1949

26. Guttmann L, Frankel H: The value of intermittent catheterization in the early management of traumatic paraplegia and tetraplegia. Paraplegia 4:63–84, 1966

27. Herr HW: Hydronephrosis and hydroureter major problem in patients with spinal cord injury. Urology 2:478–479, 1973

28. Iwatsubo E, Senoh K, Momose S: An evaluation of average flow rate in traumatic neurogenic bladder dysfunction. J Urol 114:871–873, 1975

29. Kass EH: Asymptomatic infection of the urinary tract. Trans Assoc Am Physicians 69:56–64, 1956

30. Koziol I, Hackler RH: Cutaneous ureteroileostomy in the spinal cord injured patient: A 15-year experience. J Urol 114:709–711, 1975

31. Krane RJ, Olsson CA: Phenoxybenzamine in neurogenic bladder dysfunction. I. A theory of micturition. J Urol 110:650–656, 1973

32. Kregzde J, Lambert LL, Davidson WD: Lysozymuria in renal calculosis following spinal cord injury. Urol Int 24:310–317, 1969
33. Leadbetter WF, Schaffer FG: Ileal loop diversion; its application to the treatment of neurogenic bladder dysfunction. J Urol 75:470–479, 1956
34. Manfredi RA, Leal JF: Selective sacral rhizotomy for the spastic bladder syndrome in patients with spinal cord injuries. J Urol 100:17–20, 1968
35. Marosszeky JE, Farnsworth RH, Jones RF: The indwelling urethral catheter in patients with acute spinal cord trauma. Med J Aust 2:62–66, 1973
36. McCleod JW, Mason JM, Neill RWK: Surgery of the different urinary infections which develop in the paraplegic and their relative significance. Paraplegia 3:124–143, 1965
37. McGuire EJ, Wagner FM, Weiss RN: Treatment of autonomic dysreflexia with phenoxybenzamine. J Urol 115:53–55, 1976
38. McMaster WC, Nicholas JJ, Rosen JS: Intermittent catheterization for spinal cord injury patients with chronic indwelling urethral catheters. Arch Phys Med Rehabil 53:563–567, 1972
39. Melzak A: The incidence of bladder cancer in paraplegia. Paraplegia 4:85–96, 1966
40. Morales P: Neurogenic bladder in traumatic paraplegia. NY State J Med 68:2031–2037, 1968
41. Nanninga JB, Rosen J, O'Connor VJ: Experience with transurethral external sphincterotomy in patients with spinal cord injury. J Urol 112:72–74, 1974
42. O'Flynn JD: Early management of neuropathic bladder in spinal cord injuries. Paraplegia 12:83–86, 1974
43. Ott R, Rossier AB: Urinary manometry in spinal cord injury patients. Urol Int 30:72–74, 1975
44. Owen SE, Finch EP: Bacteriological study of urine from paraplegic patients. J Urol 61:258–264, 1949
45. Patton JF, Schwartz HG: Sacral neurotomy for the spastic neurogenic bladder. J Urol 70:230–233, 1953
46. Pearman JW: Prevention of urinary tract infection following spinal cord injury. Paraplegia 9:95–104, 1971
47. Pearman JW, England EJ: The Urological Management of the Patient Following Spinal Cord Injury. Springfield, Ill., Charles C Thomas, 1973, p 243–251
48. Perkash I: Intermittent catheterization: The urologist's point of view. J Urol 111:356–360, 1974
49. Perkash I: Intermittent catheterization and bladder rehabilitation in spinal cord injury patients. J Urol 114:230–233, 1975
50. Perkash I: An attempt to understand and to treat voiding dysfunctions during rehabilitation of the bladder in spinal cord injury patients. J Urol 115:36–40, 1976
51. Retief PJM, Key AG: Urinary diversion in paraplegia. Paraplegia 4:225–235, 1967
52. Rossier AB: Neurogenic bladder in spinal cord injury. Urol Clin North Am 1:125–138, 1974
53. Rossier AB, Ott R: Urinary manometry in spinal cord injury: A follow-up study. Value of sphincterometrography as an indication for sphincterotomy. Br J Urol 46:439–448, 1974
54. Scher AT: Changes in the upper urinary tract as demonstrated on intravenous pyelography and micturating cystourethrography in patients with spinal cord injury. Paraplegia 13:157–161, 1975
55. Schoenberg HW, Murphy JJ, Young D: Electrical stimulation of the bladder. J Urol 89:820–821, 1963
56. Scott TG: The bacteriology of urinary infections in paraplegia. J Clin Pathol 13:54–57, 1960
57. Scott FB, Bradley WE, Timm GW: Treatment of urinary incontinence by implantable prosthetic sphincter. Urology 1:252–259, 1973
58. Scott FB, Bradley WE, Timm GW, Kothari D: Treatment of incontinence second-

ary to myclodysplasia by an implantable prosthetic urinary sphincter. South Med J 66:987–990, 1973

59. Stover SL, Miller JM, III, Nepomuceno CS: Intermittent catheterization in patients previously on indwelling catheter drainage. Arch Phys Med Rehabil 54:25–30, 1973
60. Tasker HJ: Pudendal neurectomy. Br J Urol 33:397–398, 1961
61. Valadka B, Cottrell TLC, Lloyd FA: Significance of vesicoureteral reflux. Am J Surg 100:527–529, 1960
62. Vivian JM, Bors E: Experience with intermittent catheterisation in the southwest regional system for treatment of spinal injury. Paraplegia 12:158–166, 1974
63. Walsh JJ: Further experience with intermittent catheterisation. Paraplegia 6:74–78, 1968

# 25

# Physical and Social Rehabilitation

## BRACING (FIGS. 1-9)

After the acute stage following cervical spine injuries, immediate and long-term immobilization may be obtained with the halo traction device[45] (Figs. 8, 9). Prolo et al.[50] recommend use of this device in the acute stage for the treatment, reduction, and stabilization of the cervical spine. Blockey and Purser,[5] Thompson,[58] and Zwerling and Riggins[62] describe successful use of the device. Use of the halo has become more widespread because the patient may be ambulatory, or at least mobility may begin with this traction device in place. Perry and Nickel[48] advised use of the halo for the treatment of scoliosis, but it has become very useful in the management of cervical spine injuries. Kerr[34] described a modification for spinal injuries. The halo traction device has also been used in infants and children,[21,35] and in the treatment of odontoid fractures. Thus it appears that the halo traction device will have a permanent place in the treatment of the acute and intermediate stages after injury, as well as in the long-term care of cervical spine fractures with instability.

When respiratory function is marginal, or the skin is anesthetized, the weight of a plaster jacket often cannot be tolerated by the patient. For these patients, Dewald and Ray[18] suggested use of the halo traction device combined with a pelvic hoop connected to rods transfixing the iliac crest, which are attached to the halo by four upright turnbuckles. A lighter weight plaster shoulder jacket may also be used. In our experience, the halo traction device works well, but it may slip, and we recorded one dislocation which recurred after the patient had been discharged from the hospital. In addition, cellulitis and osteonecrosis may occur at the pin site, pressure sores may develop in

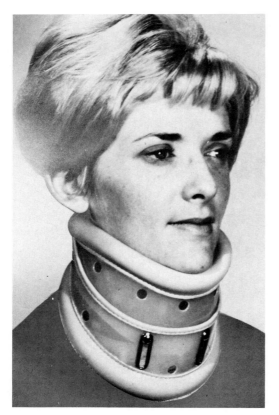

*Fig. 1.* Adjustable cervical collar (Camp).

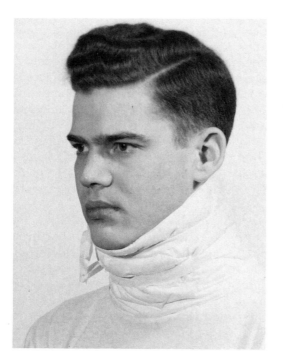

*Fig. 2.* Camp-Lewin cotton collar.

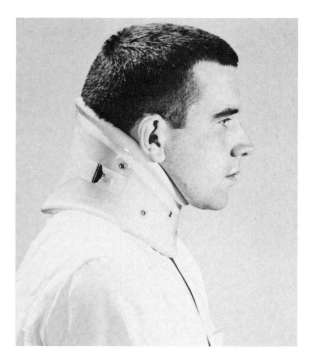

*Fig. 3.* Thomas collar.

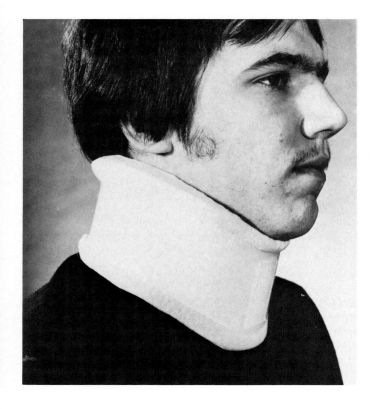

*Fig. 4.* Soft collar.

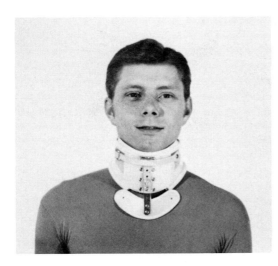

*Fig. 5.* Adjustable cervical collar with sternal plate (Camp).

the scapular and iliac areas, and if thoracic restriction is too severe, pneumonitis may result. Generally, however, such severe complications do not occur.

After a suitable period of absolute immobilization either by halo traction or in the supine position using various skeletal devices such as the Crutchfield or Cone tongs, when a patient with a cervical spine injury becomes erect he will generally require bracing to reduce movement of the cervical spine and allow bone healing.[37] There are five commonly used orthoses. A Dennison-type neck brace[54] is in essence a two-poster firm brace placed under the chin and subocciput with a chest extension. A Guilford[30] brace serves a like purpose. Others are the four-poster brace and long two-poster brace. The latter may be fitted with thoracic and abdominal supports. These braces all afford fairly good immobilization.

The plastic Thomas collar is occasionally used but provides minimal immobilization and is mainly used for pain relief. The soft cervical collar also provides only minimal immobilization but is probably the most comfortable of collars. Hartman et al.[30] demonstrated that this collar provided no restriction of motion.

Fractures of the thoracic spinal column between T1 and T10 generally require between six and eight weeks of bedrest to provide sufficient soft-tissue healing and bony union if the patient is to be treated nonoperatively. Following a sufficient period of immobilization in the supine position, a well-molded plaster body jacket from the sternum to the greater trochanters may be used. This must be carefully contoured and bivalved and must be removed almost daily to inspect the skin to prevent pressure ulcerations. Three-point fixation braces, such as a Jewett or chairback, may not have sufficient stability to provide adequate immobilization but are widely utilized (Fig. 7). Some physicians feel that a brace is not required after six to eight weeks of immobilization, but thoracolumbar spine fractures are notoriously unstable. A long

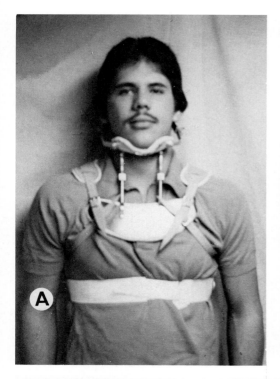

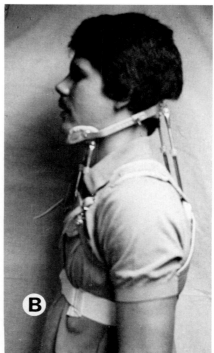

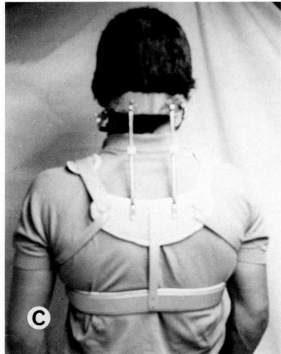

*Fig. 6A, B, C.* Four-poster cervical brace with chest extention.

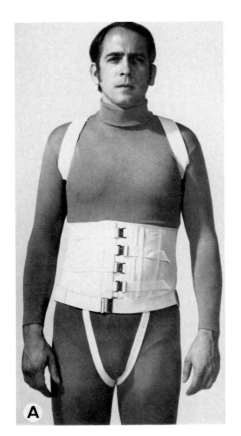
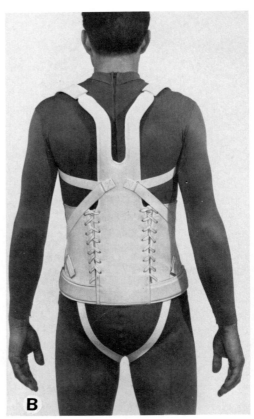

*Fig. 7A.* Thoracolumbar support (front). *B.* Thoracolumbar support (rear).

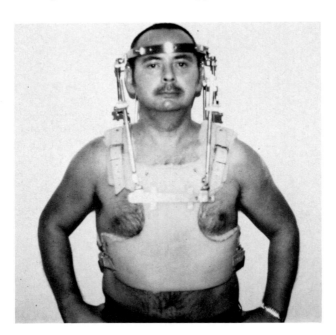

*Fig. 8.* Halo traction.

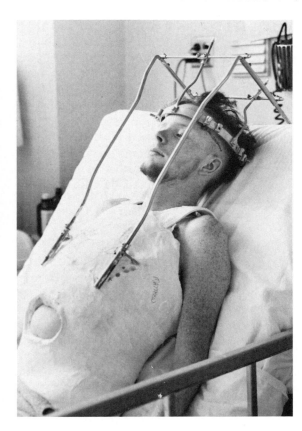

*Fig. 9.* Halo traction.

period of bedrest is required for bone healing as well as soft tissue healing, followed by gradual mobilization in a well-molded plaster jacket. Newer materials such as polyurethane foams, plastizote, and various plastics have been used, but have little advantage over a plaster of paris cast. Harrington rod internal operative stabilization can be employed.

In lumbar spine fractures immobilization is extremely difficult. Some advocate a cranial and pelvic halo in which traction is applied. This is generally insufficient for immobilization.[54]

## FUNCTIONAL SIGNIFICANCE OF SPINAL CORD LESION LEVEL

The neurologic functional level of a quadriplegic is classified according to the lowest functioning nerve root manifested by a "fair plus" muscle. A "fair plus" muscle is able to power the joint through its range of motion against gravity but requires only slight resistance to be overcome.[56]

## C4 Functional Level

The highest cervical functional level compatible with independent respiration is C4. Injuries above this level are usually fatal due to paralysis of the diaphragm for respiration and the trapezius and levator scapulae for scapular elevation. Orthoses to provide function for a C4 quadriplegic require total arm replacement devices. Electric arm motors may be controlled by tongue-operated switches or muscular electric signals. Some control of the environment may be achieved with a mouth stick. These patients have good head and neck control and can use a mouth stick adequately. Other more sophisticated environmental control manipulators can be operated by chin switches, breath control, eyebrow motion, or tongue switches.

## C5 Functional Level

The patient with a C5 functional capacity has a lesion just below the C5 myotomal segment. He has full innervation of the trapezius, sternocleidomastoid, and upper cervical paraspinal musculature. He has rhomboids, deltoids, and all major muscles of the rotator cuff, although these are only partially innervated since they share nerve supply with C6 and upper pectorals. These muscles provide scapular retraction and weak protraction, glenohumeral abduction, internal and external rotation, as well as weak flexion and extension. Elbow flexion is possible, since the biceps and brachioradialis remain partially innervated. There is no elbow extension and no function in the wrist or hand. Sensation is present over the deltoid area of the arm and the radial aspect of the thumb. To perform a prehensive pinch the patient requires electric handsplints with head, shoulder, or chin control, or a passive rachet handsplint operated by the opposite extremity. He also may require mobile arm supports to position his upper extremities in space. He cannot roll over or come to a sitting position in bed and has no use of the hands. This patient cannot push his wheelchair and his endurance is low because of reduced respiratory reserve. Ambulation is not possible, and the patient is confined to a wheelchair.[41,43]

## C6 Functional Level

A substantial functional increment is added at C6. Patients at the C6 functional level have radial wrist extensors, but no voluntary finger extensor or flexor power. This is the most common level of quadriplegia seen. Over 50 percent of all spinal cord injuries are at the C6 level or slightly lower. The upper arm rotator cuff musculature becomes fully innervated and the serratus, latissimus, and pectoralis major receive partial innervation. Nerve supply to the biceps muscle is complete. Pronation is added. At the wrist the extensor carpi radialis and sometimes the flexor carpi radialis are present.

There is good movement of the muscles about the glenohumeral joint. The biceps and brachioradialis are stronger than at the C5 level since they have gained another segment of innervation. The radial wrist extensors and flexors may be functional, but the extensor musculature of the wrist can utilize the remaining elasticity of the finger flexors to produce a weak closure of the hand through a tenodesis effect. In most cases, however, hand devices are necessary to enable prehension.

Elbow flexors can give the patient the power to sit up independently in bed, or at least to assist actively in the process. The shoulder strength of the C6 patient permits him to help in rolling over in bed. An occasional strong patient may be able to assist in lifting himself or transferring himself to a wheelchair, but an attendant is often needed for lifting the patient to and from the wheelchair.[41-43] This patient may feed himself with specific hand devices and may perform part of his toilet and dressing activites. This patient may be able to propel his own wheelchair on smooth, level surfaces. Since he has no grasp he applies his thenar eminence tightly against projections on the hand-rim for traction and uses elbow flexors and shoulder abductors and flexors to move the wheelchair.

An automatic gross grasp utilizing a tenodesis tightening of the finger

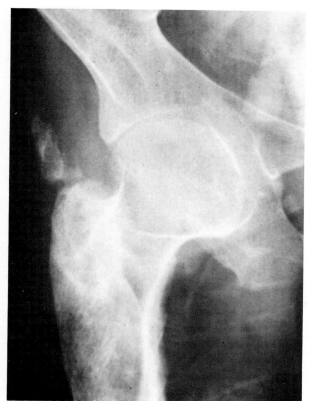

*Fig. 10.* Hip necrosis in chronic quadriplegia.

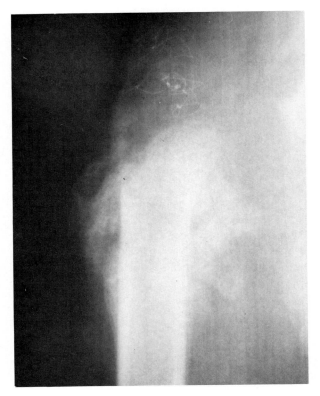

*Fig. 11.* Hip necrosis in chronic quadriplegia.

flexor and extensor muscle tendons is possible. As the wrist is extended, the thumb and fingers approximate each other in a grasp motion. As the wrist is dropped in flexion, tightness of the finger extensor muscles provides passive release. Hand splints have been devised to increase this activity.

## C7 Functional Level

The patient with sparing of the C7 segment of the spinal cord has three important functional additions: triceps, common finger extensors, and long finger flexors; occasionally these are absent owing to variations between C7 and C8. The patient can better lift his body since he can stabilize his arm with the triceps and has more shoulder girdle depression. The advantages of grasp and release afforded by finger extensors and flexors cannot be overemphasized. The intrinsic muscles of the hand are not significantly innervated so that there is no dexterity. Although some of these patients require help in transferring to and from the wheelchair, this help may consist of only a push rather than a real lift. The C7 quadriplegic is essentially confined to a wheelchair.[41-43]

## C8 and T1 Functional Levels

Patients with C8 neurologic function have finger flexors as well as extensors, but lack certain intrinsic musculature. Therefore, they are able to voluntarily grasp and release, but develop a clawhand deformity. The patient in whom T1 has been spared has full innervation of the upper extremity musculature including the essential intrinsic muscles of the hand. He therefore has strength and dexterity in grasp and release as well as fully innervated proximal musculature. The ulnar side of the wrist has its full nerve supply and crutch walking may be possible. The patient does not have trunk stability. The T1 patient may be independent in bed activities and is able to transfer to and from his wheelchair without aid. He is in most instances independent in self care. With appropriate leg braces, pelvic band, and a high spinal attachment the T1 patient can do a "drag-to" or "swing-to" gait, but this is very energy consumming and generally is not practiced.[40]

## Midthoracic Functional Level

The midthoracic paraplegic patient has a major functional gain of increased trunk control compared to the high thoracic patient. He has innervation to long muscles of the upper and midback and may use intercostals for respiration. His endurance has increased because of increased respiratory ability.

These additions enable him to be independent in all phases of self care. Full leg bracing becomes possible and the patient can stabilize his upper extremities adequately to use them to lift the pelvis in applying braces while he is recumbent. A high thoracic spinal injured patient can carry out the latter movements. He may transfer independently to and from a wheelchair using the strong upper extremities. He probably does not need an attendant.

Long leg braces can be utilized so that he is able to stand erect for a long period of time. Many physiatrists are not in favor of such bracing. Once he has reached the erect position, he can ambulate with crutches with an independent swing-through gait, although a swing-to gait remains the safer and more practical one to use. Most of these patients find ambulation tedious and laborious so that they do not use it often except to assume the standing position. The patient can drive an automobile with hand controls. It should be pointed out that some C6-spared quadriplegics can drive and an occasional C7-spared patient can transfer into a car independently.

## T12 Functional Level

The T12 functionally innervated patient has use of the rectus abdominus, the oblique muscles of the abdomen, and all muscles of the thorax. The lumbar musculature of the low back as well as hip musculature is not innervated.

The patient may use bilateral long leg braces. He can use a two-point alternate, four-point, or swing-through gait. Four-point and two-point alternate gaits are achieved through the use of the secondary hip musculature including the internal and external obliques and the latissimus dorsi. Because he can tilt his pelvis he can negotiate stairs with a handrail.

## L4 Functional Level

The patient with a lesion sparing L4 has added functional assistance of the quadratus musculature, the lower erector spinae, quadriceps, and the hip flexors. The major stabilizers of the hips are absent and the ankles are flail. Long leg bracing is unnecessary because the quadriceps extend the knee. The flail ankles must be supported by a short leg brace. With proper bracing, the patient may be independent without crutches or canes. These patients, however, do better with bilateral canes or crutches. The absence of hip extensors makes the maneuver difficult. Canes with support above the wrists, such as the Loffstrand, are advisable. Wheelchairs are necessary part of the time in some instances to conserve energy.

To predict ambulation potential with crutches and braces the patient may be classified in four neurologic level categories.

*Complete Thoracic Paraplegia.* Patients with this spinal cord injury have complete neurologic loss below T12. They do not have pelvic control, and they have no voluntary muscle or sensation in the lower extremities. These patients will generally not use crutches and braces for significant ambulation. They may, however, use long leg braces for standing activities and brief ambulation.

*Incomplete Quadriplegics and Incomplete Thoracic Paraplegics.* Patients with incomplete spinal cord injuries above the level of T12 who have sufficient sparing of muscle power to provide pelvic control and some muscle power and sensation in the lower extremities may be able to ambulate and should be fitted with long leg braces and crutches. Two long leg braces and crutches are the maximum bracing that will be functionally used. A pelvic band is rarely used to control stability of the lower extremities.

*T12–L1 Paraplegia With Pelvic Control.* Patients with T12–L1 functional levels who have pelvic control and weak hip flexors and abductors are potential ambulation candidates. They can use crutches and braces, but the energy usage is so high and the gait is so slow that most soon discard their braces and prefer wheelchair mobilization.

*Lumbar Neurologic Levels.* Those who have adequate hip flexor and knee extensor strength in one leg to warrant the use of a short leg brace on one side and either a short or long leg brace on the opposite side have excellent ambulation potential. These patients can be expected to use crutches and braces for functional walking. It appears that voluntary control of flexors of the hips and extensors of at least one knee is a key for significant ambulation.

## AMBULATION DEVICES

### Long Leg Braces

Long leg braces provide a stable post upon which the patient can balance his body weight. The braces should have a stop at the ankles and should have a locking and unlocking mechanism at the knees. Ankles are stopped in slight dorsiflexion to provide a position of slight hip extension on standing. Lacking hip extensor strength, the iliofemoral ligament and the anterior hip capsule provide anterior hip joint stability. The patient therefore can lean back at his hip joints and balance over his braces with the center of gravity behind the hip joint, in front of the ankle joint, and over the midfoot.

When the patient can be moved from bed into a standing position, he is fitted with temporary standing braces that generally incorporate the same principles as permanent braces. They are not custom fitted at this time, since the patient may lose muscle mass in his legs. After six months, he is considered a candidate for permanent braces.[25,54]

### Short Leg Braces

Short leg braces are prescribed for patients who have good knee extension and require only foot control. They should have anterior stops to compensate for deficit of the weak plantar flexors.

### Crutches

Forward- or side-opening aluminum forearm crutches are the most efficient crutches for ambulatory spinal injury patients at the lumbar level. These allow easiest rising from the wheelchair and negotiation of curbs and steps. Thoracic level patients will probably require axillary crutches.

### Wheelchairs

Most spinal cord injury patients need wheelchairs that meet certain requirements.[41-43] A folding chair allows for ease of transportation. The wheelchair must be functional, durable, versatile, collapsible, lightweight, and provide easy mobilization. The seat should be as narrow as possible for the patient.

The wheelchair should have removable desk-type armrests and removable swing-away leg rests to allow for easier patient transfer in and out of a chair or car, and on to toilets. If the patient navigates primarily indoors, solid rubber tires should be used; pneumatic tires are easier to navigate over soft grounds, sand, and grass. There should be brakes for locking the wheels. The front casters should be at least eight inches in diameter. The high cervical quadriplegic who does not have good wrist extensors will need an electric wheelchair that can be controlled by a stick on the armrests or a mouth control.

Comarr and Schwenk[10] devised a self helper interchangeable with an armrest so that the patient can help himself out of a wheelchair with greater ease. It consists of a strap elevated above the patient's head on a vertical bar. The patient can grasp it and move himself out of the chair. Letts et al.[39] described mobility aids for the paraplegic child including, for example, the caster cart which is in essence a small wheelchair. A standing frame as well as standing wheelchairs are described. Taylor and Sand[57] describe the use of the Verlo brace to assist the child in standing. The papers mentioned should be consulted for more details.

Silber et al.[53] has tested a pneumatic orthosis as a potential substitute for conventional long leg braces. It is a garment-like appliance of synthetic fabric which can be worn over underwear and under outer clothing. Pneumatic tubes can be inflated at will by the patient. In preliminary testing it was found to be very acceptable to patients with spinal cord injury. Wearing time was increased daily until the patients tolerated six to eight hours of inflation of the orthosis without harmful effects on the skin. It also appeared to prevent postural hypertension. Such orthoses have not yet achieved widespread use. These orthoses are used primarily in early phases of rehabilitation when hypotension is a problem. They are too cumbersome to use when rehabilitation is complete. The patient must carry a pump to inflate it and must deflate the orthosis to sit. Since it encloses the legs and lower trunk, heat is a problem.

## REHABILITATION POTENTIAL

Hussey[32] and Stauffer[54] studied 164 patients discharged with lower extremity function following spinal cord injury. They characterized ambulation ability at four levels: community, household, exercise, and nonambulatory. They reported that 50 percent had community function and ambulatory function. This was the best level of ambulation, and detailed muscle examinations revealed that these patients had the following characteristics: pelvic control, fair or better function of hip flexors, fair or better function of quadriceps in at least one leg, required no braces, or as a maximum, one short leg and one long leg brace, and had no fixed joint deformity or significant spasticity. Patients with similar muscle and bracing patterns but who had deformity and/or spasticity or were older achieved only household ambulation. Patients with only pelvic control rarely went beyond the exercise stage and those without pelvic control were nonambulatory. Many with only pelvic control were nonambulatory also. Hip abductors and extensors, knee flexors, and foot and ankle musculature were less important in ambulatory capability. Proprioceptive sensation was considered important because only one patient in the community ambulatory group had absent proprioception at the hips and knees, although there is considerable disagreement as to its actual importance. They felt that prediction of ambulatory potential could be made according to these criteria.

McKenzie[44] stressed the role of occupational therapy in rehabilitating spinal cord-injured patients. She stressed the prevention of contractures during the period of bedrest during the acute phase. The importance of daily range of motion exercises, both active and passive, was emphasized. Deformities can often be prevented with the proper splinting, particularly hand splinting.

One contracture is encouraged in C6 quadriplegics. That is the muscle tendon tightness that the therapist nurtures in the flexor tendons of the hand to provide a gross mechanical grasp. This tightness is fostered by using a wrist-driven, flexor-hinge hand splint, which positions the thumb, index, and long fingers so that they come together for three-point palmar prehension. The extensor carpi radialis longus and brevis supply the muscle power to operate the splint. When the splint extensors are relaxed, gravity and the weight of the hand cause the wrists to drop into flexion, opening the grasp. While the hand splint is being used to perform functional activities, it also reinforces the desire to establish a pattern of gross mechanical grasp. Many physiatrists don't encourage such contractures, even of finger flexors. The flexor hinge splint will function with or without contractures. Abramson et al.[1] discuss the mechanical substitutes necessary for hand function in the quadriplegic. Hip, knee, and ankle contractures are also worrisome. Not only range of motion is important but stretching all joints daily.

Freehafer[23,24] described transfer of the brachioradialis to enhance wrist extension and thus enhance the pincer effect of thumb, index, and long finger in a three-point prehension grasp with extension of the wrist. The brachioradialis tendon is inserted into the extensor carpi radialis brevis or into both radial wrist extensors. Following transplantation of the brachioradialis, extension of the wrist is stronger and therefore the pincer grasp is also stronger. Curtis[16] discusses various tendon transfers in the hand in patients with spinal cord injury. In all cases, depending upon the remaining forearm and hand muscles, various tendon transplants are carried out to achieve better use of the hand. Zancolli[61] classifies the forelimb of quadriplegics into four functional groups. Group 1 has only flexion of the elbow (C5). Group 2 has added extension of the wrist (C6). Group 3 has added extrinsic extension of the fingers (C7), and Group 4 has all muscle groups previously mentioned plus extrinsic flexion of the fingers and thumb extension (C8). The above-mentioned author carries out tendon transplants to improve hand function.

Many self-care and self-help devices have been devised for the quadriplegic and paraplegic patients. These include attachments to beds, wheel-chairs, and various aids to tasks of daily living, such as dressing, eating, drinking, bathing, homemaking, housecleaning, dishwashing, and so forth. The references for this chapter may be consulted for further information.

## SOCIAL ADJUSTMENT

Many studies have been made of the employability and the degree of functional independence of spinal-injured patients. While it is generally agreed that many quadriplegics can be functionally independent and be gainfully employed, unfortunately only the minority, in fact, is. This is alarming because mortality from spinal injury following World War II markedly decreased from that after World War I. During World War I, only 10 percent of those who suffered paraplegia were alive a year after onset. Following World War II, 80 percent of paraplegic persons survived, and many of these could be expected to be alive 10 years later.[7,22]

Peerless and Schweigel[47] studied the medical and economic fate of 29 industrial spinal cord injured patients and found that in the course of 12 years the cost to society per patient per year was over $2500. This is a very low figure at the present time. The total cost was $685,000, again a low estimate. Others have estimated the cost for the first year to be $28,000 to $30,000 per patient. Charles et al.[8] estimated the total cost to society of each paraplegic patient to be over $3 million. Based on statistics compiled in the state of Alabama, where 80 new cases occurred yearly and the total cost was over 25 million dollars per year, the national incidence is estimated to be 25 new patients per million per year (approximately 5000 new cases) for a total cost of one and one-half billion dollars per year.

Felton and Litman[22] studied 222 men with spinal cord injury and found that few were employed. One of the critical factors contributing to successful post-disability adjustment is the level of education or skill. Those who were employed had clerical, watchmaking, drafting, photography, carpentry, laboratory work, and other skills. Kemp[33] found that the number and type of goals expressed by the patient at the time of follow-up, what loss the patient considered to be greatest as a result of his disability, the degree of his creative thinking, and the degree of interpersonal support were the most important factors. Persons who had the greatest drive, the best vocational preparation, and the most support were most successful in making good adjustments.

Both Rosen et al.[52] and Nyboer and Johnson[46] reported electromyographic evidence of lower motor neuron disease in the lower extremities and lumbosacral erector spina muscles following cervical spinal cord trauma. Diffuse positive sharp waves and fibrillation potentials were found in 8 of 10 subjects in stages of flaccid as well as spastic paralysis. There was no preexisting motor neuron disease, no evidence of peripheral neuropathy, and the findings were not related to thoracolumbar skeletal abnormalities, previous myelography, or laminectomy. The etiologic basis of these changes could not be established. Rosen et al.[52] found similar positive electromyographic findings in patients who were still in the stage of spinal shock. Repeat electromyographic studies performed after disappearance of spinal shock revealed that previous evidence of lower motor neuron abnormality had either disappeared or was markedly diminished. They cautioned against confirming the existence of lower motor neuron disease by electromyographic evidence in patients who are still in the stage of spinal shock. They conjectured that during spinal shock functional depression of anterior horn cells causes electromyographic abnormalities that clear when spinal shock disappears.

## Disorders of Body Image

Body-image disorders have been primarily related to the parietal lobe of the brain. Many persons with parietal lobe lesions cannot sense the location of a specific body part, usually one on the side opposite the lesion. This occurs also in some peripheral nerve disorders and in spinal cord injuries. Conomy[14] studied 18 spinally injured patients and found that all experienced disordered sensation of the placement of their limbs in space early in the course of their illness, many at the time the spinal cord injury occurred. The legs were more often the site of hallucinations of limb positions than the arms. Disorders of perception of somatic bulk, size, and continuity of bodily parts were the fewest. Disorders of postured movement in the feet consisted of a curling up tonic pattern in the toes and forced plantar or palmar flexion. Similar studies were done by Arnhoff and Mehl[2] indicating that there is also body-image deterioration in long-standing paraplegics.

## Sexual Function

Female paraplegics still menstruating can conceive and give natural birth to children.[9] In this respect the female sexual function is unchanged after injury. In complete lesions there is no sensation in the vagina and although there may be some emotional satisfaction from intercourse there is little in the way of physical satisfaction. Few paraplegic women experience orgasm and it is doubtful whether a true physiologic orgasm can occur in the female with a complete lesion. During intercourse the female usually assumes the supine position. It is not necessary for her catheter to be removed.

Menses and pregnancies occur in women with spinal injury. A study by Comarr[11] established that the majority of women have a return of menses within the first six months after injury; 50 percent did not miss a single period. Durkan's[19] patients were amenorrheic. Level and extent of the lesion did not appear to play a role nor did the presence or absence of sacral reflex. Dysmenorrhea ceased after the injury. Four of Comarr's patients were pregnant at the time of injury, and five became pregnant following injury. None of the patients pregnant at the time of injury aborted, and all infants were delivered vaginally except one delivered by caesarean section. He cautioned the obstetrician to be aware of autonomic dysreflexia and to differentiate it from preeclampsia and eclampsia. Incidence of renal complications is greater in pregnancy in these patients.

Griffith and Trieschmann[27] discussed sexual function in women with spinal cord injury and indicated that they may have no greater imbalance of sex hormones than a non-spinally injured woman. They stated that the neurophysiologic responses associated with sexual activity in the cord-injured woman had not yet been adequately described. Guttmann[29] claimed that women with complete lesions do not experience orgasm. He observed that such patients may attain a state of heightened arousal or orgasm as a result of intense tactile stimulation above the sensory level of injury especially about the breasts. According to Griffith and Trieschmann,[27] the phenomenon of temporary reduction of spasticity following orgasm which has been described in men has not been documented in women. Guttmann[28] found that 46 percent of 189 women had been married before injury. Another 17 percent married after injury. The postinjury divorce rate of those married before injury was nearly the same as those married after injury (7.3 percent vs. 7.0 percent). Weiss and Diamond[60] reported that 48 percent of their subjects were married prior to disability. Two years later, 14 percent of previously single women had married, and 23 percent of those who married either before or after disability eventually divorced or separated.

Robertson and Guttmann[51] reported that the paraplegic patient can have normal pregnancy and labor, as well as normal delivery. The usual complications of the prenatal and perinatal period exist, but the incidence of complications may be somewhat higher.

Jochheim and Wahle[38] reported that among 56 male patients with spastic and flaccid paralysis the percent able to obtain erection varied between 30 and 75 percent. Very few, however, experienced ejaculation, orgasm, or libido. Jackson[36] studied male athletes who were paraplegic and found that among 20 men, 85 percent achieved erection on physical stimulus and 25 percent on mental stimulus, 75 percent were able to achieve intercourse, 35 percent had ejaculation and orgasm, 10 percent were able to conceive children. A further 10 percent had urinary problems related to sexual activity.

Comarr[12,13] found that in 150 male patients with spinal injury, 82 percent were able to obtain erections but only 1 percent could ejaculate and have orgasm. Of 35 patients with lower motor neuron lesions, approximately 35 percent had erections. Comarr stated that pin prick perception in the sacral segments of patients with incomplete upper motor neuron lesions seems to be prognostically more significant for erection and ejaculation than preservation of light touch perception or retained volitional motor function of the pelvic floor muscles. The presence of a bulbocavernosus reflex and/or anal sphincter tone indicates that the patient has upper motor neuron sexual function. Absence indicates that the patient may have lower motor neuron sexual function. Most paraplegics cannot ejaculate and therefore are unable to sire children.[9] In incomplete lesions, more patients have normal sexual function. Griffith et al.[26] provide an excellent review of the subject.

Webber[59] emphasized that fertility in men is low after spinal injury. Only 5 to 7 percent can be expected to produce offspring. Only 33 percent of those having an erection are able to maintain it long enough to have coitus. Another cause of male sterility is retroejaculation into the bladder, which occurs when the hypogastric nerve connections are lost and the internal vesicle sphincter to the bladder lacks control. As a result the semen pools in the bladder instead of being ejaculated through the urethra. The pH of the urine is rather acidic compared to the alkaline environment provided by prostatic secretions, and in the acidic solution, sperm motility is reduced or lost. Artificial insemination with this sperm will not produce pregnancy.

Another cause of infertility in males is testicular atrophy with absence of spermatogenesis. Atrophy of the testicles is common following spinal trauma, becoming evident as early as three to four months after injury. The reason for the atrophy is unknown, but it is suggested that alterations in heat regulatory mechanisms may influence the process. This could explain why ovulation continues after trauma in females, because the anatomic position of the ovaries makes them less susceptible to changes in body temperature. In quadriplegics sweating mechanisms are correlated with the extent of damage to the testes. An increase of even a few degrees in body temperature can bring about cessation of spermatogenesis. Bensman and Kottke[4] induced emission of sperm by means of electrical stimulation of the seminal vesicles and vas deferens using a rectal electrode, a technique used extensively to secure sperm for animal breeding. They successfully stimulated emission of sperm in three of five patients with spinal injury, using a continuous 2 to 10 cycle per second sinusoidal current of 20 to 30 milliamperes. Horne et al.[31] carried out fertility studies in the male with spinal cord and cauda equina injuries. They also obtained specimens by electrical stimulation.

El Ghatit[20] studied the outcome of marriages preexisting a male's spinal cord injury. Of 333 marriages, a total of 26.7 percent ended in divorce, and 1.8 percent were separated. The divorce rate among spinally injured patients did not differ significantly from that in the entire United States and was considerably lower then that found in the state of California. Most divorces occurred within five years of injury, and the divorce and separation rates were significantly higher for patients who had been married more than once at the time of their injury.

## Pain Following Spinal Injury

Pain following spinal injury is occasionally a severe problem. Davis and Martin,[17] comparing military vs. civilian cases, found a higher incidence of pain in civilian patients. Chronic pain may take several forms: pain at the site of the injury, pain radiating along the nerve roots in a radicular fashion, or pain perceived below the level of the cord lesion, such as phantom or central pain. Treatment of the pain is extremely difficult, but should consist of conservative means, such as simple analgesics and various physical therapy modalities. The transcutaneous nerve stimulator has been helpful in some cases and in some cases we have had to resort to chordotomy, albeit very reluctantly. We have carried out myelograms and serial electromyograms to identify nerve root compression, and even surgical relief of nerve root compression so demonstrated has been insufficient in many cases for pain relief. Phantom-limb pain as well as root pain are not easily treated with a transcutaneous stimulator. There is only a 20 percent response, and this is short lived in many cases.

Phantom pain is perceived by the patient as position and movement in an insensible extremity. These sensations do not correspond to the actual posture movement of the extremities and in many incidences are very painful. The pain is usually described by the patient as cramping of the extremity or as a sensation that the limb is bent into an abnormal position causing pain. Most spinally injured patients have no pain, but rather a sensation that the limbs are in abnormal positions.[14] Pollock et al.[49] found that after injuries of the spinal cord when phantom sensations are perceived from an insensible extremity, even subsequent amputation will not result in any change. They felt that the nociceptive and proprioceptive phantom sensations originate in the distal end of the proximal segment of the injured cord. Avenarius and Gerstenbrand[3] also reported several patients who had severe symptoms due to phantom pain following spinal injury. Sweet[55] felt that any sense of awareness or torsion in an area below the neural level of a total transverse lesion in the spinal canal could be described as phantom sensation. He also described an anosognostic phase following spinal injury, which is short-lived and characterized by the patient as failure to realize that he is paralyzed and attempts to walk or perform other physical activity only to find that his legs are paralyzed. Bors[6] and Cook and Druckemiller[15] also described this difficult problem. Avenarius and Gerstenbrand[3] were not able to confirm this experience in any of their 24 patients, and we have not seen it. For a more complete description the reader is referred to the paper by Sweet.[55]

## REFERENCES

1.  Abramson AS, Ebel A, Weiss AA, Bodenstein N, Orth C: Mechanical substitutes for hand function in the tetraplegic. Am J Phys Med 37:98–105, 1958
2.  Arnhoff FN, Mehl MC: Body image deterioration in paraplegia. J Nerv Ment Dis 137:88–92, 1963
3.  Avenarius von HJ, Gerstenbrand F: Phantomerlebnisse bei Ruckenmarksverletzung. Wien Klin Wochenschr 79:450–453, 1967
4.  Bensman A, Kottke FJ: Induced emission of sperm utilizing electrical stimulation of the seminal vesicles and vas deferens. Arch Phys Med 47:436–443, 1966
5.  Blockey NJ, Purser DW: Fractures of the odontoid process of the axis. J Bone Joint Surg 38B:794, 1956
6.  Bors E: Phantom limbs of patients with spinal cord injury. Arch Neurol Psychiatr 66:610–631, 1951
7.  Burke MH, Hicks AF, Robins M, Kessler H: Survival of patients with injuries of the spinal cord. JAMA 172:121–124, 1960
8.  Charles ED, Van Matre JG, Miller JM, III: Spinal cord injury—A cost benefit analysis of alternative treatment models. Paraplegia 12:222–231, 1974

9. Cole TM: Spinal cord injury patients and sexual dysfunction. Arch Phys Med Rehabil 56:11–12, 1975

10. Comarr AE, Schwenk TS: A device to help the tetraplegic patient help himself in and out of a wheel chair. Arch Phys Med Rehabil 43:576–577, 1962

11. Comarr AE: Observations on menstruation and pregnancy among female spinal cord injury patients. Paraplegia 3:263–272, 1966

12. Comarr AE: Sexual function among patients with spinal cord injury. Urol Int 25:134–168, 1970

13. Comarr AE: Sexual concepts in traumatic cord and cauda equina lesions. J Urol 106:375–378, 1971

14. Conomy JP: Disorders of body image after spinal injury. Neurology (Minneapolis) 23:842–850, 1973

15. Cook AW, Druckemiller WH: Phantom limb in paraplegic patients. Report of two cases and an analysis of its mechanism. J Neurosurg 9:508–516, 1952

16. Curtis RM: Tendon transfers in the patient with spinal cord injury. Orthop Clin North Am 5:415–423, 1974

17. Davis L, Martin J: Studies upon spinal cord injuries. II. The nature and treatment of pain. J Neurosurg 4:483–491, 1947

18. Dewald RL, Ray RD: Skeletal traction for the treatment of severe scoliosis. J Bone Joint Surg 52A:233–238, 1970

19. Durkan JP: Menstruation after high spinal cord transection. Am J Obstet Gynecol 100:521–524, 1968

20. El Ghatit AZ: Outcome of marriages existing at the time of a male's spinal cord injury. J Chron Dis 28:383–388, 1975

21. Ewald FC: Fracture of the odontoid process in a seventeen-month-old infant treated with a halo. J Bone Joint Surg 53A:1636–1640, 1971

22. Felton JS, Litman M: Study of employment of 222 men with spinal cord injury. Arch Phys Med Rehabil 809–814, 1965

23. Freehafer AA, Mast WA: Transfer of the brachioradialis to enhance wrist extension in spinal cord injury. Proc Ann Clin Spinal Cord Injury Conf 15:60–65, 1966

24. Freehafer AA: Care of the hand in cervical spinal cord injuries. Paraplegia 7:118–130, 1969

25. Garrett AL: Functional potential of patients with spinal cord injury. Clin Orthop 112:60–65, 1975

26. Griffith ER, Tomko MA, Timms RJ: Sexual function in spinal cord injured patients: A review. Arch Phys Med Rehabil 54:539–543, 1973

27. Griffith ER, Trieschmann RB: Sexual functioning in women with spinal cord injury. Arch Phys Med Rehabil 56:18–21, 1975

28. Guttmann L: Married life of paraplegics and tetraplegics. Paraplegia 2:182–188, 1964

29. Guttmann L: Clinical symptomatology of spinal cord lesions. In Vinken PJ, Bruyn GW (eds): Handbook of Clinical Neurology, vol 2. Amsterdam, North Holland, 1969, pp 178–216

30. Hartman JT, Palumbo F, Hill BJ: Cineradiography of the braced normal cervical spine. Clin Orthop 109:97–102, 1975

31. Horne HW, Paull DP, Munro D: Fertility studies in the human male with traumatic injuries of the spinal cord and cauda equina. N Engl J Med 239:959–961, 1948

32. Hussey RW: Spinal cord injury requirements for ambulation. Arch Phys Med Rehabil 54:544–547, 1973

33. Kemp BJ: Productivity after injury in a sample of spinal cord injured persons: A pilot study. J Chronic Dis 24:259–275, 1971

34. Kerr FWL: A brace for the management of fracture dislocation of the cervical spine: Traction, immobilization, and myelography. J Neurosurg 30:97–101, 1969

35. Kropits SE, Steingass MH: Experience with the "halo-cast" in small children. Surg Clin North Am 50:935–943, 1970

36. Jackson RW: Sexual rehabilitation after cord injury. Paraplegia 10:50–55, 1972
37. James JIP: Fracture dislocation of cervical spine. J Coll Surg Edinburgh 5:232–233, 1960
38. Jochheim KA, Wahle H: A study on sexual function in 56 male patients with complete irreversible lesions of the spinal cord and cauda equina. Paraplegia 8: 166–172, 1970
39. Letts RM, Fulford R, Hobson DA: Mobility aids for the paraplegic child. J Bone Joint Surg 58A:38–41, 1976
40. Long C, II, Lawton EB: Functional significance of spinal cord lesion level. Arch Phys Med 36:249–255, 1955
41. Lowman EW, Rusk HA: Self-help devices: Selection of wheel chairs. Postgrad Med 28:308–311, 1960
42. Lowman EW, Rusk HA: Self-help devices: Selection of wheel chairs. General considerations. Postgrad Med 29:124–127, 1961
43. Lowman EW, Rusk HA: Self-help devices: Selection of wheel chairs. Consideration of specific disabiltities. Postgrad Med 29:219–223, 1961
44. McKenzie MW: The role of occupational therapy in rehabilitating spinal cord injured patients. Am J Occup Ther 24:257–263, 1970
45. Nickel VL, Perry J, Garrett A, Heppenstall M: The halo. J Bone Joint Surg 50-A:1400–1409, 1968
46. Nyboer VJ, Johnson HE: Electromyographic findings in lower extremities of patients with traumatic quadriplegia. Arch Phys Med Rehabil 256–259, 1971
47. Peerless SJ, Schweigel JF: The medical and economic fate of twenty-nine industrial spinal cord injured patients. Paraplegia 12:145–150, 1974
48. Perry J, Nickel VL: Total cervical spine fusion for neck paralysis. J Bone Joint Surg 41A:37–60, 1959
49. Pollock LJ, Boshes B, Arieff AJ, et al: Phantom limb in patients with injuries to the spinal cord and cauda equina. Surg Gynecol Obstet 104:407–415, 1957
50. Prolo DJ, Runnels JB, Jameson RM: The injured cervical spine. JAMA 224:591–594, 1973
51. Robertson DNS, Guttmann L: The paraplegic patient in pregnancy and labor. Proc R Soc Med 56:381–387, 1963
52. Rosen JS, Lerner IM, Rosenthal AM: Electromyography in spinal cord injury. Arch Phys Med Rehabil 50:271–273, 1969
53. Silber M, Chung TS, Varghese G, et al: Pneumatic orthosis: Pilot study. Arch Phys Med Rehabil 56:27–32, 1975
54. Stauffer ES: Orthotics for spinal cord injuries. Clin Orthop Rel Res 102:92–99, 1974
55. Sweet WH: Phantom sensations following intraspinal injury. Neurochirurgia 18: 139–154, 1975
56. Symington DC, Mackay DE: A study of functional independence in the quadriplegic patient. Arch Phys Med Rehabil 47:378–392, 1966
57. Taylor N, Sand P: Verlo brace use in children with myelomeningocele and spinal injury. Arch Phys Med Rehabil 55:231–235, 1974
58. Thompson H: The "halo" traction apparatus. A method of external splinting of the cervical spine after injury. J Bone Joint Surg 44:655–661, 1962
59. Weber DK: A review of sexual function following spinal cord trauma. Phys Ther 51:290–295, 1971
60. Weiss AJ, Diamond MD: Sexual adjustment, identification, and attitudes of patients with myelopathy. Arch Phys Med Rehabil 47:245–250, 1966
61. Zancolli E: Surgery for the quadriplegic hand with active, strong wrist extension preserved. A study of 97 cases. Clin Orthop Rel Res 112:101–113, 1975
62. Zwerling MT, Riggins RS: Use of the halo apparatus in acute injuries of the cervical spine. Surg Gynecol Obstet 138:189–193, 1974

# 26

## Biomechanics

### SPINAL CORD

The spinal cord is immersed in fluid contained in a relatively elastic dural sac, which is encased in the solid vertebral canal. White matter and gray matter are semifluid cohesive masses having the potential for plastic deformation in response to stress. Cerebrospinal fluid and the vertebral column provide hydraulic and mechanical protection to the spinal cord under ordinary circumstances; however, these two substances can also transmit damaging external forces to the spinal cord.[5,6]

The pons, spinal cord, and nerve roots constitute a continuous unit, anchored cephalad at the brain stem and along the spinal cord by nerve roots leaving the spinal canal. Forceful deformation of tissue results in changes determined by the force itself and by other factors, such as fixation of the cord, the dorsoventral diameter of the canal, and changes in the length of the spinal column.[45] In the erect neutral position, axial tension on the cord is neutral. Hyperextension shortens the spinal canal, causing slackening and thickening of the cord. Flexion increases physiologic tension on spinal tracts because of axial anchorage and the restraining effects of the dentate ligaments. In ventroflexion, plasticity, elasticity, and cord diameter are reduced because of the maximal lengthening of the spinal canal.[5] Spinal stenosis, spondylolisthesis, and spondylosis further reduce the margin of safety by narrowing available space; constriction of the anteroposterior diameter by more than 15 to 20 percent invariably results in damage to nerve fibers and injury to blood vessels.

Since the spinal cord is fixed cephalad and caudad, injury at either end can be caused by abrupt lengthening of the spinal canal resulting from acute flexion. Trauma to the vertex of the skull causes retropulsion of the brain and brain stem, followed by rebound of the cerebral and cerebellar hemispheres.[45,46] The upper cervical spinal cord is relatively fixed and anchored by dentate ligaments above which mobility is maximal. Impact stress to the cord at this level results in linear and reticular hemorrhages in gray matter and white matter pathways with the possibility of respiratory failure. Gosch et al.,[21] in 1970, demonstrated in the monkey the tethering effect of the dentate ligaments and their inhibition of longitudinal motion of the spinal cord. When the dentate ligaments were sectioned, trauma was better tolerated by the mobile, relaxed cord. The dentate ligaments do not restrict ventrodorsal movements to any great extent. Trauma to the cervical medullary junction is not well tolerated because of poor collateral circulation from posterior radicular vessels.[53,54] Compression of venous sinuses and distortion of the freely mobile brain in vertex injury increases stress on the relatively fixed spinal cord, leading to acute edema complicated by tentorial or tonsillar herniation.

Schmaus,[47] in 1890, was probably the first to study the effect of a force applied to the spinal canal. He attached wooden boards to the backs of rabbits that were suspended vertically. Following blows to the boards, he noted areas of degeneration and cavitation within the spinal cord. Many other animal models of spinal injury were employed over the next several decades because investigators felt a need for standardization of experimental spinal injury so that effects of treatment could be scientifically evaluated.[14] Among early experimentors were Spiller,[49] Stcherbak,[51] and D'Abundo.[11] For a historical review, the reader is directed to Dohrmann.[12]

Allen,[3,4] in 1911 and 1914, was among the first to directly injure the cord following removal of the posterior vertebral column. The lesion he created by dropping a weight a known distance on the dura-invested spinal cord is the lesion most often used today for the study of experimental spinal cord injury. McVeigh[36] found that regardless of the point of impact, the worst spinal cord injury occurs at the point of least resistance, i.e., the central gray matter dorsal to the central canal. Hung et al.[28] used the same technique for causing injury and, by using high-speed cameras taking 1500 to 3000 frames per second, found that the cord itself is compressed to half its posterior-anterior diameter 7 milliseconds after impact with a 300 g/cm force. This is equivalent to a 20 g mass falling 15 cm. The peak impact force averaged 1.21 lb and the corresponding stress acting on the dural surface reached 421 lb per square inch (or 2200 mm Hg). Positive and negative pressure waves were observed to be propagated in cerebrospinal fluid.

At impact, vertebrae may be fractured and pushed into the spinal canal damaging cord substance. Bulging of the vertebral endplate and fracture-dislocation are commonly observed in cervical spine trauma. The importance of the reduction of the cross-sectional area of the spinal canal caused by forward bulging of the ligamentum flavum on the cord has been emphasized in studies of cervical spondylosis. Breig and El-Nadi[6] analyzed detrimental forces with respect to contact pressure, axial tension, and radial tension due to disc protrusion in the cervical area and emphasized the difficulty of extrapolating from histologic data the individual affects of various forces within cord substance after trauma. Breig[5] suggested that mechanical deformation caused by pressure on the spinal cord was the primary mechanism of paralysis. Damage to the spinal cord depends on impact velocity, the relative dimensions of the impacted structure, and characteristics of the elastic wave which takes place in a relatively liquid substance (spinal cord) encased in a hard, bony material (the vertebral column). The damaging effect of the impact stress wave on spinal cord may be more closely related to impulse, since the response of the cord is probably slower than the duration of impact loading. Otherwise, the wave resembles an applied static pressure that often produces stress quite different from that due to dynamic loading.

Dohrmann and Panjabi[13] employed a weight-dropping technique at the T5–T6 level using 400 g/cm on the open dura-invested feline spinal cord. Results of five different combinations of weight/distance, all totaling 400 g/cm were studied. They found that the lesion volume varied in each of the groups. In all groups, a linear relationship was apparent between lesion volume and impulse, while the relation between lesion volume and energy was sigmoid-shape and nonlinear. The amount of energy transferred to the spinal cord was dependent upon mass height, energy mass, and velocity. Energy absorbed by the spinal cord in the group subjected to 40 g dropped 10 cm was approximately 100 times that resulting from a drop of 5 g for 80 cm.

The dentate ligaments and nerve roots offer considerable stabilization to the spinal cord. If the impact force is of short duration, any vibratory motion in cerebrospinal fluid, white matter and gray matter, and the dural sac tends to subside quickly. The possibility of spinal injury due to vibratory motion of the cord either in the transverse or longitudinal direction is believed therefore to be small.

Spinal cord damage may occur without demonstrable skeletal injury.[52] Hyperextension can result in temporary dislocation with rupture of the anterior longitudinal ligament. The ligamentum flavum may bulge forward during forced hyperextension of the cervical spine such as that occurring in automobile accidents in which the body is thrown forward while the head is arrested by a fixed object such as the dashboard or window. The commonest site of bulging of the ligamentum flavum is thought to be between C3 and C6, and the segmental level at which cord damage occurs in this type of injury is usually C5 through C7. More often in young children than in infants, and occasionally in adults, dislocation of the vertebrae may be reduced spontaneously without physical deformity on x-ray but with residual spinal cord damage.

Unterharnscheidt and Higgins[54] caused rotational traumatic lesions of the monkey's head by nondeforming angular acceleration of the head. Although the spinal cord was not primarily subjected to impact force, in except only a few animals, the cord had small hemorrhages in various segments throughout its length, extending to the cauda equina. Since such nondeforming rotational acceleration produced lesions not only in the brain but also throughout the entire length of the spinal cord, they suggested that in persons subjected to severe rotational acceleration of the head, the spinal cord as well as the brain should be examined histopathologically. Such injuries are uncommon.

In hyperextension injury, vascular insufficiency of the upper cervical spinal cord may be caused by compression of the vertebral arteries between the occipital condyles and first cervical lamina. Because of the confined course of the vertebral arteries in the foramina transversia, vascular compression causing ischemia of the brain stem can occur. Injury to the vertebral artery may also occur by torsion and pressure transmitted to the bony cervical skeleton. Chiropractic manipulation and karate blows to the lateral cervical spine can cause vertebral artery insufficiency and loss of consciousness. The main point of impaction is at the level of the atlas.

## THE INTERVERTEBRAL DISC

The intervertebral disc has both liquid and elastic properties and can withstand great stress. The nucleus itself is mostly liquid in nature and therefore is not compressible. Compression of the disc takes place in the annulus, which is very resilient. The intervertebral disc has the ability to absorb large amounts of water, and the essential compound involved in this process is a protein/polysaccharide gel that can bind almost 90 times its own volume of water.

Actual pressure measurements have been obtained by inserting transducers into the third lumbar disc. Nachemson[38] indicated that the internal intervertebral disc pressure increases from 100 kg in a standing position with the spine straight to 150 kg when the trunk is bent forward, and to 220 kg when a 70 kg man lifts a 50 kg weight. In the sitting position, identical maneuvers caused a pressure of 350 kg within the third lumbar disc.

Brown et al.[8] and Roaf[41] noted that during slow vertebral column compression, there is a decrease in disc volume which ranges between 1 and 2.5 cu cm before one of the adjacent vertebral endplates fractures. Recognizing the fluid-retaining capabilities of the disc annulus and the structural porosity of the endplates, these investigators postulated that this diminishing disc volume was due to two sequentially occurring events. Early during spinal compression, sinuses, fissures, and microspaces normally present in adult discs collapse. Disc fluid displaced during this process is then forced across the vertebral endplates. As compression continues, and as endplate bulging is occurring, the fluid within the cancellous bone of the vertebral body is forced into paravertebral sinuses. With spinal compression above the energy-dissipating capability of this fluid-transfer mechanism, vertebral endplate bulging increases to the point of fracture. Both Brown et al.[8] and Roaf[41,42] noted that only after endplate fracture did compressive vertebral body damage occur. Whether a disc was normal or degenerated made no difference in this sequence.

In a cadaver study of biomechanics of spinal injury, Roaf[41] observed that vertical compression of the spine resulted in collapse of the vertebral endplate with rupture of the nucleus pulposus into the cancellous portion of the vertebra and subsequent disintegration of the body. There was no significant bulging of the annulus until the intervertebral disc lost all its turgor because of nuclear displacement. Vertical compression in older persons, in whom the nucleus was no longer fluid, resulted in tearing of the annulus because of transmitted pressure, and general vertebral collapse due to buckling and/or plateau fracture. In younger persons, mechanical removal of the fluid nucleus pulposus resulted in abnormal mobility between vertebral bodies. Since absorption of stress by the vertebral endplate could no longer occur, annular prolapse was common.

## LIGAMENTS

We recognize that it is not possible to separate the various anatomic segments of the vertebral column. Nevertheless, to some extent, vertebral ligaments can be discussed as a unit.

Hyperflexion injuries to the normal spine result in crushing of the vertebral bodies before posterior ligaments rupture. There is no significant alteration in position or shape of the nucleus pulposus nor any buckling of the annulus. After removal of the nucleus pulposus, bulging becomes significant and is posterior on extension and anterior on flexion.[43]

It is very difficult to rupture the anterior longitudinal ligament in the cervical spine by hyperextension. Crush fracture of the neural arch must occur first. While cervical discs, joints, and ligaments are resistant to compression, distraction, flexion, and extension, they are vulnerable to rotation and horizontal shearing forces.[43] Therefore, cervical fracture dislocation attributed to flexion or hyperextension injuries are probably caused primarily by complicating rotational factors.

With loss of turgor of the nucleus pulposus, rotation and horizontal shear forces can produce considerable vertebral displacement and subluxation without rupture of the anterior longitudinal ligament.[24] Spontaneous reduction can then occur, and radiologic examination may not show bony damage and vertebral instability.[43]

Fielding[16] used a cadaver model to define the mechanism of injury to the transverse ligament in anterior atlantoaxial subluxation. The anterior shift of the first cervical vertebra at the instant of rupture of the transverse ligament ranged from 3 to 5 mm. In no case did odontoid process fracture occur prior to failure of ligamentous stability. Following rupture of the transverse ligament, the auxiliary alar ligaments were shown to be inadequate for prevention of further displacement of the first on the second cervical vertebra when a force similar to that which ruptured the transverse ligament was applied. Although the alar ligaments appear thick and stong, they stretch with relative ease and permit significant motion.

Johnson et al.[31] concluded that ligaments are the major stabilizing components in the cervical spine and are critical for spinal stability. By cadaver dissection, they identified eight different, intrinsic ligaments of the lower cervical spine. Largest and most rigid are the annulus fibrosis, the posterior longitudinal ligament, and the capsular ligament. Other ligaments play a secondary role. For example, the intertransverse ligaments, although thin and frail, appear to limit rotation and lateral bending. The anterior longitudinal ligament limits extension, and the intraspinous and supraspinous ligaments limit spinal flexion. Under physiologic conditions, the elastic ligamentum flavum permits extension of the spine without impinging upon spinal cord or nerve roots.

## VERTEBRAL COLUMN

The spine is capable of rotation, extension, flexion, and lateral motion. Its most important function is to protect the spinal cord, and secondly, to provide support for the trunk and appendages. Because vertebral motions are carried out at multiple joints, there is little vulnerability and functions are performed efficiently.

The atlanto-occipital joints permit flexion and extension with only limited lateral or rotational movement. The atlanto-axial joints allow only horizontal rotation without much flexion and extension. The remainder of the cervical spine is capable of flexion and extension with some rotation. Lateral flexion in the cervical spine is limited by the articular facets and pedicles, as well as numerous ligaments.

The anteroposterior diameter of the ring of the atlas is about 3 cm. Both the spinal cord and the odontoid process are 1 cm in diameter, leaving 1 cm of reserve to absorb pathologic displacement. If the ring of the atlas is greater than 3 cm in diameter, there is less danger of cord injury, while if it is narrower, there is more. There seems less danger of cord injury if the odontoid process is fractured and is carried forward with the atlas. If not, direct impingement on cord can occur.

Fracture of the odontoid process with backward projection, an unusual fracture, can result in compression of the cranial portion of the pyramidal decussation in the lower medulla oblongata. Fibers functionally related to arm movements cross above those related to leg movements, so that midline injury can result in cruciate paralysis of the upper extremities without involvement of the lower extremities. This is a presentation similar to that of central cord injury and is most unusual.

King et al.[33] proposed a mechanism of spinal injury due to cephalocaudal acceleration, using a cadaver model and strain gauges. Axial compressive forces alone did not cause anterior wedge fractures of the vertebrae because articular facets acted as motion limiters. When the vertebral column was subjected to eccentric loading and a significant amount of bending with flexion of the head on the torso, anterior wedge fractures resulted. Moderate hyperextension of the vertebral column, using a half-inch block placed in the lumbar area at L1, resulted in decrease in strain along the posterior aspect of the lower thoracic and lumbar vertebrae with fewer fractures and injuries.

Marar,[35] analyzing 126 cases of cervical spine trauma, stated that the injury causing the greatest neurologic deficit was the flexion-compression fracture with bilateral facet dislocation. He found that unrecognized instability could result in sudden tetraplegia hours or days after an accident; thus, he recommended that follow-up x-rays be made in controlled flexion and extension.

Hyperextension produces a clinical picture of acute central cervical cord injury. The vertical compression, or tear-drop, fracture seen after acute anterior flexion injuries is associated with an anterior spinal cord syndrome caused by displacement of bone and disc fragments into the ventral portion of the spinal canal. In both cases there may be no visible fracture or dislocation. Lateral forces combined with rotation can rupture supporting ligaments and cause instability. In pure flexion injuries, dislocation of the vertebral body is forward, and disc and bone fragments may be displaced anteriorly. In hyperextension injuries with bilateral articular process dislocation, the spinal cord is compressed in its anteroposterior diameter.

Hyperextension of the neck may rupture the disk and anterior ligaments with dislocation. Posterior ligaments may be unaffected and the dislocation almost always reduces spontaneously, making the radiographic diagnosis difficult. This dislocation is stable only in flexion and can be demonstrated by stress films.

In Burke's[7] report of 52 cases of diving accidents, 88 percent were vertical compression or burst fractures. Vertical compression could not explain all pathologic findings, since only 4 patients showed evidence of hitting bottom. The remainder had no objective signs of impact, and slightly less than half denied it. A mechanism resulting from the resistance of the water partially counteracting the momentum of the falling body must be considered along with the position of the head on entry.[32]

Henzel[24] emphasized that endplate fractures occur at load levels significantly below those required to produce compressive vertebral fractures. Roaf[41] stressed that compression forces are absorbed mainly by the vertebral body. He suggested that the nucleus pulposus, being liquid, is not compressible, and the tense annulus bulges very little. On compression, the vertebral endplate bulges and blood is forced out of the cancellous bone of the vertebral body into the paravertebral sinuses. This appears to be the normal energy-dissipating mechanism on compression. He found that the vertebral body always fractures before normal disc gives way. The vertebral endplate bulges and then breaks, leading to a vertical fracture. If the nucleus pulposus has lost its turgor, there is abnormal mobility between vertebral bodies. He could not produce rupture of normal spinal ligaments in experimental cadaver spine by rapid hyperextension or hyperflexion. Before rupture occurred, the bone sustained a compression fracture. Horizontal shear and rotation forces easily caused ligamentous rupture and dislocation. Roaf stated that a combination of rotation and compression can produce almost every variety of spinal injury. In the cervical region, subluxation with spontaneous reduction can be produced easily by rotation. If intravertebral turgor is impaired, this may occur in the presence of an intact anterior longitudinal ligament and may explain tetraplegia without radiologic changes or a torn anterior longitudinal ligament. The anterior longitudinal ligament is easily ruptured by rotation, and he suggested that hyperextension and hyperflexion injuries are in reality primarily rotation injuries.

Alexander et al.[2] emphasized the importance of the sagittal diameter of the cervical spinal canal on x-ray in relation to the severity of cervical hyperextension injuries. It cannot be emphasized too strongly that a narrow cervical spinal canal increases the possibilities of severe spinal cord damage. They felt that surgical intervention is indicated if continued compression of the spinal cord is demonstrated by radiograph, myelogram, or manometric block of the cerebrospinal fluid on lumbar puncture.

Webb et al.[55] described seven patients who developed late vertebral deformity months after flexion injury of the cervical spine. They ranged in age from 12 to 20 years, and in all, the severity of the injury was not initially appreciated. Late vertebral deformity, as well as pain and instability of the cervical spine, was found months later.

Injuries to the cervical spine when the patient has facial or frontal injuries are usually termed hyperextension injuries.[26] Roaf[41] points out that a wide variety of anatomic lesions may occur and may require different modes of management. Many cervical spine lesions are attributed to flexion, yet pathologic hyperflexion cannot occur unless either the mandible or a manubrium sterni is fractured, as the mandible normally impinges upon the sternum before the limit of cervical flexion is reached. Cervical flexion injuries, therefore, are probably due to the rapidity rather than to the extent of flexion. Also, there is room for deformity of both jaw and sternum. Roaf[41] stated that experiments on isolated vertebrae show that hyperflexion injuries produce compression of vertebral bodies and/or disc but not tearing of intraspinous ligaments. He suggested that hyperflexion injuries are examples of either vertical compression or rotation or lateral flexion with forward displacement or distraction.

Diving accidents are commonly the cause of cervical spine injury resulting in quadriplegia. Albrand and Walter[1] analyzed 25 such patients and felt that vertical compression, hyperextension, and hyperflexion were primarily responsible. In a study of experienced divers, they found that the impact was broken by the arms and hands rather than the head and neck. Schneider et al.[46] studied Acapulco's high divers. Radiographs of the cervical spine showed chronic bone changes in four of six divers, one having minimal bone encroachment on the cervical spine by spurs or ridges posteriorly. The greatest bone changes were in those divers who had slightly longer, less heavily muscled necks and who struck the water with hands outstretched, thus absorbing the shock of impact directly upon their heads. Divers who clasped their hands over their heads upon impact with the water did not have severe cervical spondylosis. Momentum on impact varied between 11,170 and 16,760 ft-lb per second. The study of Gosch et al.[21] suggested that muscular tone at the time of impact has a profound affect on ability to withstand injury.

Penning and van der Zwagg[40] discussed biomechanical aspects of spondylotic myelopathy and stressed that injury to the spinal cord is more frequent in patients with spondylosis. Both flexion and extension contributed to spondylotic myelopathy rather than extension alone, as is commonly thought.

Marar[34] studied hyperextension injuries of the cervical spine in 45 patients and at autopsy in 4 patients who died with this injury. He also studied 7 cadavers in which hyperextension injury was induced. He demonstrated that the spinal cord is damaged in an anterior-posterior direction by the squeezing effect produced between a backward subluxating vertebral body at the disc space level, or through a complete fracture of the vertebral body just below the pedicle anteriorly and an infolded ligamentum flavum posteriorly. The mechanism of injury, he felt, was a combination of hyperextension and backward shearing forces. He indicated that hyperextension alone does not produce damage to the cervical cord, but addition of a large backward displacement force will produce damage. Maximum inward bulging of the ligamentum flavum was produced when the spine in the cadaver was extended 30 degrees. Therefore, it appears unlikely that an infolded ligamentum flavum by itself damages the cord.

Severe hyperextension injury can produce either a complete transverse fracture of a lower cervical vertebral body below the pedicular level or disc disruption with posterior subluxation. Because of spontaneous reduction of dislocation due to the elasticity of the soft tissue, the fracture or disc space disruption may not be seen unless stress roentgenograms are made or myelography is carried out.

White et al.[56] analyzed biomechanical aspects of clinical stability in the cervical spine in cadavers by quantitative analysis of the behavior of the spine upon systematic destruction of various anatomic elements, including sectioning of ligaments and removal of facets. They concluded that after sectioning of ligaments, stress produced small increments of change followed without warning by sudden, complete disruption of the spine. Removal of facets alters motion segments in such a way that in flexion there is less angular but more horizontal displacement. In extension, anterior ligaments contribute more to stability than do posterior ligaments, and in flexion the reverse is true. They concluded that the adult cervical spine is unstable, or on the brink of instability, when any of the following conditions is present: all anterior or all posterior bony elements are destroyed or are unable to function; more than 3.5 mm of horizontal displacement of one vertebra in relation to an adjacent vertebra can be measured on lateral x-ray in either neutral position or in flexion-extension; more than 11° of rotation difference exists in any vertebra to that of either adjacent vertebra, measured on resting lateral or flexion-extension x-ray films.

Panjabi et al.[39] studied 17 cadaver motion segments of the human cervical spine. A motion segment consists of two adjacent vertebrae with interconnecting soft tissue. A constant load of 25 percent of the body weight was applied to the upper vertebra while the lower vertebra was fixed. Various ligaments, the intervertebral disc, and facet joints of the motion segments were dissected in two predetermined patterns: anterior to posterior, and posterior to anterior. The load was then applied to stimulate flexion or extension. Motion was measured in the sagittal plane at each stage of transection. In general, elastic deformation was small even when a large part of the structural components were destroyed. Failure, however, was sudden and there was no consistent prefailure phase.

Hangman's fracture results from hyperextension of the upper cervical spine. The axis breaks symmetrically across its pedicle or lateral masses, and the fracture may extend across the posterior part of the body. Contrary to popular belief, the dens always remains intact and never contributes to cord injury or death in this condition. The pedicles are the thinnest part of the bony ring of the axis, weakened by the foramen transversarium on each side. The lateral masses bearing the superior articular facets straddle the vertebral body and the inferior facet in the lateral view, and therefore take the brunt of forces transmitted from the modified upper two cervical vertebrae to the cervical spine below. The fracture occurs because the pedicles and lateral masses are at the point of greatest leverage between the upper portion, including skull, atlas, dens, and body of the axis, and the relatively fixed lower cervical spine, to which the neural arch of the axis is anchored by inferior facets, stout spinous processes, and strong nuchal muscles.

Glasauer and Cares[20] described biomechanical aspects of traumatic paraplegia in infancy. The structure of the spinal column in infants differs anatomically from that in adults in that the vertebral bodies are a series of elastic cartilages surrounded by inelastic connective tissue. At autopsy, the infant vertebral column can be stretched two inches, but the spinal cord stretches to a lesser degree. There is actual elongation of the spinal cord in flexion and shortening in extension of the spine. The spinal cord does not move up and down in the canal. Nerve roots are also capable of similar elongation and shortening. The dentate ligaments stretch only in flexion and not on extension, and thus tend to stabilize the spinal cord. Flaccidity is limited by the pia mater and axons, so that once the maximal length of the cord is reached, further axial tension fails to increase its length. Therefore, in further flexion of the spinal column, the cord is pulled forward in the canal and any existing pathologic changes, such as disc protrusion, spondylitic ridges, or dislocations, will indent the anterior surface of the spinal cord. Under these circumstances, flexion of the neck may cause widening and flattening in the anteroposterior diameter of the spinal cord.

Cervical spine ligaments in children are lax, and a normal degree of subluxation, up to 4 mm at C2–C3 or C3–C4 can occur. In breech deliveries a longitudinal force can separate the vertebral bodies sufficiently to result in anatomic transsection of the spinal cord without fracture or dislocation. Cervical musculature is poorly developed in the infant, providing no specific checking factor in distraction and displacement. Also, articular facets in the infant are oriented more horizontally than in the adult, so that subluxation can occur with the application of a small amount of force followed by spontaneous reduction of the dislocation.[19]

Morris et al.[37] pointed out the role of the trunk in stability of the thoracolumbar spine, emphasizing that the trunk structures, namely the thorax and abdomen and its muscles, provided considerable stability for the vertebral column. The thoracic region has limited mobility because of the attachment of the ribs as well as the anatomy of the thoracic vertebral column. Mobility is greater in the lower thoracic area where the ribs are not present and here, in fact, is where most injuries occur. Flexion, lateral flexion, and extension occur in the lumbar area where there is less rotation than in the cervical spine. Stauffer and Neil[50] tested three different methods of internal fixation for flexion-rotation thoracolumbar spinal fractures in a cadaver model. Each was tested for mechanical strength, motor failure, and ease of application. The compression rod system was clearly superior to the spring device in strength and rotational stability, but it was more difficult to apply. A distraction rod system exhibited intermediate strength and adequate rotational stability.

## Mechanism of Seat-Belt Injuries

There can be no doubt that lap and shoulder strap seat belts and restraining harnesses are effective in reducing severity of injury and number of fatalities in automobile accidents, because the forces of collision are dissipated on the skull, thorax, or extremities of an unrestrained passenger. The lap-type seat belt centers collision forces on the pelvis and lower torso, which, because of rugged construction, are better able to absorb applied forces without structural failure. Although shoulder straps restrain the torso, the neck and head remain movable, and injuries can be caused by this circumstance. The head rest may prevent certain flexion-extension injuries, or mitigate them to some extent. However, it is inevitable that some fractures are caused by the restraining force of straps and belts, and reports of abdominal visceral injuries despite restraining belts have been common, though in some cases they are associated with improper seat-belt application. Restraining devices do prevent the passenger from being thrown out of the automobile where perhaps most serious injuries occur.

Saldeen[44] described three patients with fatal neck injuries caused by diagonal safety belts. In all three, he felt that the neck injury resulted when the lower jaw was caught in the belt as the victim slipped out of the belt and was ejected from the car. Thoracic and intra-abdominal injuries have also been associated with use of these belts, although most experts agree that trauma caused by belts is minimal, compared with the frequency with which they have saved passengers from injury.

Lap seat belts can cause injuries to the vertebral column by disruption of posterior elements, compression fracture, and dislocation either anteriorly or laterally, with a visible contusion on the abdomen. The disruption most commonly occurs between the first and third lumbar vertebrae, according to Smith and Kaufer.[48]

In 1948, Chance[9] described a type of flexion fracture seen in lap-belt injuries, which causes horizontal splitting of the vertebral body including the spinous process, laminae, and vertebral body. It is possible that horizontal shear is a mechanism for this so-called Chance fracture, but the absence of forward or lateral displacement of the fragments and avulsion of bone suggests that it may be a tension injury.

Fractures and fracture-dislocations of the lumbar spine may result from compression, shear, or torsion stresses occurring singly or in combination. The most common lumbar fracture is the compression fracture and the most common location is the T12–L1 junction. It is produced by a combination of vertical load and hyperflexion; if the lumbar spine is subjected to a vertical load it is forced into flexion. In lap-type seat-belt injuries, spinous processes are pulled apart. Disruption of the posterior ligamentous structures strongly suggests that flexion injury with tension causes the distraction. In Smith and Kaufer's series,[48] a few patients had a vertical-loading-type fracture, and this type of injury is more likely to occur in unbelted passengers. In most cases the pattern of injury was consistent, characterized by separation of the posterior elements without the expected decrease in height of the anterior portion of the vertebral bodies. Smith and Kauffer suggested that tension stress is primarily responsible for such patterns.

Greenbaum et al.[22] reported that visceral injuries can occur and that seat-belt contusions may be visible on the abdomen in lap-type belt injuries. They stated that seat-belt injuries may present with gross separation of the posterior elements due to rupture of lumbar dorsal fascia, interspinous ligaments, ligamentum flavum, and the posterior longitudinal ligament. This results in widening of the interspinous distance the increase in height of the intervertebral foramen. The difference between this type of fracture and the Chance fracture, in which the force is directed entirely through the osseous structure, causing a splitting fracture of the vertebral body and posterior elements but sparing ligamentous structures, was stressed. Friedman et al.[18] reported a patient with lap-type seat-belt injury who had fractures of L1, L2, and L3.

Fletcher and Brogdon[17] stressed that improperly positioned or inadequately tightened lap-type seat-belts may act as a central fulcrum to produce transverse fractures of the lumbar vertebrae upon sudden deceleration. Bandolier belts, also known as the shoulder-type safety belt, prevent acute flexion of the spine, but may be responsible for fractures of the sternum, rib cage, and intrathoracic viscera rupture, as well as cervical spine fracture.

Huelke and Kaufer[27] emphasized that seat-belt-related lumbar fracture-distraction injuries do not involve neural structures, unless accompanied by anterior or lateral displacement of the injured segment. They suggested that lap seat belts are not necessarily the cause of lumbar fractures, since they occur in passengers without seat belts. For a complete review of the role of seat belts in spinal injury, consult this paper.

### Other Thoracolumbar Injuries

Roberts et al.[43] reported an increased incidence of vertical-loading vertebral fractures associated with the use of snowmobiles and discussed the biomechanics. Most patients have compression fractures, but other injuries can occur. They suggested that snowmobiles be redesigned to include adequate suspension systems.

Hoff and Chapman[25] discussed vertebral fractures incurred in suicide attempts. Of 204 patients treated for traumatic vertebral body fractures in a seven-year period, 12 sustained injury during a suicide attempt. All but 2 had significant psychiatric illness, and 10 of the 12 abused drugs or alcohol. All injuries were sustained in jumps from heights between 10 and 40 feet, and most persons landed feet-first. The thoracolumbar area is most vulnerable, and all 12 had at least one fracture between T12 and L2. No intraspinal bony fragments were evident radiographically in any patient. Fractures of the feet were common because of the drop from a height, as were other somatic injuries. Neurologic deficits ranged from complete paraplegia to no spinal cord injury in 5 patients.

Chubb et al.[10] studied 729 ejections from aircraft. Of 44 compression fractures, 28 were believed to have occurred during ejection, and 16 during parachute landings. Compression fractures of one or more vertebrae are attributable to the G forces generated by the ejection seat. These injuries usually heal without residual disability, but they result in temporary disability lasting usually six weeks or longer. Sitting in the erect position with hips and head firmly against the seat was the most significant factor in prevention of compression fractures. In a study of naval aircraft accidents, Ewing[15] found that 60 percent of all vertebral fractures occurred in jets (104 accidents), and 60 percent (62) of vertebral fractures in jet aircraft accidents occurred in ejections. Italiano[30] studied two types of vertebral fractures sustained in ejections by pilots, a fracture of the anterior superior margin of the vertebrae and a wedge-shaped fracture of the vertebrae. Both are considered stable, and in both cases, the pilot need not be disqualified from further jet flight. Italiano[29] also commented on vertebral fractures occurring after helicopter accidents, the mechanism of which is vertical loading of the vertebral body on impact.

King et al.[33] stressed that during pilot ejection the commonly observed wedge fractures are due to caudocephaladic acceleration and both axial compression and bending, which occurs because of the eccentricity of the articular facets in relation to the spine and is enhanced by forward rotation of the head and torso. In the erect mode, the facets tend to unload and go into tension, causing the vertebral bodies to sustain greater compressive load than the total spinal load. This occurs when the head and torso undergo maximal forward flexion. Anterior wedge fractures are therefore the result of eccentric compression coupled with unloading of facets. In the hyperextended mode, facets relieve the vertebral bodies of some compressive load, and thus the fracture level is raised to a higher vertebral body. Henzel[24] discussed biodynamic implications of human ejection from aircraft. They developed an accurate probability of injury by static loading from experimental data on vertebral breaking loads, and suggested that application of this concept could refine the estimate of safe acceleration profiles and aid designers of ejection systems to minimize risk of vertebral injury. It has become apparent that injury to the spinal column represents a significant percent of the morbidity associated with aircraft ejection.

Decompression sickness is an illness of healthy young people resulting from a reduction of the environmental pressure sufficient to cause formation of bubbles from gases dissolved in tissues. Deep-sea divers and tunnel construction workers are most often affected. Hallenbeck et al.[23] studied the mechanisms underlying spinal cord damage in decompression sickness. The conventional view of the cause of paraplegia in decompression sickness ascribes damage to the spinal cord to systemic arterial embolization by bubbles with consequent capillary and precapillary obstruction. The brain is not a prime target, whereas the spinal cord is. Hallenbeck et al. pointed out that in other embolization disorders, such as subacute bacterial endocarditis, fat embolism, and others, the brain, not the spinal cord, is the major target organ. They suggested that the reason the spinal cord is involved in decompression sickness is that the epidural vertebral venous system becomes obstructed and spinal cord infarction results. Infarction is caused by obstruction of cord venous drainage at the epidural vertebral venous level. They concluded that acute pulmonary hypertension followed by central venous obstruction with consequent obstruction of epidural vertebral venous system was the cause of the spinal injury.

## REFERENCES

1. Albrand OW, Walter J: Underwater deceleration curves in relation to injuries from diving. Surg Neurol 4:461–464, 1975
2. Alexander E, Davis CH, Field CH: Hyperextension injuries of the cervical spine. Arch Neurol Psychiatr 79:146–150, 1958
3. Allen AR: Surgery of experimental lesion of spinal cord equivalent to crush injury of fracture dislocation of spinal column: A preliminary report. JAMA 57:878–880, 1911
4. Allen AR: Remarks on the histopathological changes in the spinal cord due to impact. An experimental study. J Nerv Ment Dis 41:141–147, 1914
5. Breig A: Biomechanics of the Central Nervous System. Stockholm, Almqvist & Wiksell, 1961
6. Breig A, El-Nadi AF: Biomechanics of the cervical spinal cord. Acta Radiol 4:602–624, 1964
7. Burke DC: Spinal cord injuries from water sports. Med J Aust 2:1190–1194, 1972
8. Brown T, Hansen RV, Yorra AS: Some mechanical tests on the lumbosacral spine with particular reference to the intervertebral discs. A preliminary report. J Bone Joint Surg 39:1135–1164, 1957
9. Chance GQ: Note on a type of flexion fracture of the spine. Br J Radiol 21:452–453, 1948
10. Chubb RM, Detrick WR, Shannon RH: Compression fractures of the spine during USAF ejections. Aerosp Med 36:968–972, 1965
11. D'Abundo G: Alterazioni nel sistema nervoso centrale consecutive a particolari commozioni traumatiche. Riv Ital Neuropat 9:145–171, 1916
12. Dohrmann GJ: Experimental spinal cord trauma. Arch Neurol 27:468–473, 1972
13. Dohrmann GJ, Panjabi MM: Spinal cord deformation velocity, impulse, and energy related to lesion volume in "standardized" trauma. Surg Forum 27:466–468, 1976

14. Dohrmann GJ, Panjabi MM: "Standardized" spinal cord trauma: biomechanical parameters and lesion volume. Surg Neurol 6:263–267, 1976
15. Ewing CL: Vertebral fracture in jet aircraft accidents: A statistical analysis for the period 1959 through 1963, US Navy. Aerosp Med 37:505–508, 1966
16. Fielding JW: Tears of the transverse ligament of the atlas. J Bone Joint Surg 56-A:1683–1691, 1974
17. Fletcher BD, Brogdon BG: Seat-belt fractures of the spine and sternum. JAMA 200:167–168, 1967
18. Friedman MM, Becker L, Riechmister JP, Neviaser JS: Seat belt spinal fractures. Am Surg 35:617–618, 1969
19. Gaufin LM, Goodman SJ: Cervical spine injuries in infants. J Neurosurg 42:179–184, 1975
20. Glasauer FE, Cares HI: Biomechanical features of traumatic paraplegia in infancy. J Trauma 13:166–170, 1973
21. Gosch HH, Gooding E, Schneider RC: An experimental study of cervical spine and cord injuries. J Trauma 12:570–576, 1972
22. Greenbaum E, Harris L, Halloran WX: Flexion fracture of the lumbar spine due to lap-type seat belts. Calif Med 113:74–75, 1970
23. Hallenbeck JM, Bove AA, Elliott DH: Mechanisms underlying spinal cord damage in decompression sickness. Neurology 25:308–316, 1975
24. Henzel JH: Reappraisal of biodynamic implications of human ejections. Aerosp Med 39:231–240, 1968
25. Hoff J, Chapman M: Vertebral fractures associated with suicide attempts. Proc VA Spinal Cord Injury Conf 18:53–55, 1971
26. Holdsworth F: Fractures, dislocations, and fracture dislocations of the spine. J Bone Joint Surg 52A:1534–1551, 1970
27. Huelke DF, Kaufer H: Vertebral column injuries and seat belts. J Trauma 15:304–318, 1975
28. Hung T-K, Albin MS, Brown TD, et al: Biomechanical responses to open experimental spinal cord injury. Surg Neurol 4:271–276, 1975
29. Italiano P: Interpretation of the mechanism of fractures in jet plane pilots. Rivista de Medicina Aeronautica 29:407–410, 1966
30. Italiano P: Evolution of vertebral fractures caused by ejection. Rivista de Medicina Aeronautica 30:307–323, 1967
31. Johnson RM, Crelin ES, White AA, Panjabi MM, Southwick WO: Some new observations on the functional anatomy of the lower spine. Clin Orthop 3:192–200, Sept 1975
32. Kewalramani LS, Taylor RG: Injuries to the cervical spine from diving accidents. J Trauma 15:130–142, 1975
33. King AJ, Prasad P, Ewing CL: Mechanism of spinal injury due to caudocephalad acceleration. Orthop Clin North Am 6:19–31, 1975
34. Marar BC, Orth MC: Hyperextension injuries of the cervical spine. The pathogenesis of damage to the spinal cord. J Bone Joint Surg 56A:1655–1662, 1974
35. Marar BC: The pattern of neurological damage as an aid to the diagnosis of the mechanism in cervical spine injuries. J Bone Joint Surg 56A:1648–1654, 1974
36. McVeigh JF: Experimental cord crushes with especial reference to the mechanical factors involved and subsequent changes in the areas of the cord affected. Arch Surg 7:573–600, 1923
37. Morris JM, Lucas DB, Bresler B: Role of the trunk in stability of the spine. J Bone Joint Surg 43A:327–335, 1961
38. Nachemson A: The load on lumbar discs in different positions of the body. Clin Orthop 45:107–122, 1966
39. Panjabi MM, White AA, III, Johnson RM: Cervical spine mechanics as a function of transection of components. J Biomech 8:327–336, 1975

40. Penning L, van der Zwaag P: Biomechanical aspects of spondylotic myelopathy. Acta Radiologica 5:1090–1102, 1966
41. Roaf R: A study of the mechanics of spinal injuries. J Bone Joint Surg 42B:810–823, 1960
42. Roaf R: International classification of spinal injuries. Paraplegia 10:78–84, 1972
43. Roberts VL, Noyes FR, Hubbard RP, McCabe J: Biomech of snowmobile spine injuries. J Biomech 4:569–577, 1971
44. Saldeen T: Fatal neck injuries caused by use of diagonal safety belts. J Trauma 7:856–862, 1967
45. Schneider R: Vascular insufficiency and differential distortion of brain and spinal cord caused by cervico-medullary football injuries. J Neurosurg 33:363–375, 1970
46. Schneider RC, Papo M, Alvarez CS: The effects of chronic recurrent spinal trauma in high-diving. J Bone Joint Surg 44A:648–656, 1962
47. Schmaus H: Beiträge zur pathologischen Anatomie der Rückermarkserschütter-ung. Virchows Arch 122:470–495, 1890
48. Smith WS, Kaufer H: Patterns and mechanisms of lumbar injuries associated with lap seat belts. J Bone Joint Surg 51A:239–254, 1969
49. Spiller WG: A critical summary of recent literature on concussion of the spinal cord with some original observations. Am J Med Sci 118:190–198, 1899
50. Stauffer ES, Neil JL: Biomechanical analysis of structural stability of internal fixation in fractures of the thoracolumbar spine. Clin Orthop 112:159–164, 1975
51. Stcherbak A: Des altérations de la moelle épinière chez le lapin sous l'influence de la vibration intensive: Valeur diagnostique du clonus vibratoire: Contribution à l'étude de la commotion de la moelle épinière. Encephale 2:521–535, 1907
52. Tarlov IM: Spinal Cord Compression: Mechanism of Paralysis and Treatment. Springfield, Ill, Charles C Thomas, 1957
53. Turnbull IM, Brieg A, Hassler O: Blood supply of cervical spinal cord in man. A microangiographic cadaver study. J Neurosurg 24:951–965, 1966
54. Unterharnscheidt F, Higgins LS: Traumatic lesions of brain and spinal cord due to nondeforming angular acceleration of the head. Texas Reports Biol Med 27:127–166, 1969
55. Webb JK, Broughton RBK, McSweeney T, Park WM: Hidden flexion injury of the cervical spine. J Bone Joint Surg 58B:322–327, 1976
56. White AA, Johnson RM, Panjabi MM, Southwick WO: Biomechanical analysis of clinical stability in the cervical spine. Clin Orthop 109:85–96, 1975

# 27

# Catecholamines in Spinal Injury

There is considerable controversy over the role of catecholamines in the genesis of secondary destruction in spinal injury. One prevailing theory to explain the observed neurologic deficit accompanying spinal cord injury centers around a catecholamine-mediated, spreading ischemia of the lateral white matter. This theory is based in large part on Osterholm's[14-17] reports concerning elevated norepinephrine levels in the injured spinal segment after experimental spinal cord injury. Osterholm hypothesized that trauma to the spinal cord could possibly induce an excessive or perverted metabolic response in tissue leading to elaboration and release of transmitter substances. Toxic concentrations of these materials, given access to spinal cord smooth muscle vascular sites as a result of trauma, might produce vasospasm, hypoxia, and subsequent tissue necrosis. He further suggested that the neurotransmitter substance might be norepinephrine (noradrenalin).[1]

Osterholm and Mathews injected norepinephrine into the spinal cord and observed lesions resembling those seen in spinal trauma. Injection of anti-catecholamine drugs produced improvement in the lesions.[14] Controls injected with saline were lesion free. Schoultz and DeLuca[19] also reported increases in noradrenalin at the lesion site. Vise et al.[21] suggested that if a catecholamine-like substance were indeed responsible for hemorrhagic necrosis in the injured spinal cord, it was probably blood-borne and was not a result of axonal transport mechanisms. They hypothesized and demonstrated by fluorescence microscopy a breakdown in the blood-brain barrier with leakage of a catecholamine-like substance. It was postulated that known catecholamine axonal transport was too slow to account for the great damage, hence the breakdown of the blood-brain barrier as a more reasonable explanation of the accumulation of catecholamines.

Osterholm's findings could not be substantiated by other laboratories. One might observe that the experimental designs were dissimilar. Nevertheless, Rawe et al.[18] attempted to repeat the work of Osterholm and found no significant change in the norepinephrine content in the post-traumatic spinal cords of cats.[18] Hedeman et al.[7] measured norepinephrine, dopamine, and 5-hydroxytryptamine levels in traumatized spinal cords of dogs and found a decrease, rather than an increase in norepinephrine content in the injured segment. Naftchi et al.[13] measured levels of norepinephrine, dopamine, serotonin, and histamine in the traumatized spinal cord of cats and found an elevated histamine level. De la Torre et al.[4] measured norepinephrine levels in spinal cords of cats and dogs following severe spinal cord injury and did not demonstrate a significant rise. Bingham et al.[2] measured the norepinephrine content of the spinal cords of monkeys and found a progressive decrease in norepinephrine activity following experimental trauma. However, according to Zivin et al.[23] concentrations of norepinephrine and dopamine in normal spinal cord are at the lower limits of detectability by methods based on fluorimetric estimation of amines and thus cannot be reliably detected.

Blood flow measurements after experimental spinal cord injury tend to cast further doubt on the catecholamine theory. Kobrine et al.,[10] using the hydrogen clearance method of blood flow measurement, demonstrated hyperemia in the lateral white matter of monkeys following experimental injury sufficient to render the animals permanently paraplegic. Griffiths,[5] using a similar method, demonstrated a lack of ischemia and occasionally a hyperemia in the lateral funiculus of dogs after experimental trauma. Bingham et al.[2] measured focal blood flow with the antipyrine autoradiographic method, and also demonstrated a hyperemia in the lateral white matter. Kobrine[9] has advocated primary damage to the neural structures as a cause of spinal dysfunction rather than either ischemia or increase in catecholamines.

Moskowitz and Wurtman[12] provide an excellent review of the role of catecholamines in neurologic disease. They discuss synthesis and fate, localization, storage and metabolism, and pharmacology of the catecholamines. They do not discuss the problem of catecholamines in spinal trauma. Zivin et al.[22] investigated spinal cord serotonin, norepinephrine, and dopamine concentrations in rabbit spinal cord trauma. Within five minutes after trauma, norepinephrine and serotonin in gray matter decreased considerably at the lesion center, while in white matter norepinephrine decreased only slightly or was unchanged. At the lesion edges in the white matter serotonin increased. No change in dopamine concentration was detected. The fact that platelets cause increase of serotonin should be kept in mind. In another study methysergide, a serotonin antagonist, was not found effective in ameliorating spinal cord injury.[8]

Gurden and Feringa[6] inhibited production of norepinephrine in rats after spinal transection by use of alpha methyl tyrosine and dibenamine. None of the rats showed any evidence of long motor tract regeneration which could not be expected. Cystic change at the injury site was identical in control and treated groups.

The site from which the specimen is taken from the spinal cord is important. For example, Zivin et al.[23] combined highly sensitive radiometric assays for biogenic amines with microdissection methods to localize and quantitate amines in various areas of the spinal cord. The highest concentration of biogenic amines was found in the lateral and ventral horns, slightly less was found around the central canal, and a relatively low concentration was found in white matter.

Stanton et al.[20] and Carlsson et al.[3] indicated that several days following a high or midthoracic transection of the spinal cord, biogenic amines, including noradrenaline, dopamine, and serotonin, fell. The fall occurred between 7 and 10 days. Their results indicated that there is active distal axonal transport of the monoamines. Anatomic severance of transport fibers cause buildup at the cut and decrease distally. Species variations exist. Bingham et al.[2] found that levels of norepinephrine and dopamine in the monkey were double those found in the dog. Both norepinephrine (NE) and dopamine (DA) increased at descending cord levels and showed a direct correlation with amount of grey matter present in the segment.

Magnusson[11] found that 15 days after transection in the rat spinal cord, levels of noradrenaline, dopamine, and serotonin increased at sites above the level of injury. Noradrenaline and dopamine decreased markedly below the lesion site. These results emphasize that an axonal transport mechanism is involved.

The above emphasize that there is at present controversy over the role of catecholamines in the genesis of secondary destruction in spinal injury.[1] If true, it might have considerable impact on treatment of spinal injury where fiber systems are still intact. In cases where anatomic severance has occurred regeneration is the only hope.

## REFERENCES

1. Anden NE, Fuxe K: A new dopamine-$\beta$-hydroxylase inhibitor: effects on the noradrenaline concentration and on the action of L-Dopa in the spinal cord. Br J Pharmacol 43:747–756, 1971
2. Bingham WG, Ruffolo R, Goodman JH, Knofel J, Friedman S: Norepinephrine and dopamine levels in normal dog and monkey spinal cord. Life Sci 16:1521–1526, 1975
3. Carlsson A, Magnusson T, Rosengren E: 5-Hydroxytryptamine of the spinal cord normally and after transection. Experienta 19:359, 1963
4. de la Torre JC, Johnson CM, Harris LH, et al: Monoamine changes in experimental head and spinal cord trauma: failure to confirm previous observations. Surg Neurol 2:5–12, 1974
5. Griffiths IR: Spinal cord blood flow in dogs: the effect of blood pressure. J Neurol Neurosurg Psychiatr 36:914–920, 1973
6. Gurden GG, Feringa ER: Effects of sympatholytic agents on CNS regeneration, cystic necrosis after spinal cord transection. Neurology 24:187–191, 1974
7. Hedeman LS, Shellenberger MK, Gordon JH: Studies in experimental spinal cord trauma. J Neurosurg 43:37–43, 1974

8. Howitt WM, Turnbull IM: Effects of hypothermia and methysergide on recovery from experimental paraplegia. Can J Surg 15:179–186, 1972

9. Kobrine AI: The neuronal theory of experimental traumatic spinal cord dysfunction. Surg Neurol 3:261–265, 1975

10. Kobrine AI, Doyle TF, Martins AN: Local spinal cord blood flow in experimental traumatic myelopathy. J Neurosurg 40:144–150, 1975

11. Magnusson T: Effect of chronic transection of dopamine, noradrenaline and 5-hydroxytryptamine in the rat spinal cord. Naunyn-Schmiedeberg's Arch Pharmacol 278:13–22, 1973

12. Moskowitz MA, Wurtman RJ: Catecholamines and neurologic diseases. N Engl J Med 293:274–280, 332–338, 1975

13. Naftchi NE, Demeny M, DeCrescito V, et al: Biogenic amine concentrations in traumatized spinal cords of cats. J Neurosurg 40:52–57, 1974

14. Osterholm JL, Mathews GJ: Altered norepinephrine metabolism following experimental spinal cord injury. Part I. Relationship to hemorrhagic necrosis and post-wounding neurological deficits. J Neurosurg 36:386–394, 1972

15. Osterholm JL, Mathews GJ: Altered norepinephrine metabolism following experimental spinal cord injury. Part 2. Protection against traumatic spinal cord hemorrhagic necrosis by norepinephrine synthesis blockade with alpha methyl tyrosine. J Neurosurg 36:395–401, 1972

16. Osterholm JL: The pathophysiological response to spinal cord injury. J Neurosurg 40:5–33, 1974

17. Osterholm JL: Noradrenergic mediation of traumatic spinal cord autodestruction. Life Sci 14:1363–1384, 1974

18. Rawe SE, Roth RH, D'Angelo CM, et al: Norepinephrine levels in experimental spinal cord trauma. Presented at the American Association of Neurological Surgeons Annual Meeting, St. Louis, Mo. April 1974

19. Schoultz TW, DeLuca DC: Alterations in spinal cord norepinephrine levels following experimentally produced trauma in normal and adrenalectomized cats. Life Sci 15:1485–1495, 1974

20. Stanton ES, Smolen PM, Nashold BS, Dreyer DA, Davis JN: Segmental analysis of spinal cord monoamines after thoracic transection in the dog. Brain Res 89:93–98, 1975

21. Vise WM, Yashon D, Hunt WE: Mechanisms of norepinephrine accumulation within sites of spinal cord injury. J Neurosurg 40:76–82, 1974

22. Zivin JA, Reid JL, Saavedra JM, Kopin IJ: Quantitative localization of biogenic amines in the spinal cord. Brain Res 99:291–301, 1975

23. Zivin JA, Doppman JL, Reid JL, et al: Biochemical and histochemical studies of biogenic amines in spinal cord trauma. Neurology 26:99–107, 1976

# 28

## Regeneration in the Central Nervous System

Regeneration in the central nervous system has been an enigma to researchers for many years, but recent research has led to renewed hope that the process will be clarified. Adult nerve cells once destroyed are never replaced. Regrowth from partially damaged nerve cells of axons and dendrites does occur in the form of sprouting.[34] In the peripheral nervous system, damaged axons will regrow and reestablish functionally useful connections, but this is not true in the central nervous system (CNS). In the CNS nerve fiber, outgrowth (sprouting) is abortive and large numbers of nonneuronal cells and scar tissue accumulate at the site of damage causing mechanical obstruction and compression of any fibers that might find their way through the damaged region.[34]

Historically the long record of the problem of traumatic paralysis goes back to the Egyptian surgeons of the twelfth to eighteenth dynasties who provided a lucid account of symptoms following spinal damage at different levels.[22] Brown-Sequard[23] transected the spinal cord of pigeons in 1849, and believed he had evidence of regeneration. A classic report was that of a young Philadelphia woman whose thoracic spinal cord had been severed by a bullet and was surgically reunited at the Pennsylvania Hospital in 1901. The surgeons, Stewart and Harte,[104] reported evidence of partial functional restitution several months later. The most noteworthy of many experiments were those of Ramon y Cajal, who used puppies and kittens between 1906 and 1911.[26,91,92] His concept of abortive regeneration in the transected spinal cord was reported in 1914. Severed nerve fibers of the spinal cord sprouted growths much as did severed peripheral nerves, but growth in the CNS was abortive and actually regressed after a few weeks. Freeman[40-43,108] described some functional return of hind limb movement in adult rats and dogs after complete transection of the cord. He suggested growth of neural elements. Wolman[117] studied 76 cases of traumatic paraplegia in man. Evidence of well-developed regeneration was found in 12 cases, but the origin of most of these nerve fibers was the posterior nerve roots and spinal ganglia.

Experiments with lower vertebrates, notably fish and amphibia,[101] began to shed light on the problem of CNS regeneration since some functional CNS regeneration of the optic nerve segments takes place in those species. The spinal cord of fish[6,11-13,55] and amphibia[68,87] can be functionally reconstituted after surgical transection whereas that of most mammals including man[60,96, 114-116] cannot. Regeneration of axons in the severed spinal cord of the larval chordate lamprey occurred rapidly resulting in recovery of function in less than 20 days.[55] Within 30 days following transection of the spinal cord of the goldfish, function was restored completely.[6,11-13]

Holtzer[56] unilaterally ablated a portion of the larval amphibian urodele spinal cord and showed not only axon regeneration across the site of the lesion but reconstitution of the gray matter itself. Thus, in addition to nerve fiber regeneration, a new complement of cells appeared in the regenerated gray matter. Similar findings were reported by Butler and Ward[25] who removed a 4-mm segment of spinal cord and showed regeneration to be accompanied by the return of function. Such mechanisms are lacking in adult higher vertebrates, but recently a CNS system in adult mammals has been found capable of regenerative growth. This is the aminergic system of the brain.[1,17] Monoamine systems seem to be exceptions to the general rule that several axons do not regenerate inside the CNS.[95] This failure may be related to the ability of serotonin to block, or mask, the immune response to transmitter substances which leak into brain tissue after damage.[17]

Two forms of axonal growth which can be demonstrated are regenerative and collateral sprouting. Regenerative sprouting along previously intact axon cylinders in the peripheral nervous system has long been recognized as a common event. Collateral sprouting of intact axons into nearby regions that had been damaged or that had a loss of afferent input was described by Cajal.[26,91,92]

The mammalian central nervous system has been shown to regenerate axonal complements after injury by the process of sprouting of normal intact axons into zones of tissue damage or partial neuronal deafferentation.[7-10, 14-16,46,69,70,95,102,103] Regenerated axons and axonal sprouts in synaptic complexes have been demonstrated in the mammalian septum[88-90] and spinal cord.[7-11] In the spinal cord of rat and monkey, nerve fibers grow into the ventral horn proximal to the site of a spinal cord hemisection and reinnervate partially denervated neurons in the horn.[7-11] Collateral sprouting following CNS trauma occurs primarily in young animals but has recently been described in mature animals.[27] At present there is little evidence that sprouting is of functional benefit to the organism.[36]

Damage to the axon results in metabolic changes throughout the entire nerve cell. Some of these changes are supportive of axonal regrowth while others cause increased degradation of cell constituents.[118] Central nervous system neuron systems are capable of outgrowth as evidenced by the sprouting of intact nerve fibers near or within a CNS lesion. Although this collateral sprouting[35] usually results in functionally inappropriate connections, study of the phenomenon provides useful insights into mechanisms involved in the initiation of axonal outgrowth and establishment of synaptic terminals.[110] Moreover, the fact that axonal sprouting does occur reveals that CNS fibers do have regrowth capability.[24]

Axonal sprouting has been reasonably well established as a phenomenon that occurs in the mammalian central nervous system. Liu and Chambers[67] demonstrated the phenomenon in the cat. It has also been demonstrated in the visual system, limbic system, thalamus, and spinal cord of the rat.[18–21,32, 45,46,58,67,69–71,80,82,88,102] These morphologic observations have been supported by electrophysiologic,[28,74] pharmacologic, and behavioral evidence.[45,80,99,100] This type of reorganization within the central nervous system may underly not only some of the recovery observed after insult to central neural structures (for a review see Rosner et al.[94]) but also some of the deficits observed.[28]

The important question remains whether collateral axonal sprouting is a significant factor in determining the pattern of recovery following spinal cord trauma, and whether inhibition of anomalous sprouting and stimulation of proper growth might increase the probability of recovery after CNS trauma. These questions are prompted by studies in the cat by Liu and Chambers,[67] and by Goldberger and Murray[45] investigating the relation of axonal sprouting to spasticity and hyperreflexia following cord transections. Liu and Chambers,[67] using the Nauta degenerating axon silver stain, demonstrated that after spinal cord transection, dorsal root axons sprout to take over synaptic sites previously occupied by descending tracts. They argue that this increase in input from the dorsal roots is the basis of the spasticity and hyperreflexia observed after cord transections.[28] Goldberger and Murray[45,80] repeated the experiments, added to the findings by using both silver stains and autoradiography, and performed an extensive behavioral analysis. They demonstrated that the time interval for the development of hyperreflexia of intrinsic reflexes following partial cord transections is correlated with the time interval of sprouting of dorsal root afferents. They also examined cats with chronic deafferentation of the hind limb (dorsal rhizotomy) and observed axonal sprouting of descending tracts to occupy those regions previously occupied by dorsal root afferents. And in these cases they observed hyperreflexia of descending reflexes.

Particularly relevant to recovery from spinal cord trauma, then, is the fact that the spasticity observed after transections is suggested to depend to a significant degree upon takeover of synaptic sites by dorsal root afferents. If this anomalous sprouting were prevented, thereby permitting sprouting of remaining suprasegmental axons, would a more normal reflex pattern develop in patients with partial paraplegia? McCouch and his coworkers[72–74] reported that selected dorsal rhizotomies in two patients with partial paraplegia resulted in a decrease in spasticity and improvement in motor function.

Transection of the mammalian spinal cord results in abortive regeneration of but a few of the transected nerve fibers through the site of the lesion.[30, 31,114] However, axonal regeneration could be induced by the administration of drugs,[76] such as piromen,[30,31,114–116] nerve growth factor,[97] and ACTH.[75] Use of specific fluorescences and microspectrophotometry demonstrated that the regenerated central nervous system nerve fibers contain catecholamines, 5-hydroxytryptamine, or an unidentified monoamine.[18–20,58]

In addition, the mammalian nervous system can regenerate collateral sprouts of normal intact nerve fibers into zones of tissue damage. The axonal sprouts grow varying distances and may even cross the midline in the spinal cord to reinnervate neurons in the hemisected rat and monkey spinal cord.[6–11,14] It appears that one of the requirements for the activation of axonal sprouts in the central nervous system is the partial deafferentation of neurons by the sparing of a portion of the normal intact synaptic input innervating a cell. Sprouting of intact nerve fibers has been demonstrated in the peripheral nervous system.[35] The sprouting is activated after partial deafferentation of a muscle.[51] Thus, after transection of the L4 root of the sciatic nerve, the L5 root to the muscle will sprout nerve fibers increasing muscle strength over that accomplished by L4 innervation alone. Following partial deafferentation of the cervical sympathetic ganglion by the crushing of one of the roots that innervate the cervical sympathetic trunk, the remaining nerve fibers innervating the ganglion will sprout and take over the function of the denervated cells.[52] Crushing the T1 nerve root results in T4 control of pupillary dilation, a function in which it is not normally involved. Nathaniel and Nathaniel,[81] using the electron microscope, observed regeneration of dorsal root fibers in the adult rat spinal cord. The astrocytic response subsided as regeneration progressed.

The administration of drugs[76] such as piromen,[30,114] nerve growth factor,[65,97] and ACTH[75] enhance collateral sprouting. Without drug induction[77] few of the total CNS fibers available are regenerated.[30,114]

Gurden and Feringa[48] studied two groups of rats subjected to spinal cord transection. One group received apha methyl tyrosine to block norepinepherine production and the second group received dibenamine to block the effect of excess norepinepherine on blood vessels. Neither group showed improved regenerative capabilities determined by electrophysiologic and histologic (hematoxylin and eosin) criteria over controls. O'Callaghan and Speakman[83] suggested that in transected adult rat spinal cords, methyl prednisolone diminishes the formation of collagen fibers and retards organization of the scar. Intraperitoneal injection of a nervous tissue homogenate prolonged the interval when regenerating neurofibrils at the transection site were observed. Five of 35 rats maintained longer than six weeks developed coordinated walking. Five additional rats developed walking ability by the eighth week after transection. Histologic studies showed a complete scar densely infiltrated with axons. Conversely, rats receiving piromen showed no increase in regeneration compared to controls.

Regeneration in the frog and toad (Anura) was enhanced by the use of weak electric currents.[98-100] Spontaneous limb regeneration was not observed. The degree of regeneration in the normally nonregenerating system depends upon the strength and duration of the electrical current and the location of the electrodes. Once initiated, regeneration will proceed without continuation of the electrical current. Becker[3] and Becker and Spadaro[4] showed a similar phenomenon in the rat.

Landolt[61] found the human pituitary capable of considerable regeneration without mitotic figures in patients who had pituitary ablation for widespread metastatic disease and who survived longer than 252 days. In patients who survived 24 to 219 days after ablation, there were mitotic figures and signs of regeneration.

Nerve growth factor (NGF) is a chemically defined protein that promotes the growth of sensory and autonomic neurones both in tissue culture and in intact animals. It may be one factor that participates in certain trophic interactions. Stoeckel and Thoenen[105] demonstrated that NGF could be transported retrogradely with a high selectivity for adrenergic and sensory but not motor neurons. Nerve growth factor was originally defined by Levi-Montalcini[65] in terms of a bioassay in which material from a mouse sarcoma stimulated growth and differentiation of some embryonic sensory and all sympathetic neurons. Mouse submaxillary gland also contains NGF activity. Nerve growth factor, in small amounts, has been found in many other vertebrates.[30,57] A number of snake venoms have also been found to be high in NGF.[55] This substance may in the future enhance regenerative capacity in man.

Trophic interactions, including the immune response and chemical influences, are among factors promoting the growth of nerve cells. Glial cells play a role not only in maintaining the nerve cell but in determining specific patterns of association among neurons. Trophic interactions among nerve cell structures are evidenced by an increase in size of the cells when one cell makes contact with another. It has been suggested that a local autoimmune response occurs in the traumatized spinal cord which may interfere with axonal regeneration.[17,37-39,44] Paterson[86] provides a review of the overall problem.

Piromen (Pseudomonas polysaccharide complex), a bacterial extract, appears by its febrile action to retard the development of scar tissue in the area of spinal cord transection.[31,66,106] It is postulated that the immune response is inhibited. The same mechanism is postulated as the reason that steroids diminish scar formation.

Although significant central nervous system regeneration is thought not to occur in the adult, there is considerable evidence for central nervous system regeneration in newborn and young mammals. There are reports of functional regeneration of the severed spinal cord in young rats,[40,41,107] newborn rats, and kittens and puppies.[40-43,78] Such findings in newborn and young mammals are not completely consistent with those of Ramon y Cajal,[26,91,92] and Barnard and Carpenter[2] report only abortive regeneration in newborns, similar to that found in adult mammals.

Several explanations have been proposed for better regenerative capabilities in young mammals. It is said that less dense glial scarring occurs in the newborn and young mammal and therefore a less effective barrier is formed.[49-54,114-116] This theory is widely accepted. Berry and Riches[17] suggest that after injury to the adult, CNS axonal growth is inhibited by immunologic mechanisms activated against CNS autoantigens. Because this autoimmune mechanism is developed late in mammals, neonates may regenerate better. Reinis'[93] work reinforces this concept. The presence of plasma cells, lymphocytes, and macrophages, all cells of the immune response, lends support to this hypothesis.[111]

Feringa et al.[37-39] postulated that the well-known autoimmune reaction to their own brain antigens that occurs in mammals may be responsible, in part, for excessive scar tissue formation and lack of regeneration. They attempted to demonstrate that regeneration in the mammalian spinal cord is inhibited by the allergic reaction of the animals to CNS antigens released by traumatic interruption of the integrity of the blood–brain barrier. Administration of immunosuppressive agents yielded only slight electrophysiologic evidence of regeneration.[39]

Still another explanation for CNS regeneration in neonates by Clark[29] was based on the postulation that posttransection growth of new spinal fibers in neonates may be due simply to continuing growth and development whereas no such growth occurs in adult forms.

There has been no satisfactory explanation as to why central axons can regenerate in fish, amphibia, and reptiles but not in birds and mammals.[110] Cell-mediated allergic responses are weak in the first species and thus may account for regeneration. The central part of a severed dorsal root will regenerate only as far as the glial-neurilemmal cell boundary.[72,79,113]

Axonal transport[112] consists of the movement of materials from their sites of synthesis in the cell body to their sites of utilization in the outlying portions of the nerve cell. In the regenerating cell, axonal transport plays a key role in conveying materials necessary for formation of the new axon and may also be involved in sending information to the cell body about the status of the axon. Fast axonoplasmic transport has been estimated at $410 \pm 50$ mm per day.[84] Osterholm[85] postulates axonal transport as one mechanism by which catecholamines move to the site of a spinal lesion. Vise et al.[109] on the other hand feel that catecholamine-like substances may enter the site of injury in a damaged blood–brain barrier.

In order to demonstrate directly the movement of materials along the axon, methods were devised to incorporate radioactive tracers within nerve cell bodies and to observe the movement of the tracers toward the periphery.[33,47,63] It was found, for example, that radioactive amino acids were taken up by the neuron and incorporated into a protein, that radioactive fucose was incorporated into glycoprotein, and that radioactive glycerol was incorporated into phospholipid. After formation of these substances in the neuron cell body, the resulting macromolecules were then transported distally toward the periphery. It was found that not all substances are transported at the same rate. Some material is transported at the rate of 1 to 5 mm/day, which is equivalent to the rate of nerve regeneration, while other materials travel at rates previously indicated.[84] The variable rates of movement indicate that the simple contractile or peristaltic action of the neural perikaryon and axon, possibly accounting for slow axonal flow and regeneration, does not account for fast flow.

The demonstration of retrograde transport[59,64] by which certain proteins can be taken up by nerve terminals and transported toward the cell body is evidence that an active transport system must be involved. Thus a distinction may be drawn between axoplasmic flow and axonal transport. Axoplasmic flow is the slow proximodistal movement of substances and may represent perpetual growth of the axon. Axonal transport is an active, energy-dependent transport of macromolecules at various rates, usually rapid, in both anterograde and retrograde directions along the axonal axis-cylinder. It is possible that the movement of materials along the axon is dependent on the presence of contractile elements in the axon comparable to those in muscle. An actomycin-like protein has been isolated from neural tissue[5] which, like actomycin in muscle, may convert chemical to mechanical energy.

The formation of a new synaptic junction during regeneration requires a modification of both the nerve ending and the cell with which it makes a connection. In the superior cervical sympathetic ganglion of the cat, the preganglionic fibers deriving from spinal level T1 form synapses solely on postganglionic cells whose fibers innervate the pupil, while fibers from level T4 synapse solely on postganglionic cells that innervate blood vessels. These relationships are restored following transection and regeneration of the cervical sympathetic trunk.[49,52,62] Thus the reestablishment of synapses in the sympathetic ganglion of mammals is a highly selective process and follows the same regenerative principles as the central nervous system in amphibia.

The mechanism of neurite (axonal) elongation has been studied in tissue culture with time lapse photomicrography during axonal outgrowth. Elongation has been modified by changing the composition of the medium in which growth is occurring. This indicates the importance of the environment to the growing nerve. For further details see Guth.[49]

## REFERENCES

1. Bachman CH, Slaughter W: The longitudinal direct current gradients of spinal nerves. Nature 196:675–676, 1962
2. Barnard JW, Carpenter W: Lack of regeneration in spinal cord of rat. J Neurophysiol 13:223–228, 1950
3. Becker RO: Stimulation of partial limb regeneration in rats. Nature 235:109–111, 1972
4. Becker RO, Spadaro JA: Electrical stimulation of partial limb regeneration in mammals. Bull NY Acad Med 48:627–641, 1972
5. Berl S, Puszkin S, Nicklas WJ: Actomysin-like protein in brain. Science 179:441–446, 1973
6. Bernstein JJ: Anatomy and physiology of the central nervous system. In Hoar WS, Randall DJ (eds): Physiology of Fishes. New York, Academic, 1970, pp 1–89

7. Bernstein JJ, Bernstein ME: Alteration of neuronal synaptic compliment during axonal sprouting and regeneration of rat spinal cord. In Guth L, Windle W (eds): The Enigma of the Central Nervous System. Exp Neurol 45:634–637, 1975
8. Bernstein JJ, Bernstein ME: Formation of synapses proximal to the site of lesion following regeneration in the rat spinal cord. Anat Res 169:278, 1971
9. Bernstein JJ, Bernstein ME: Neuronal alteration and reinnervation following axonal regeneration and sprouting in mammalian spinal cord. Brain Behav Evol 8:135–161, 1973
10. Bernstein JJ, Bernstein ME: Neuronal alteration and reinnervation following axonal regeneration and sprouting in the mammalian spinal cord. In Bernstein JJ, Goodman DC (eds): Neuromorphological Plasticity. Brain Behav Evol 8:135–161, 1973
11. Bernstein JJ, Gelderd JB: Regeneration of the long spinal tracts in the goldfish. Brain Res 20:33–38, 1970
12. Bernstein JJ, Gelderd JB: Motor neuron synaptic compliment following regeneration of goldfish spinal cord. Anat Res 175:272, 1973
13. Bernstein JJ, Gelderd J: Synaptic reorganization following regeneration of goldfish spinal cord. Exp Neurol 41:402–410, 1973
14. Bernstein JJ, Gelderd J, Bernstein ME: Alteration of neuronal synaptic compliment during regeneration and axonal sprouting of rat spinal cord. Exp Neurol 44:470–483, 1974
15. Bernstein JJ, Goodman DC: Overview in neuromorphological plasticity. Brain Behav Evol 8:162–164, 1973
16. Bernstein ME, Bernstein JJ: Regeneration of axons and synaptic complex formation rostral to the site of hemisection in the spinal cord of the monkey. Int J Neurosci 5:15–26, 1973
17. Berry M, Riches AC: An immunological approach to regeneration in the central nervous system. Br Med Bull 30:135–140, 1974
18. Bjorklund A, Katzman R, Stenevi U, West KA: Development and growth of axonal sprouts from noradrenaline and 5-hydroxytryptamine neurons in the rat spinal cord. Brain Res 31:21–33, 1971
19. Bjorklund A, Stenevi U: Growth of central catecholamine neurons into smooth muscle grafts in the rat mesencephalon. Brain Res 31:1–20, 1971
20. Bjorklund A, Stenevi U: Nerve growth factor: stimulation of regenerative growth of central noradrenergic neurons. Science 175:1251–1253, 1972
21. Bogdassarian R, Goodman D: Axonal sprouting in intact retinofugal neurons as a consequence of opposite eye removal: homotypic compared to heterotypic axonal sprouting. Anat Res 166:280, 1970
22. Breasted JH: The Edwin-Smith Surgical Papyrus, vol 1. Chicago, University of Chicago Press, 1930, pp 323–332
23. Brown-Sequard CE: Experiences sur les plaies de la moelle epiniere. Compt Rend Soc Biol 1:17–18, 1849
24. Bunge MB: Fine structure of nerve fibers and growth cones of isolated sympathetic neurons in culture. J Cell Biol 56:713–735, 1973
25. Butler EG, Ward MB: Reconstitution of the spinal cord after ablation in adult Triturus. Dev Biol 15:464–486, 1967
26. Cajal RY: Degeneration and Regeneration of the Nervous System, vol 2. RM May (trans). London, Oxford University Press, 1928
27. Campbell JB, Bassett CAL, Husby J, Noback CR: Regeneration of adult mammalian spinal cord. Science 126:939, 1957
28. Chambers WW, Liu CN, McCouch GP, et al: Reflexes involving triceps surae from the ankle joint of the cat. Exp Neurol 39:461–468, 1973
29. Clark SL: Innervation of blood vessels of medulla and spinal cord. J Comp Neurol 48:247–265, 1929
30. Clemente CD: Regeneration in the vertebrate central nervous system. In Pfeiffer

CC, Smythies JR (eds): Internation Review of Neurobiology. New York, Academic, 1964, p 476

31. Clemente CD, Windle WF: Regeneration of severed nerve fibers in the spinal cord of the adult cat. J Comp Neurol 109:123–151, 1954
32. Cunningham TJ: Sprouting of the optic projection after cortical lesions. Anat Res 172:298, 1972
33. Droz B, Leblond CP: Axonal migration of proteins in the central nervous system and peripheral nerves as shown by radioautography. J Comp Neurol 121:325–346, 1963
34. Druckman R, Mair WGP: Aberrant regenerating nerve fibres in injury to the spinal cord. Brain 76:448–454, 1953
35. Edds MV, Jr: Collateral nerve regeneration. Q Rev Biol 28:260–276, 1953
36. Eggar MD, Wall PD: The plantar cushion reflex circuit: an oliosynaptic cutaneous reflex. J Physiol (London) 216:483–501, 1971
37. Feringa ER, Gurden CG, Strodel W, Chandler W, Knake J: Descending spinal motor tract regeneration after spinal cord transection. Neurology 23:599–608, 1973
38. Feringa ER, Johnson RD, Wendt JS: Spinal cord regeneration in rats after immunosuppressive treatment. Arch Neurol 32:676–683, 1975
39. Feringa ER, Wendt JS, Johnson RD: Immunosuppressive treatment to enhance spinal cord regeneration in rats. Neurology 24:287–293, 1974
40. Freeman LW: Experimental observation upon axonal regeneration in the transected spinal cord of mammals. Clin Neurosurg 8:294–319, 1962
41. Freeman LW: Return of function after complete transection of the spinal cord of the rat, cat, and dog. Ann Surg 136:193–205, 1952
42. Freeman LW: Return of function after complete transection of the spinal cord of the rat, cat and dog. Ann Surg 136:206–210, 1952
43. Freeman LW, MacDougall J, Turbes CC, Bowman DE: The treatment of experimental lesions of the spinal cord of dogs with trypsin. J Neurosurg 17:250–265, 1960
44. Gilson BC, Stensaas LJ: Early axonal changes following lesions of the dorsal columns in rats. Cell Tiss Res 149:1–20, 1974
45. Goldberger M, Murray M: Restitution of functional and collateral sprouting in cat spinal cord: the deafferented animal. J Comp Neurol 158:37–54, 1974
46. Goodman DC, Horl JA: Sprouting of optic tract projections in the brain stem of the rat. J Comp Neurol 127:71–88, 1966
47. Grafstein B: Axonal transport: Communication between soma and synapse. In Costa E, Greengard P (eds): Advances in Biochemical Psychopharmacology, vol 1. New York, Raven Press, 1969, pp 11–25
48. Gurden CG, Feringa ER: Effects of sympatholytic agents on CNS regeneration, cystic necrosis after spinal cord transection. Neurology 24:187–191, 1974
49. Guth L: Axonal regeneration and functional plasticity in the central nervous system. Exp Neurol 45:606–654, 1974
50. Guth L: History of central nervous system regeneration research. Exp Neurol 48, No 3 (part 2):3–15, 1975
51. Guth L: Neuromuscular function after regeneration of interrupted nerve fibers into partially denervated muscle. Exp Neurol 6:129–141, 1962
52. Guth L, Bernstein JJ: Selectivity in the re-establishment of synapses in the superior cervical sympathetic ganglion of the cat. Exp Neurol 4:59–69, 1961
53. Guth L, Windle WF: The enigma of central nervous regeneration. Exp Neurol 28(suppl 5):1–43, 1970
54. Guth L, Windle WF: Physiological, molecular and genetic aspects of central nervous system regeneration. Exp Neurol 39:3–16, 1973
55. Hibbard E: Regeneration in the severed spinal cord of chordate larvae of petromyzon marinas. Exp Neurol 7:175–185, 1963

56. Holtzer H: Reconstitution of the urodele spinal cord following unilateral ablation. J Exp Zool 117:523–558, 1951
57. Johnson DG, Gorden P, Kopin IJ: A sensitive radioimmunoassay for 7S nerve growth factor antigens in serum and tissues. J Neurochem 18:2355–2362, 1971
58. Katzman R, Bjorklund A, Owman CH, Stenevi U, West KA: Evidence for regenerative axon sprouting of central catecholamine neurons in the rat mesencephalon following electrolytic lesion. Brain Res 25:579–596, 1971
59. Kristensson K, Olsson Y, Sjostrand J: Axonal uptake and retrograde transport of exogenous proteins in the hypoglossal nerve. Brain Res 32:399–406, 1971
60. Lance JW: Behavior of pyramidal axons following section. Brain 77:314–324, 1954
61. Landolt AM: Regeneration of the human pituitary. J Neurosurg 39:35–41, 1973
62. Langley JN: On the regeneration of pre-ganglionic and of post-ganglionic visceral nerve fibers. J Physiol (London) 22:215–230, 1897
63. Lasek RJ: Protein transport in neurons. Int Rev Neurobiol 13:289–321, 1970
64. LaVail JH, LaVail MM: Retrograde axonal transport in the central nervous system. Science 176:1416–1417, 1972
65. Levi-Montalcini R, Angeletti PU: Nerve growth factor. Physiol Rev 48:534–569, 1968
66. Littrell JL: Apparent functional restitution in piromen treated spinal cats. In Windle WF (ed): Regeneration in the Central Nervous System. Springfield, Ill, Charles C Thomas, 1955, pp 219–228
67. Liu CN, Chambers WW: Intraspinal sprouting of dorsal root axons. Arch Neurol Psychiatr 79:46–61, 1958
68. Lorente de No R: Comments on the relation of age to capacity for regeneration in amphibians. In Windle WF (ed): Regeneration in the Central Nervous System. Springfield, Ill, Charles C Thomas, 1955, pp 77–80
69. Lund RD, Lund JS: Reorganization of the retinotectal pathway in rats after neonatal retinal lesions. Exp Neurol 40:377–390, 1973
70. Lund RD, Lund JS: Synaptic adjustment after deafferentation of the superior colliculus of the rat. Science 171:804–807, 1971
71. Lynch GS, Deadwyler S, Cotman CW: Postlesion axonal growth produces permanent functional connections. Science 180:1364–1366, 1973
72. McCouch GP: Comments on Regeneration of Functional Connections. In Windle WF (ed): Regeneration in the Central Nervous System. Springfield, Ill, Charles C Thomas, 1955, pp 171–180
73. McCouch GP, Austin GM: Site of origin and reflex behaviour of postsynaptic negative potentials recorded from spinal cord. Yale J Biol Med 28:372–379, Dec 55–Feb 56
74. McCouch GP, Austin GM, Liu CN, Liu CY: Sprouting as a cause of spasticity. J Neurophysiol 21:205–216, 1958
75. McMaster RE: Regeneration of the spinal cord in the rat. Effects of piromen and ACTH upon the regenerative capacity. J Comp Neurol 119:113–116, 1962
76. Magenis TP, Freeman LW, Bowman DE: Functional recovery following spinal cord hemisection and intrathecal use of hypochlorite treated trypsin. Fed Proc 11:99, 1952
77. Matinian LA, Andreasian AS: Enzymotherapy in organic lesions of the spinal cord. (In Russian, English summary). In Akademia Nauk Armenian SSR 1–94, 1973
78. Migliavacca A: Richerche sperimentali sulla rigenerazione del middlo spinale nei feti e nei neonati. Arch 1st Biochem Ital 2:201–236, 1930
79. Moyer EK, Kimmel DL, Winborne LW: Regeneration of sensory spinal nerve roots in young and in senile rats. J Comp Neurol 98:283–307, 1953
80. Murray M, Goldberger ME: Restitution of functional and collateral sprouting in cat spinal cord: the partially hemisected animal. J Comp Neurol 158:19–36, 1974

81. Nathaniel EJH, Nathaniel DR: Regeneration of dorsal root fibers into the adult rat spinal cord. Exper Neurol 40:333–350, 1973
82. Nygren L, Olson L, Seiger A: Regeneration of monoamine containing axons in the developing and adult spinal cord of the rat following 6-OH-dopamine injections or transections. Histochemistry 28:1–15, 1971
83. O'Callaghan WJ, Speakman TJ: Axon regeneration in the rat spinal cord. Surg Forum 14:410–411, 1963
84. Ochs S, Jersild RA, Jr: Fast axoplasmic transport in nonmyelinated mammalian nerve fibers shown by electron microscopic radioautography. J Neurobiol 5:373–377, 1974
85. Osterholm JL: The pathophysiological response to spinal injury. The current status of related research. J Neurosurg 40:3–33, 1974
86. Paterson PY: Immune processes and infectious factors in central nervous system disease. Ann Rev Med 20:75–100, 1969
87. Piatt J: Regeneration of the spinal cord in the salamander. J Exp Zool 129:177, 1955
88. Raisman G: A comparison of the mode of termination of the hippocampal and hypothalamic afferents to the septal nuclei as revealed by the electron microscopy of degeneration. Exp Brain Res 7:317–343, 1969
89. Raisman G, Field P: A quantitative investigation of the development of collateral reinnervation after partial deafferentation of the septal nuclei. Brain Res 50:241–264, 1973
90. Raisman G, Matthews MR: Degeneration and regeneration of synapses. In Bourne G (ed): The Structure and Function of Nervous Tissue. New York, Academic, 1972, pp 61–104
91. Ramon y Cajal S: Degeneration and Regeneration of the Nervous System, vol 2, May RM (trans). Reprinted by Hafner, New York, 1959 (originally published in Madrid, 1928)
92. Ramon y Cajal S: Studies on Vertebrate Neurogenesis, Guth L (trans). Springfield, Ill, Charles C Thomas, 1960
93. Reinis S: Contribution to the problems of the regeneration of nerve fibers in the CNS after operative damage in the early postnatal period. Acta Anat 60:165–180, 1965
94. Rosner J, Wiegandt H, Rahmann H: Sialic acid incorporation into gangliosides and glycoproteins of the fish brain. J Neurochem 21:655–665, 1973
95. Schneider D: Regenerative phenomena in the central nervous system. A symposium summary. J Neurosurg 37:129–136, 1972
96. Scott D, Clemente CD: Regeneration of spinal cord fibers in the cat. J Comp Neurol 102:633–669, 1955
97. Scott D, Liu CN: Factors promoting regeneration of spinal neurons: Positive influence of nerve growth factor. Prog Brain Res 13:127–150, 1964
98. Smith SD: Effects of electrical fields upon regeneration in the Metazoa. Am Zool 10:133–140, 1970
99. Smith SD: Effects of electrode placement on stimulati of adult frog limb regeneration. Ann NY Acad Sci 238:500–507, 1974
100. Smith SD: Induction of partial limb regeneration in Rana pipiens by galvanic stimulation. Anat Rec 158:89–98, 1967
101. Sperry RW: The problem of central nervous reorganization after nerve regeneration and muscle transposition. Q Rev Biol 20:311–369, 1945
102. Stenevi U, Bjorklund A: Regenerative sprouting of central monoamine neurons. Acta Physiol Pol 24:193–203, 1973
103. Steward O, Cotman C, Lynch G: Histochemical detection of orthograde degeneration in the central nervous system of the rat. Brain Res 54:65–73, 1973
104. Stewart FT, Harte RH: A case of severed spinal cord in which myelorrhaphy

was followed by partial return of function. Philadelphia Med J 1902:1016–1020, June 2, 1902

105. Stoeckel K, Thoenen H: Retrograde axonal transport of nerve growth factor: specificity and biological importance. Brain Res 85:337–341, 1975

106. Stuart EG: Tissue reactions and possible mechanisms of piromen and desoxycorticosterone acetate in central nervous system regeneration. In Windle WF (ed): Regeneration in the Central Nervous System. Springfield Ill, Charles C Thomas, 1955, pp 162–170

107. Sugar O, Gerard RW: Spinal cord regeneration in the rat. J Neurophysiol 3:1–19, 1940

108. Turbes CC, Freeman LW: Apparent spinal cord regeneration following intramuscular trypsin. Anat Rec 117:288, 1953

109. Vise WM, Yashon D, Hunt WE: Mechanisms of norepinephrine accumulation within sites of spinal cord injury. J Neurosurg 40:76–82, 1974

110. Wakefield CL, Eidelberg E: Electron microscopic observations of the delayed effects of spinal cord compression. Exp Neurol 48:637–646, 1975

111. Weiss L: The Cells and Tissues of the Immune System. Foundation of Immunology Series. Englewood Cliffs, NJ, Prentice-Hall, 1972

112. Weiss P, Hiscoe HB: Experiments on the mechanism of nerve growth. J Exp Zool 107:315–396, 1948

113. Westbrook WHL, Jr, Tower SS: Analysis of problem of emergent fibers in posterior spinal roots, dealing with rate of growth of extraneous fibers into roots after gangionectomy. J Comp Neurol 72:383–397, 1940

114. Windle WF (ed): Regeneration in the Central Nervous System. Springfield, Ill, Charles C Thomas, 1955

115. Windle WF, Chambers WW: Regeneration in the spinal cord of· cat and dog. J Comp Neurol 93:241–258, 1950

116. Windle WF, Clemente CD, Chambers WW: Inhibition of formation of a glial barrier as a means of permitting a peripheral nerve to grow into the brain. J Comp Neurol 96:359–370, 1952

117. Wolman L: Axon regeneration after spinal cord injury. Paraplegia 4:175–188, 1966

118. Yu RC-P, Bunge RP: Damage and repair of the peripheral myelin sheath and node of Ranvier after treatment with trypsin. J Cell Biol 64:1–14, 1975

# 29

## Evoked Potentials in the Assessment of Spinal Function

Electrical assessment of the functional integrity of the spinal cord has both practical and theoretical value. It is clinically significant in the injured unconscious patient and its intraoperative use has great potential. It also may provide subtle information as to remaining functioning pathways even when the patient has no neurologic function detectable by examination. Electrical assessment is also an aid in the adjudication of spinal long tract function after various treatment regimens.

Recording of somatosensory cortical evoked potential (CEP) in man or in experimental animals is accomplished by stimulating a peripheral nerve, usually the common peroneal or sural, and recording responses with either the electroencephalograph or with appropriately placed cortical depth electrodes. No CEP is recorded if there is a block in conduction because of a partial or complete functional transection of either the peripheral nerve or spinal cord.

In 1947, Dawson[7] demonstrated that CEP following peripheral nerve stimulation could be recorded from the primary somatosensory area of the cortex. The tibial nerve stimulus and cortical activity are monitored by electroencephalogram and by oscilloscope. The CEP is then averaged and analyzed by computer. Donaghy and Numoto[9] suggested that the prognosis for recovery in acutely paralyzed dogs is poor if a CEP cannot be recorded within four hours of the injury. Croft et al.[4] described the loss of the CEP following spinal cord compression and showed that elevation of systemic blood pressure made such changes reversible.

Because the CEP is thought to be carried almost exclusively in the posterior column in man, theoretically a ventral lesion could go undetected. D'Angelo et al.[5] recorded the CEP following tibial nerve stimulation over a four-hour period in cats sustaining 100, 300, and 500 g-cm impact injury to the posterior spinal cord and found that the time required for return of the evoked response could be correlated with the severity of the damage to the spinal cord. The CEP returned almost immediately in animals sustaining only gray matter petechial hemorrhages, was delayed one hour in animals with peri-gray-white matter hemorrhages, and did not return at all in animals with central cavitation and posterior column fragmentation. Similar experiments were carried out following administration of nitrous oxide and halothane anesthesia as well as the paralyzing drug succinyl choline.

Gilbin[12] reported a CEP study on seven patients with spinal lesions involving the posterior column. He could not obtain cortical CEPs from distal nerve stimulation and concluded that the spinal CEP pathway lies in the posterior spinal cord. Halliday and Wakefield[13] further documented this observation in the Brown-Sequard syndrome with unilateral position sense loss. Normal evoked brain responses were recorded from the cortex contralateral to the normal side, but CEPs were diminished or absent from the cortex on the abnormal side of the body.

Gelfan and Tarlov[11] reported electrophysiologic measurements across experimental spinal cord compression. A pressure of 200 mm Hg by means of a cuff about a 5-mm cord segment caused failure of impulse transmission. To distinguish the role of mechanical compression versus that of hypoxia they compared the cuff data to data obtained after hypoxia induced by nitrogen inhalation or by ascending aorta ligation. They concluded that inhibition of the CEP resulted from cord compression and that hypoxia was a minor factor.

The "H" reflex has been advocated as a useful measurement of spinal gray matter integrity by VanGilder,[26] who suggests that the absence of this segmental reflex after trauma indicates considerable disruption of the central internuncial pool by traumatic hemorrhage.

Perot[20] found CEPs to be of great assistance in management of patients with spinal cord injury. The procedure provided a sensitive and early distinction of incomplete versus complete lesion and served as well as a valuable monitoring device during treatment under anesthesia.

Singer et al.[25] subjected monkeys to acute cervical cord trauma by flexion-extension. They found that the CEP was still present immediately following injury but began to disappear 20 to 90 seconds after injury and did not reappear until 24 hours after injury. Loss of CEP was thought to coincide with the onset of primary spinal cord hemorrhage and edema. Transection of the spinal cord itself has a great influence on cerebral cortical electrical activity, as was shown by Lavy and Herishanu.[14] After complete transection they noted fusiform spindle bursts of two to five seconds' duration. In addition, long, symmetrical runs of regular fast and low amplitude activity were intermingled with the electrical background patterns.

Martin and Bloedel[18] carried out experiments to determine if CEP activity could be used to aid in prognosis following spinal injury. Severe irreversible neurologic deficits occurred in cats in which the CEP disappeared. In animals in which the CEP did not disappear, only mild neurologic loss was evident after six weeks.

Deecke and Tator[8] used a somewhat different electrical recording technique to test afferent and efferent conduction in spinal-injured monkeys. Using sciatic nerve stimulation, they recorded afferent electrical volleys in the dorsal column above a spinal lesion. An isoelectric line rostral to the lesion site indicated a complete afferent conduction block. Efferent conduction was tested by stimulating the pyramidal tract in the cord above the injury site and observing distal nerve limb movements. They found that the more severe the injury the less was the capability to record movements.

Bremer,[1] in 1941, first described spontaneous electrical activity of the spinal cord. The electrospinogram (ESG) offers yet a third method of electrically studying the spinal cord. Impulses recorded by ESG are thought to arise from segmental neurones and to be composed of low-voltage background activity tonically maintained by afferent impulses from the periphery and larger sharp waves with amplitudes influenced by supraspinal centers. Pool recorded the ESG in a paralyzed patient in 1946. Sawa[23] used electrodes introduced into the spinal cord itself and Magladery et al.[17] employed electrodes introduced intrathecally. Shimoji et al.[24] recorded the ESG through the intact skin in infants. Sarnowski et al.[22] recorded summated evoked potentials from surface electrodes placed over the skin of cats. They credited Gasser and Graham[10] with first having recorded evoked potentials over the spinal cord after dorsal root stimulation. Liberson et al.[15] and Liberson and Kim[16] used computer averaging techniques to record summated evoked potentials to peripheral nerve stimulation from skin surface electrodes placed over the spine. Failure of transmission rostral to a spinal cord lesion was observed by Cracco.[2,3] Morrison et al.[19] studied the ESG after spinal cord compression in cats. They attributed the increase in amplitude and frequency of the ESG potentials in the segment caudal to the lesion as being due to loss of rostral inhibitory influences. Whether such studies as these will some day be of clinical value remains to be seen.

## REFERENCES

1. Bremer E: Spontaneous electrical activity of the spinal cord. Arch Int Physiol Biochem 51:51–84, 1941
2. Cracco RQ: Spinal evoked response: peripheral nerve stimulation in man. Electroenceph Clin Neurophysiol 35:379–386, 1973
3. Cracco JB, Cracco RQ, Graziani LJ: Spinal evoked response in infants and children. Neurology (Minneapolis) 25:31–36, 1975
4. Croft TJ, Brodkey JS, Nulsen FE: Reversible spinal cord trauma: a model for electrical monitoring of spinal cord function. J Neurosurg 36:402–406, 1972
5. D'Angelo CM, VanGilder JC, Taub A: Evoked cortical potentials in experimental spinal cord trauma. J Neurosurg 38:332–336, 1973
6. Dawson GD: Cerebral responses to electrical stimulation of peripheral nerve in man. J Neurol Neurosurg Psychiatr 10:137–140, 1947

7. Dawson GD: A summation technique for the detection of small evoked potentials. EEG Clin Neurophysiol 6:65–84, 1954

8. Deecke L, Tator CH: Neurophysiological assessment of afferent and efferent conduction in the injured spinal cord of monkeys. J Neurosurg 39:65–74, 1973

9. Donaghy RMP, Numoto M: Prognostic significance of sensory evoked potential in spinal cord injury. Proceedings of the Seventeenth Veterans Administration Spinal Cord Injury Conference. Bronx, New York, pp 251–257

10. Gasser HS, Graham HT: Potentials produced in the spinal cord by stimulation of dorsal roots. Am J Physiol 103:303–320, 1933

11. Gelfan S, Tarlov IM: Physiology of the spinal cord, nerve roots and peripheral nerve compression. Am J Physiol 185:217–229, 1956

12. Gilbin DR: Somatosensory evoked potentials in healthy subjects and in patients with lesions in the nervous system. Ann NY Acad Sci 112:93–142, 1964

13. Halliday AM, Wakefield GS: Cerebral evoked responses in patients with dissociated sensory loss. Neurophysiol 14:786 (abstract), 1962

14. Lavy S, Herishanu Y: The effect of complete transection of thoracic spinal cord on cat's electrocorticogram. Epilepsia 12:117–122, 1971

15. Liberson WT, Gratzer M, Zales A, et al: Comparison of conduction velocities of motor and sensory fibers determined by different methods. Arch Phys Med Rehabil 47:17–23, 1966

16. Liberson WT, Kim KS: Mapping evoked potentials elicited by stimulation of the median and peroneal nerves. Electroenceph Clin Neurophysiol 15:721, 1963

17. Magladery JW, Porter WE, Park AM, Teasdall RD: Electrophysiological studies of nerve and reflex activity in normal man. IV. Two-neurone reflex and identification of certain action potentials from spinal roots and cord. Bull Johns Hopkins Hosp 88:449–519, 1951

18. Martin SH, Bloedel JR: Evaluation of experimental spinal cord injury using cortical evoked potentials. J Neurosurg 39:75–81, 1973

19. Morrison G, Lorig RJ, Brodkey JS, Nulsen FE: Electrospinogram and spinal and cortical evoked potentials in experimental spinal cord trauma. J Neurosurg 43:737–741, 1975

20. Perot PL, Jr: The clinical use of somatosensory evoked potentials in spinal cord injury. Clin Neurosurg 20:367–381, 1973

21. Pool JL: Electrospinogram—spinal cord action potentials recorded from a paraplegic patient. J Neurosurg 3:192–198, 1946

22. Sarnowski RJ, Cracco RQ, Vogen HB, Mount F: Spinal evoked response in the cat. J Neurosurg 43:329–336, 1975

23. Sawa H: Spontaneous electrical activities obtained from human spinal cord. Folia Psychiatr Neurol Japan 2:165–179, 1947

24. Shimoji K, Kano T, Higashi H, Morioka T, Henschel EO: Evoked spinal electrograms recorded from epidural space in man. J Appl Psychol 33:468–471, 1972

25. Singer JM, Russell GV, Coe JE: Changes in evoked potentials after experimental cervical spinal cord injury in the monkey. Exp Neurol 29:449–461, 1970

26. VanGilder J: Data presented to the National Paraplegia Foundation, Milwaukee, June 1972

# 30

## Centers for Total Care

In many countries, spinal cord centers for the care of the spinally injured patient from the acute stage through rehabilitation have been established during the last several decades. The United States has lagged somewhat in implementing this concept, but gradually such centers are being developed. The patient in a general hospital geared to care for spinally injured patients and to which a rehabilitation center is accessible probably receives care identical in quality. However, the focus in such a hospital is not on the spinally injured patient but on all types of neurosurgical, orthopedic, and physiatric problems.

It is estimated that there are 4000 to 10,000 new cases of spinal injury per year in the United States,[14] so perhaps more attention should be concentrated on their care because of the enormous cost. In 1970, Young[14] estimated costs for the first year of care to average $25,000, even to be as high as $35,000. Since medical costs have risen since 1970, the expense of caring for these patients has also risen. Young estimated the cost per year for care of all spinally injured patients in the United States to be $2 billion. A large part of this represents medical waste in treatment of preventable complications and payment for unneccessary custodial care. He suggested that a combined systems approach, preventing complications such as bedsores and urinary tract infection, could reduce the expense by 20 percent to 30 percent.

Young suggested that a population of 3 to 5 million might support one spinal injury center of 50 to 100 beds. These figures probably represent the minimum and the maximum in size for such a unit. In such a spinal injury center, the patient is given the optimum in early care and in later training to equip him for living with this disability. He is taught how to prevent or minimize future medical complications that impair his rehabilitation, reduce his potential level of function, and compound the expense of his future care.

At present in the United States, facilities for the care of spinally injured patients are supported by localities, by the state government, or by the federal government, but in most instances, municipal, county, and state support is haphazard and no spinal injury center exists. Some states do support rehabilitation facilities. In many cases, the National Guard assists in transporting acutely injured patients via helicopter.

Federal programs for the care of spinal injury fall under four related but separately financed agencies: the Department of Defense, the Department of Health, Education, and Welfare, the Veterans Administration, and the National Institutes of Health. The Department of Defense, composed of the Army, Navy, and Air Force, is generally concerned with the immediate care of acute wartime injuries. It has sponsored the National Spinal Cord Injury Registry, and in conjunction with the Department of Transportation has established a program for helicopter transport of injured civilians known as MAST (Military Assistance to Traffic and Safety). The Department of Defense also sponsors research programs concerning acute spinal cord injury. In a sense, the patient sustaining a service-connected injury receives care equivalent to that given in a spinal cord injury center, in that he is transported as quickly as possible to experts for immediate treatment and is rehabilitated as quickly as possible through the Veterans Administration.

The Veterans Administration currently supports 14 or more regional spinal cord injury centers, having a total of approximately 1200 beds with an average of 90 to 100 beds per hospital. At any given time, 1000 service and nonservice personnel are being treated. Care of the service-related injury is delegated to the Veterans Administration and by and large an excellent job of rehabilitation is accomplished. Bors[2] described the spinal cord injury center at the Veterans Administration Hospital in Long Beach, California, which cares for subacute and chronically ill patients. In addition to providing care, such centers also carry out some measure of basic research relating to spinal injury.

The social and rehabilitation services of the Department of Health, Education, and Welfare are specifically involved in spinal cord injury programs. The Rehabilitation Services Administration cooperates with state or private programs to provide vocational rehabilitation for all disabled persons including about 1400 with spinal cord injuries. Rehabilitation programs begin four to eight weeks after the injury and continue for six months to three years. This program also provides partial support to seven state owned and operated facilities with patients ranging in number from 30 to 100. In addition, the Bureau of Research and Demonstration is developing several model centers for spinal cord injury rehabilitation.[9]

The National Institute of Neurological Diseases and Stroke under the Department of Health, Education, and Welfare supports basic research into spinal cord injury. Large numbers of individual research grants have been made, and acute spinal injury research centers have been developed for investigating amelioration, or reversal of the effects of spinal cord injury in the acute stages.

However, in England, 85 percent of paraplegics are enabled to return to gainful employment (54 percent full time) because of the long-term results of care at the National Spinal Injury Center of the Stokes Mandeville Hospital and other similar centers. Guttmann[7] organized this unit in 1944 and it has continued to expand and to provide total care for spinal cord injury patients in Great Britain. Other centers have developed in Great Britain in a similar fashion. Harris[8] described organization of centers in Great Britain which have been emulated by other countries.

For example, Cheshire[3] described the unit in Victoria, Australia, where complete and centralized treatment of paraplegia takes place. Australia is virtually the same size as the United States, and consists of six sovereign states joined in a federation relationship with a federal government comparable to that in the United States. Likewise, there is a system of private and public hospitals. The latter include all teaching hospitals that are dependent upon the state government for the major part of their financial support and that are subservient to the State Hospital and Charities Commission in matters of public policy.

Today, Australia has four well-developed spinal cord injury centers. Of these, the center in Perth was first developed in 1954, followed by that in Victoria in 1956. Bedbrook[1] described the unit at Perth initiated in 1953, as a cooperative venture by the medical community, which recognized that spinal cord injuries are a special problem that can be better handled in a center than elsewhere. By 1957, with the aid of the Australian Medical Association, all cases of spinal injury were directed to the unit in the Royal Perth Rehabilitation Hospital. The cooperative venture has expanded to a 40-bed, air-conditioned unit that today cares for all groups in need of rehabilitation, and provisions have been made for acute care.

The spinal injury center in Melbourne, on the other hand, has been more concerned with acute injuries. This center serves a population of 4 million people within a 400 mile radius of Melbourne; 50 percent of spinally injured patients treated there have been involved in automobile accidents. Since 70 percent of the injuries occur in the outlying countryside, an air ambulance system has been developed so that most patients are seen within eight hours of injury. The two fundamental concepts underlying their philosophy of health care delivery are (1) all unnecessary movement of the patient must be avoided, and (2) optimum primary treatment requires the immediate participation of a team of several specialists, all of whom are aware of the special problems of spinal cord injury. The organization of the 64-bed unit is tripartite. There is a 14-bed acute ward which provides care for not only acute spinal cord trauma but also other problems of spinal cord injury. The 14-bed acute ward provides care for not only acute spinal cord trauma but also the problems of major resuscitation and serious multiple injuries. Once the patient has achieved spinal stability and has been up in a wheelchair for about four hours a day, he is transferred to a 24-bed rehabilitation ward. Yet a third ward is occupied by patients who have been readmitted for complications of their initial injury or for routine checkups. The Melbourne Center handles about 478 new admissions every year. Upon completion of treatment, the patient is discharged to his home whenever possible. By that time he will have achieved maximum rehabilitation, his family will have been educated, his home modified, and his employment arranged. Thereafter, the Paraplegic Association meets any social welfare needs, including paraplegic sports activities. As is the case at Stokes Mandeville Center in England, a residential hostel for working paraplegics has been established in the metropolitan area of Melbourne with convenient access to industry. All who have been patients at this center remain under the same care for the duration of their lives. Thus, permanent systematic follow-up is ensured.

Spinal injury units have been developed in many parts of the world, among them are Bochum[12] and Heidelberg,[13] Germany, Italy,[10] Great Britain,[11] Spain,[4,5] and Ireland.[6]

It seems desirable to have a definite systematic program for spinal-injured patients beginning with acute care and extending through the rehabilitation phase. Whether this should be carried out in one physical facility as is emphasized in this chapter or in more than one is debatable. What is important is that each patient receive expert care, and this can be rendered only by experienced persons acting as a team.

## REFERENCES

1. Bedbrook GM: The organisation of a spinal injuries unit at Royal Perth Hospital, Perth, Western Australia. Paraplegia 5:150–158, 1967
2. Bors E: The spinal cord injury center of the Veterans Administration Hospital, Long Beach, California, USA. Paraplegia 5:126–130, 1967
3. Cheshire DJE: The complete and centralised treatment of paraplegia. Paraplegia 6:59–73, 1968
4. Domingo MS: Organisation of an autonomous spinal injuries unit. Paraplegia 5:170–176, 1967
5. Domingo MS: Development of an autonomous spinal injuries unit. Paraplegia 7:217–219, 1969
6. Gregg TM: Organisation of a spinal injury unit within a rehabilitation centre. Paraplegia 5:163–166, 1967
7. Guttmann L: Organisation of spinal units. History of the National Spinal Injuries Centre, Stoke Mandeville Hospital, Aylesbury. Paraplegia 5:115–126, 1967
8. Harris P: Organisation of spinal units. Paraplegia 5:132–137, 1967
9. Heyl HL: Federal programs for the care and study of spinal cord injuries. J Neurosurg 36:379–385, 1972
10. Maglio A: Organisation of an autonomous spinal unit as part of a national accident insurance organisation. Paraplegia 5:176–178, 1967
11. McSweeney T: The Midland Spinal Injury Unit at the Robert Jones and Agnes Hunt Orthopaedic Hospital, Oswestry. Paraplegia 5:142–146, 1967
12. Meinecke FW: The situation of a spinal unit in an accident hospital. Paraplegia 5:147–150, 1967
13. Paeslack DV: Organisation of a spinal injuries unit within a university hospital. Paraplegia 5:140–142, 1967
14. Young JS: Development of systems of spinal injury management with a correlation to the development of other esoteric health care systems. Arizona Med 27:1–6 1970

# 31

## Whiplash,
## Soft Tissue Injuries,
## and Functional Disorders

The term "whiplash," said to have been coined by Crowe in 1928,[3,13] is given to a syndrome consisting of pain in the area of the neck and suboccipit following rapid flexion-extension occurring in an automobile accident in which the vehicle is struck either from the rear or the front. It implies few, if any, objective findings, but is characterized by a complaint of pain either transient or long lasting. Gay and Abbott[6] used the term "whiplash injuries of the neck" in probably the first published report in 1953.

Gates and Cento[5] studied a series of 612 patients with whiplash injury who were engaged in litigation. Questionnaires were answered by 95 patients, 105 were returned undelivered, and 412 were not answered. The authors questioned whether those 412 patients (66 percent) could be considered recovered and not interested. Of the 95 patients who replied, 70 stated that they had not recovered from their injuries. All had been injured 3 years or more prior to the study, so that presumably litigation had been concluded. The authors stated that no group of patients have more complaints with fewer objective findings. They also stated that of all the patients they treated, only one patient requested further treatment for the whiplash syndrome after all litigation had been settled.

Jackson[8] defined the possibly related cervical strain as a condition occurring in joint structures that have a certain degree of elasticity having a definite range of active voluntary motion but a limited range of passive motion. If, by trauma, motion is forced beyond the range of passive mobility, joint structures suffer a strain injury that leaves no permanent damage. Joints so injured may be painful for a few days or for two to three weeks, but they recover to the pretraumatic state.

Jackson[8] defined a sprain as a condition in which the cervical joint structures are forced far beyond their range of passive motion so that they are stretched, torn, or avulsed from their attachments. Hemorrhages and traumatic inflammation occur. Healing of the sprained ligamentous structures takes place by formation of scar tissue that is less elastic and less functional than normal tissue. Therefore, she stated, sprains result in some degree of permanent damage. We cannot quarrel with Jackson's definition of cervical sprain or strain, but we believe that permanent sequelae are uncommon.

Symptoms of a patient who alleges vertebral injury as a result of an accident include onset of pain immediately or even several hours or days later. The patient may be amnesic for the immediate postaccident symptoms. He may liken onset of the pain in the neck and head to having been "hit by a sledgehammer." The patient may complain of stiffness or limitation of motion. Jackson described clinical findings as an observed tendency to protect movements of the neck. In a patient with severe pain, there is limitation of movement of the neck, including lateral motion, flexion, and hyperextension.

The head compression test consists of application of pressure to the top of the head with the head tilted to either side and forward and backward as a test for increase of pain. Injury of the joints is indicated if the pain response is confined to the neck; if radicular pain occurs, nerve root irritation is present.

A shoulder depression test may be carried out with the patient's head tilted to one side and downward pressure applied to the opposite shoulder. If this test increases radicular pain, irritation or compression of nerve roots is indicated. Jackson recommends examining shoulder motion and looking for deep tenderness and muscle spasm in the areas in question.

Braaf and Rosner[2] surveyed over 6000 patients with chronic recurring headache observed for 2 to 25 years. As a cause of headache, they suggested that trauma to the cervical spine is probably the most important single factor and that the cervical area should be suspected in every headache of nonspecific origin. They recommended cervical traction as specific therapy for headaches of cervical origin. If conservative methods of treatment failed to give their patients adequate relief of headache, myelography was advised, followed by cervical laminectomy if indicated. Laminectomy or spinal fusion as treatment of headaches, even after documented cervical spine injury, has little physiologic basis. Most neurologists, neurosurgeons, and orthopedists do not recommend such procedures.

Hohl[7] studied 146 patients with only soft tissue injuries to the neck resulting from automobile accidents. He found that symptomatic recovery occurred in 57 percent, while degenerative changes appeared on x-ray after the injury in 39 percent of patients. Five years or more after the accident, there were significant changes on x-ray, and many patients still had symptoms. X-ray signs included reversal of normal cervical lordosis and restricted motion at one interspace observed on flexion-extension stress views.

The term "malingering" encompasses fraud relating to matters of health. After injury to the area of the vertebral column, malingering includes simulation of diseases or disabilities not present, and, more commonly, gross exaggeration of minor disabilities. It also includes a conscious and deliberate attribution of disability to an injury or accident that did not in fact cause it, for personal, usually financial, advantage.

Miller and Cartlidge[10] reviewed malingering related to brain and spinal cord injuries. Many others have distinguished between conscious simulation, or malingering, and unconscious or semiconscious simulation, known as hysteria. Miller and Cartlidge stated that the prevalence of malingering following injury is clearly related to the degree of development of insurance and welfare services. It is usually impossible to prove malingering, even when it is strongly suspected. Confrontation rarely leads to an admission of pretense and is probably not advisable. Occasionally an opportunity arises to verify the disappearance of a visible disability when the complainant does not know he is under observation. Also, some nonorganic and nonanatomic findings, particularly on sensory examination, assist in the presumption of malingering or hysteria. Fallik[4] found it difficult to distinguish between malingering and neurotic reaction. The monograph by Weintraub[12] includes an excellent review of the diagnosis of hysteria.

Toglia[11] examined 309 patients whose chief complaint was dizziness following a flexion-extension type of acceleration neck injury. He utilized electronystagmography and searched for latent and positional nystagmus as well as abnormal responses to calorics and rotation. Latent nystagmus was present in 29 percent of patients, and caloric tests were abnormal in 57 percent. Rotatory tests were abnormal in 51 percent. These findings suggest that many patients had a verifiable objective vestibular disturbance causing dizziness, even though neurologic examination was normal. He suggested that such testing for organicity in patients with unexplainable complaints might be of value. However, his report lacked a control group so that data concerning patients without symptoms but perhaps with similar abnormalities were not available.

Kirgis[9] reviewed the subject of low back injury due to industrial claims. He stated that most injuries to the lower back are specific enough so that controversy regarding diagnosis and degree of disability is unwarranted. To the contrary, in our view, such injuries are nonspecific, and objectivity is lacking. He did point out that the insurer selects physicians known for expeditious medical clearance rather than those who are more critical of the patient's ability to return to work. The choice of an objective physician is difficult for that reason.

Albright et al.[1] reported incidence of nonfatal neck injuries in 104 active high school and 75 college freshmen football players. Half the players who volunteered a history of significant neck pain had abnormal x-ray films. The incidence of x-ray evidence of neck injuries was as high as 32 percent and was related to the number of years of playing. This seems to us a very high incidence of x-ray abnormality and raises the question of interpretation of the cervical spine x-ray films. They found injuries more common in linebackers or defensive halfbacks who tackled the ball carrier. The incidence of neck pain in the presence of mild, moderate, or severe cervical osteoarthritis seems higher in individuals who have a background of contact sports or similar athletic activity.

# REFERENCES

1. Albright JP, Moses JM, Feldick HG, Dolan KD, Burneister LF: Nonfatal cervical spine injuries in interscholastic football. JAMA 236:1243–1245, 1976
2. Braaf MM, Rosner S: Trauma of cervical spine as cause of chronic headache. J Trauma 15:441–446, 1975
3. Crowe HE: A new diagnostic sign in neck injuries. The continuing revolt against whiplash. Monograph. The Defense Research Institute Inc, Milwaukee, Feb 1964
4. Fallik A: Simulation and malingering after injuries to the brain and spinal cord. Lancet 1:1126, 1972
5. Gates EM, Cento D: Studies in cervical trauma. Part I. The so-called "whiplash." Int Surg 46:218–222, 1966
6. Gay JR, Abbott KH: Common whiplash injuries of the neck. JAMA 152:1698, 1953
7. Hohl M: Soft-tissue injuries of the neck in automobile accidents. Factors influencing prognosis. J Bone Joint Surg 56A:1675–1681, 1974
8. Jackson R: The positive findings in alleged neck injuries. Am J Orthop 6:178–187, 1964
9. Kirgis HD: The problem of industrial injuries to the lower back. J Louisiana Med Soc 116:439–442, 1964
10. Miller H, Cartlidge N: Simulation and malingering after injuries to the brain and spinal cord. Lancet 1:580–585, 1972
11. Toglia JU: Acute flexion-extension injury of the neck. Neurology 26:808–814, 1976
12. Weintraub MI: Hysteria, a clinical guide to diagnosis. Clin Sympos (CIBA) 29:1–31, 1977
13. Weir DC: Roentgenographic signs of cervical injury. Orthop Dig 2:17–27, 1974

# Index